Principles of Pediatric Neurosurgery

Series Editor: Anthony J. Raimondi

Principles of Pediatric Neurosurgery

Head Injuries in the Newborn and Infant

The Pediatric Spine I: Development and Dysraphic State
The Pediatric Spine II: Developmental Anomalies
The Pediatric Spine III: Cysts, Tumors, and Infections

Cerebrovascular Diseases in Children

Edited by Anthony J. Raimondi, Maurice Choux,
and Concezio Di Rocco

Cerebrovascular Diseases
in Children

Edited by Anthony J. Raimondi,
Maurice Choux, and Concezio Di Rocco

With 163 Figures

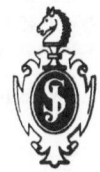

Springer-Verlag

New York Berlin Heidelberg London Paris
Tokyo Hong Kong Barcelona Budapest

ANTHONY J. RAIMONDI, M.D., Professor of Surgery (Neurosurgery), Northwestern University Medical School, Chicago, Illinois, U.S.A.

MAURICE CHOUX, M.D., Hôpital des Enfantes de la Timone, Rue Sainte Pierre, 13005 Marseille, France

CONCEZIO DI ROCCO, M.D., Istituto di Neurochirurgia, Università Cattolica del Sacre Cuore, Largo Gemelli 8, 00168 Rome, Italy

Library of Congress Cataloging-in-Publication Data
Cerebrovascular diseases in children

   p.   cm. — (Principles of pediatric neurosurgery)
   Includes bibliographical references and index.
   ISBN-13: 978-1-4612-7676-0   e-ISBN-13: 978-1-4612-2800-4
   DOI: 10.1007/978-1-4612-2800-4

   1. Cerebrovascular disease in children.   I. Raimondi, Anthony J.,
   1928–   . II. Choux, M. (Maurice)   III. Di Rocco, C. (Concezio)
   IV. Series.
   [DNLM: 1. Cerebrovascular Disorders—in infancy & childhood.   WL
   355 C41344]
   RJ496.C45C48   1991
   618.92′81—dc20
   DNLM/DLC
   for Library of Congress   91-4944

Printed on acid-free paper.

Typeset by Techset Composition Ltd, Salisbury, United Kingdom.

9 8 7 6 5 4 3 2 1

Series Preface

It is estimated that the functionally significant body of knowledge for a given medical specialty changes radically every 8 years. New specialties and "sub-specialization" are occurring at approximately an equal rate. Historically, established journals have not been able either to absorb this increase in publishable material or to extend their readership to the new specialists. International and national meetings, symposia and seminars, workshops, and newsletters successfully bring to the attention of physicians within developing specialties what is occurring, but generally only in demonstration form without providing historical perspective, pathoanatomical correlates, or extensive discussion. Page and time limitations oblige the authors to present only the essence of their material.

Pediatric neurosurgery is an example of a specialty that has developed during the past 15 years. Over this period neurosurgeons have obtained special training in pediatric neurosurgery and then dedicated themselves primarily to its practice. Centers, Chairs, and educational programs have been established as groups of neurosurgeons in different countries throughout the world organized themselves respectively into national and international societies for pediatric neurosurgery. These events were both preceded and followed by specialized courses, national and international journals, and ever-increasing clinical and investigative studies into all aspects of surgically treatable diseases of the child's nervous system.

Principles of Pediatric Neurosurgery is an ongoing series of publications, each dedicated exclusively to a particular subject, a subject which is currently timely either because of an extensive amount of work occurring in it, or because it has been neglected. The two first subjects, "Head Injuries in the Newborn and Infant" and "The Pediatric Spine," are expressive of those extremes.

Volumes will be published continuously, as the subjects are dealt with, rather than on an annual basis, since our goal is to make this information available to the specialist when it is new and informative. If a volume becomes obsolete because of newer methods of treatment and concepts, we shall publish a new edition.

The chapters are selected and arranged to provide the reader, in each instance, with embryological, developmental, epidemiological, clinical, therapeutic, and psychosocial aspects of each subject, thusly permitting each specialist to learn what is most current in his field and to familiarize himself with sister fields of the same subject. Each chapter is organized along classical lines, progressing from introduction through symptoms and treatment, to prognosis for clinical material; and introduction through history and data, to results and discussion for experimental material.

Contents

Contributors

PIER ANTONIO BATTISTELLA
Department of Pediatrics, University of Padua Medical School, Padua, Italy

A. BELTRAMELLO
Service of Neuroradiology, Verona University Hospital, Verona, Italy

MASSIMO CALDARELLI
Institute of Neurosurgery, Section of Pediatric Neurosurgery, Catholic University School of Medicine, Rome, Italy

MAURICE CHOUX
Hôpital des Enfants de la Timone, Marseille, France

FEDERICO COLOMBO
Department of Neurosurgery, City Hospital, Vicenza, Italy

CONCEZIO DI ROCCO
Institute of Neurosurgery, Section of Pediatric Neurosurgery, Catholic University School of Medicine, Rome, Italy

KAZUMASA EHARA
Department of Neurological Surgery, Kobe University School of Medicine, Kobe, Japan

PHILIPPE FARNARIER
Hôpital des Enfants de la Timone, Marseille, France

RICARDO GARCIA-MONACO
Unité de Neurologie Vasculaire Diagnostique et Theraputique, Hopital Bicetre, Universite Paris Sud, Paris, France

LORENZO GENITORI
Hôpital des Enfants de la Timone, Marseille, France

ALAN HILL
Division of Neurology, Department of Paediatrics, University of British Columbia, British Columbia's Children's Hospital, Vancouver, British Columbia, Canada

W. ISLER
Kinderspital Zurich, Zurich, Switzerland

CLAUDE LAPRAS
Hôpital Neurologique, Lyon, France

PIERRE LASJAUNIAS
Unité de Neurologie Vasculaire Diagnostique et Theraputique, Hopital
Bicetre, Universite Paris Sud, Paris, France

K. STUART LEE
Barrow Neurological Institute, Phoenix, Arizona, USA

GABRIEL LENA
Hôpital des Enfants de la Timone, Marseille, France

CARLO MARCELLETTI
Department of Cardiovascular Surgery, Bambino Gesu Hospital,
Rome, Italy

SHIZUO OI
Department of Neurosurgery, Kobe University School of Medicine,
Kobe, Japan

IGNACIO PASCUAL-CASTROVIEJO
Service of Child Neurology, La Paz Hospital, Madrid, Spain

PIERO A. PELLEGRINO
Department of Pediatrics, University of Padua School of Medicine,
Padua, Italy

SERGIO PICARDO
Department of Cardiovascular Surgery, Bambino Gesu Hospital,
Rome, Italy

ANTHONY J. RAIMONDI
Villa Monteleone, Gargagnago, Italy

HAROLD L. REKATE
Barrow Neurological Institute, Phoenix, Arizona, USA

KIYOSHI SATO
Department of Neurosurgery, The Juntendo University Hospital,
Tokyo, Japan

TAKEYOSHI SHIMOJI
Department of Neurosurgery, The Juntendo University Hospital,
Tokyo, Japan

NORIHIKO TAMAKI
Department of Neurological Surgery, Kobe University School of
Medicine, Kobe, Japan

KAREL TERBRUGGE
Unité de Neurologie Vasculaire Diagnostique et Theraputique, Hopital Bicetre, Universite Paris Sud, Paris, France

JOSEPH J. VOLPE
Washington University School of Medicine, St. Louis, Missouri, USA

LUIGI ZANESCO
Department of Pediatric Oncohematology, University of Padua School of Medicine, Padua, Italy

MICHEL ZERAH
Unité de Neurologie Vasculaire Diagnostique et Theraputique, Hopital Bicetre, Universite Paris Sud, Paris, France

CHAPTER 1

Dynamics of Changes from Fetal to Postnatal Circulation

Carlo Marcelletti and Sergio Picardo

Introduction

In the first few minutes after birth tremendous and dramatic changes occur in the circulation. During birth, constriction of the umbilical vessels removes the very low-resistance placental vascular bed, which is associated with an increase in systemic vascular resistance and results in a marked reduction of the inferior vena cava return. Simultaneously with the cessation of the umbilical–placental flow, the gas-exchange function is transferred from the placenta to the lungs, with a rapid reduction in pulmonary vascular resistance and a marked increase of the pulmonary blood flow associated with expansion of the lungs with air. Following these changes, which are essential for immediate survival, many other cardiocirculatory adaptations occur during the postnatal period with continuous adjustment. In this chapter we propose a brief review of our current knowledge of fetal circulation and the changes that occur postnatally.

Fetal Circulation

Knowledge of the course and distribution of the fetal circulation is very important to the understanding of the normal adaptations at the time of birth. Most of the information regarding the fetal circulation has been derived from fetal lambs,[1-3] and despite differences in species, degree of maturity, and body proportions, preliminary observations indicate that the course and the distribution of the circulation are quite similar in fetal lambs and in human fetuses. Although studies in fetal lambs have produced

varying results in terms of the relative distribution of fetal blood flow, the course of the flow is certain. Blood is oxygenated in the placenta and returns to the fetus through the umbilical veins (Fig. 1.1). The blood splits at the liver, so that approximately 50% perfuses the liver and returns to the inferior vena cava via the hepatic veins. The remaining 50% of the umbilical blood flow bypasses the liver via the ductus venosus and directly enters the inferior vena cava.[4,5] The

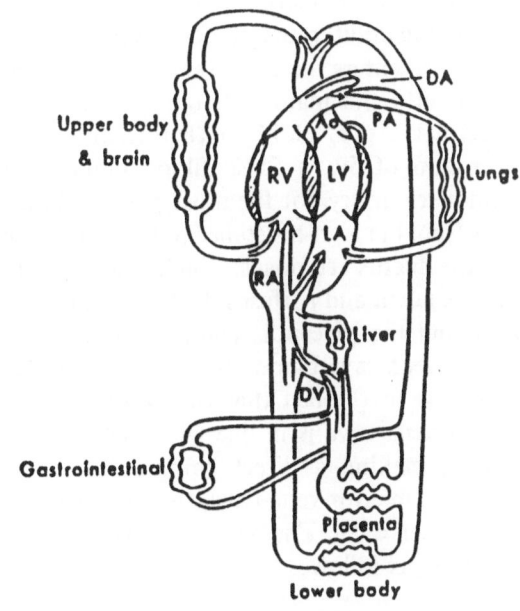

Figure 1.1. Fetal circulation. RV, right ventricle; LV, left ventricle; RA, right atrium; LA, left atrium; DA, ductus arteriosus; DV, ductus venosus; Ao, aorta; PA, pulmonary artery. (From Rudolph AM: Congenital Diseases of the Heart. Chicago, Year Book Medical, 1974, p. 2, with permission.)

factors that control this split are not well understood. The ductus does not appear to be particularly sensitive to changes in pO_2, pCO_2, or pH; the ductus flow is independent of the total umbilical blood flow; and there is not any relationship with different gestational ages. The ductus venosus could serve as a low-resistance shunt and could be effective in lowering the total umbilical–placental resistance, thus decreasing the vascular impedance to the fetal ventricles. The inferior vena cava carries the oxygenated blood from the umbilical vein and the desaturated blood from the lower part of the body. Approximately one-third of the blood from the inferior vena cava, or 25% or the total venous return, is shunted through the foramen ovale into the left atrium. The inferior vena cava blood has a pO_2 of 28 to 30 torr and an O_2 saturation of 70%. Here it is joined by the pulmonary blood flow, which is about 9% of the venous return, and pO_2 is lowered to 26 to 28 torr with an O_2 saturation of 65%. Then this blood goes to the left ventricle, it is ejected into the ascending aorta, and perfuses the coronary circulation and the upper part of the body. The remaining two-thirds of the inferior vena cava blood, plus most of the desaturated blood from the superior vena cava, enters the right ventricle and is then ejected into the main pulmonary artery. This blood has a pO_2 of 16 to 18 torr and an O_2 saturation of 50 to 55%. Blood entering the pulmonary artery, for the most part, is shunted away from the high-resistance pulmonary circuit into the ductus arteriosus, which enters the descending aorta and perfuses the lower part of the body and the placenta. The separation of the inferior vena cava blood into two streams is felt to be due to the fact that the entrance of the inferior vena cava is in line with the interatrial septum, making a direct communication between the inferior vena cava, the two atria, and the foramen ovale. The results of this fetal circulation are as follows:

1. The right ventricle ejects against a high-resistance district (lungs district), and so blood is shunted to the low-resistance pathway at the ductus arteriosus. The left ventricle, on the other hand, ejects into a low-resistance district that supplies the blood to the upper

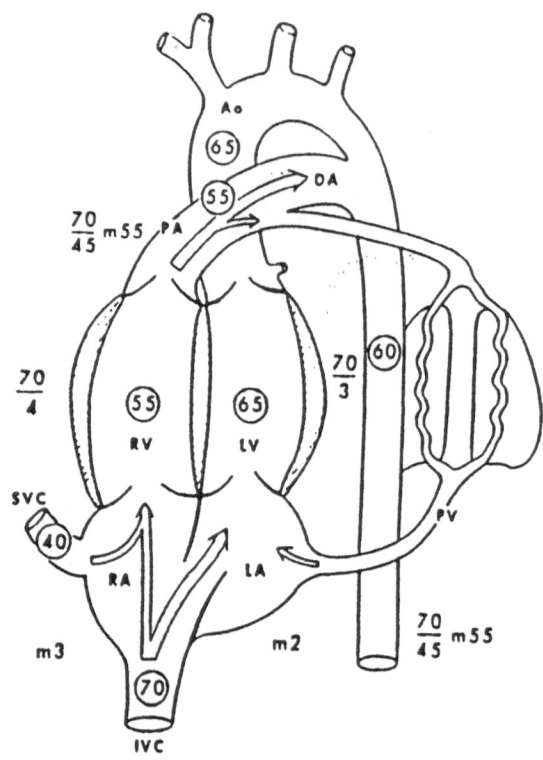

Figure 1.2. Fetal pressures and oxygen saturations. Circled numbers are the oxygen saturations. The ventricular and vascular pressures are shown: m, mean pressure; RV, right ventricle; LV, left ventricle; RA, right atrium; LA, left atrium; DA, ductus arteriosus; Ao, aorta,; PA, pulmonary artery; SVC, superior vena cava; IVC, inferior vena cava; PV, pulmonary vein. (From Rudolph AM: Congenital Diseases of the Heart. Chicago, Year Book Medical, 1974, p. 3, with permission.)

body. Therefore, although the ventricles function in parallel, the fact that there is an intercommunication at atrial level and at the level of the great arteries results in a right-to-left shunt at both sites during fetal development.

2. The lower part of the body and the placenta are supplied with blood of a lower pO_2 than the upper part of the body (Fig. 1.2).

Cardiac Output

The fetal cardiac output is expressed by the term *combined ventricular output* (CVO). This is defined as the total volume of blood ejected by both the right and the left ventricles and includes the coronary and pulmonary circulations. The cardiac output in the newborn is represented, instead, by the output of one ventricle, because in the normal postnatal circulation the ventricular outputs are similar. The CVO of fetal lambs is about 500 ml/kg/min, the cardiac output of newborn lambs is about 200 ml/kg/min, if one ventricle is considered, and 400 ml/kg/min if both ventricles are taken into account.[6] Approximately 35 to 55% of the CVO passes to the placenta, where the gaseous exchange occurs, while only 7% passes through the lungs because of the extremely high resistance. The proportions of CVO distributed to fetal organs and the placenta change with advancing gestation. There is a gradual reduction in the proportion of CVO distributed to the placenta, and this is associated with an increase of brain, lung, and gut flow. Although the myocardium receives a large flow throughout gestation,[7] and it is reasonable considering that it is the most active organ metabolically in the fetus, the flow per unit of mass does not change during fetal growth. On the other hand, the increase in flow that goes to the brain, gut, and lungs could be related to an increase in vascularity of these organs, or to an increase in metabolic activity, or both. Because the proportions of blood shunted through the major fetal communications do not change with gestation, it may be convenient to consider flows in terms of proportion of CVO. The right ventricle ejects about 60 to 65% and the left ventricle only 35 to 40% of CVO. The lungs receive 7 to 8% of CVO, and the remaining 55% of CVO ejected by the right ventricle passes through the ductus arteriosus. The left ventricle provides 3% of CVO to the myocardium, 20% to the head, neck, upper body, and forequarters, and only 10 to 15% passes into the descending aorta. The placenta receives 40% of CVO. The difference in output of the left and right ventricles in the fetus is of considerable interest, particularly considering that these differences disappear immediately after birth. In the fetus the left and right ventricles are subjected to the same filling pressures because the atrial pressures are almost identical, as a result of the presence of the large foramen ovale. Also, the free walls of the two

ventricles are similar in thickness. The aortic and pulmonary trunk systolic and diastolic pressures are similar. However, although the pressures are equal, the resistances against which the two ventricles eject are apparently different. The aortic isthmus is the narrower part of the aorta, thus its cross-sectional area is only about half that of the descending aorta. Although the pressures in descending and ascending aorta are equal, there is some evidence that the aortic isthmus represents a site of functional separation. The difference in outflow resistance of the two ventricles has been shown in a study using flow transducers around the aorta and pulmonary trunk. In conclusion, in spite of similar filling pressures and equal systolic and diastolic pressures, the two ventricles eject different amounts of blood.

Regulation of Fetal Cardiac Output

The factors that influence CVO are

1. Heart rate
2. Preload
3. Afterload
4. Myocardial contractility

Heart Rate

During sleep state, or fetal activity, spontaneous changes in fetal heart rate occur. In particular, spontaneous increases in heart rate are associated with an increase in CVO, whereas decreases in heart rate are associated with a considerable fall in CVO.[8] The limited ability to increase CVO suggests that the fetal heart is functioning near its maximum performance.

Preload

The end-diastolic pressure in both ventricles is similar, and in the fetal lamb in utero it is about 3 to 5 mm Hg above intraamniotic pressure. Reducing ventricular filling pressure below its resting value results in a dramatic fall in CVO, while increasing end-diastolic pressure produces only small increases in CVO.[9] These findings suggest that the fetal ventricle normally functions near the acme of its functional curve, having very little reserve to increase its output further. The lack of response to increasing filling pressure could indicate that the fetal myocardium does not have the ability to increase its force of contraction, but it could possibly be related to poor compliance of the ventricle. In conclusion, from several experimental studies it is evident that CVO is near its maximum level in the fetus at resting atrial filling pressure, and volume loading further increases output to a limited extent, possibly because the heart is very sensitive to the increased afterload created by the rise in arterial pressure. It could also be that ventricular compliance is relatively low, because ability to increase myocardial contractility is limited, or it could be due to a combination of these factors.

Afterload

The inflation of a balloon in the fetal descending aorta produces a dramatic decrease in CVO, indicating that the fetal heart is very sensitive to increases in afterload. The relative influence of afterload change on CVO at different gestational ages and different postnatal ages is yet to be assessed.

Myocardial Contractility

The fetal myocardium presents, from a morphological point of view, considerable differences from adult myocardium.[10] Relative to tissue volume, the myofibrillar content is less, so that the fetal myocardium has less contractile tissue. Ultrastructural studies of fetal myocardium have shown a paucity of sarcoplasmic reticulum and a poorly developed or absent T-tubule system as compared with adult myocardium. After birth, the relationship between sarcoplasmic reticulum and sarcolemma in regulating excitation–contraction coupling may change, with a resultant modification of intracellular calcium cycling. In fetal heart, the increase in cytosolic calcium following excitation may be provided largely by transsarcolemmal movement of calcium.

Control of the Fetal Circulation

In the adult, the circulation is regulated by nervous and hormonal influences, and the Frank–Starling mechanism is responsible for maintaining a balance between left and right ventricle output. In the fetus, because of the presence of large communications between the left and right sides of the heart, the ventricles function as a common chamber, and there is no need for a balancing of ventricular output, so the Frank–Starling mechanism is not essential.[11] The neuronal control of the circulation is mediated by the autonomic nervous system. This regulation needs maturation of the nervous system, development of the receptor sites, and development of the reflex response. Although several studies have shown that the neural and reflex mechanisms are developed in the fetus, it is not known whether they are important in fetal circulation. Since the fetus has a limited ability to increase CVO, a baroreflex stimulation results in a decrease in heart rate and in CVO, with a decrease in umbilical flow, and fetal asphyxia. Thus, it is possible that the baroreflexes are developed for postnatal adaptation. Hormonal control of the circulation is dependent on the ability of the endocrine organs to secrete the hormones on the development of the receptor, and on the ability of the effector cells to respond. Although it has been shown that there is some α- and β-adrenergic activity, it is not clear whether the adrenergic activity is due to circulating catecholamines or to autonomic circulation; there is some evidence favoring a dominance of parasympathetic and α-adrenergic activity at earlier gestational periods, and that β-adrenergic activity matures later.

Transitional Circulation

The fundamental adaptation to postnatal life depends upon a change from the placenta to the lungs as the oxygenating organ (Fig. 1.3). The rapid transition to adult circulation at birth depends on four factors:

1. Removal of the low-resistance circuit (placenta) from systemic circulation
2. Reversal of the relative pressure between the right and the left atrium, leading to closure of the foramen ovale
3. Muscular constriction of the ductus arteriosus
4. Decrease in pulmonary vascular resistance

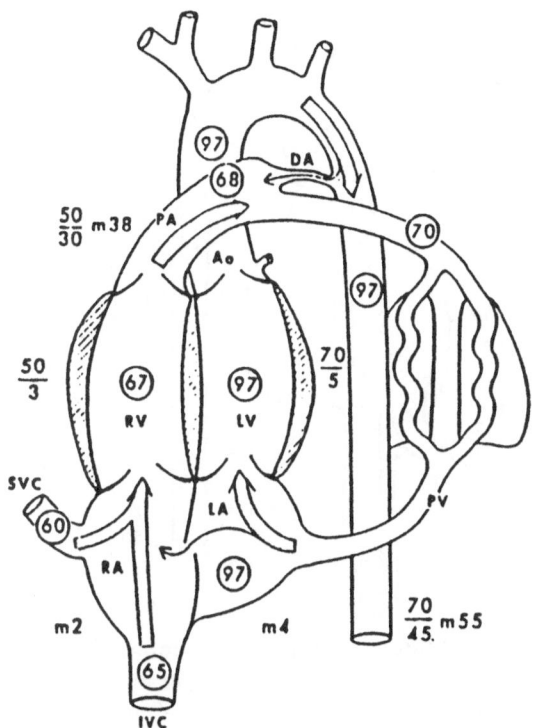

Figure 1.3. Transitional circulation. Ao, Aorta; LV, left ventricle; RV, right ventricle; RA, right atrium; LA, left atrium; DA, ductus arteriosus; PA, pulmonary artery; PV, pulmonary vein; SVC, superior vena cava; IVC, inferior vena cava; m, mean pressure. Circled numbers are oxygen saturations. (From Rudolph AM: Congenital Diseases of the Heart. Chicago, Year Book Medical, 1974, p. 18, with permission.)

Interruption of the Umbilical Cord

The separation of the infant from the umbilical–placental circulation results in the sudden cessation of a flow of about 40% of CVO from the descending aorta to the placenta. The removal of this low-resistance circulation results in an increase in systemic vascular resistance. The inferior vena cava return falls dramatically, because only the venous return of the lower part of body is now returning to the heart. Also, the blood flow from the portal vein through the liver is reduced, and the blood flow through the ductus venosus falls immediately; this channel closes after birth. It is possible that the ductus venosus is closed passively, as a result of the decrease of the portal venous pressure. As a result of this decrease in the inferior vena cava

blood flow there is a small decrease in inferior vena cava pressure.

Closure of the Foramen Ovale

The foramen ovale is held open in the fetus by the large flow from the inferior vena cava, but after birth, due to the decrease in pulmonary vascular resistance, there is a large increase in pulmonary blood flow, and thus in left atrium venous return. The simultaneous increase in left atrium venous return and the decrease of the inferior vena cava venous return result in opposition of the valve of the foramen ovale against the crista dividens, with functional closure of the foramen ovale.

Closure of the Ductus Arteriosus

In the fetus, the ductus arteriosus is a very large channel. It has a thick medial muscular coat that is capable of constriction, mainly in response to changes in pO_2. The rise in systemic pO_2 immediately after birth is the main factor responsible for closure of the ductus arteriosus. In the normal mature infant the ductus closes within 10 to 15 hr after birth, but it can be reopened if systemic pO_2 is reduced. Although pO_2 is the main factor responsible for the closure of the ductus, there is the possibility that either neurologic mechanisms or vasoactive substances may exert some constrictor response.

Changes of the Pulmonary Circulation

Pulmonary vascular resistance falls precipitously after birth, in association with breathing. The immediate change must be due to active vasodilation, or the lack of a vasoconstricting agent, or both. The exact mechanisms responsible for the postnatal fall in resistance are not known, but at the least, increase in arterial pO_2 release of vasodilator agent, and expansion of the lungs play an important role. It has been shown that an increase in systemic O_2 saturation decreases pulmonary vascular resistance, but it is not known if this effect is the direct result of factors acting on the pulmonary vasculature or stimulates release of a vasodilator agent. It has been shown that the lungs release vasodilator hormones into the circulation, and recently it has been suggested that some agents, such as angiotensin and bradykinin, stimulate local production of prostaglandin I_2 (PGI_2). In addition, infusion of inhibitor of leukotriene causes an increase in pulmonary blood flow. Distension of the lungs causes release of prostaglandin E, and more recently it has been shown that the ventilated lung produces PGI_2. Finally, two phases of fall in pulmonary vascular resistance were noted after ventilation. An initial drop occurs within 30 sec, and it is not influenced by indomethacin; and, a second phase, which occurs over 10 to 20 min, is impaired by indomethacin.

Change in Cardiac Output

After birth, left ventricular output increases considerably from the fetal level of about 150 ml/min/kg of body weight to 300 to 400 ml/min/kg. Postnatally, resting cardiac output decreases progressively in relation to body weight.[12] Since the fetal heart has a reduced reserve for increased CVO, it is of interest to assess the factors responsible for the increase in the myocardial performance. One of these could be an increase in myocardial contractility immediately after birth, which then disappears within the first week. Another factor could be thyroid hormones, since they have been shown to influence the relationship between the α and β heavy-chain myosins in ventricular myocardium.[13,14]

In conclusion, the transitional circulation consists of a low-resistance pulmonary circuit and a high-resistance systemic circuit only functionally, but not anatomically, separated.

Mature Circulation

Within a few days after birth, the infant circulation is similar to the adult circulation (Fig. 1.4). The pulmonary vascular resistance, which drops dramatically at the time of birth, is still somewhat higher than in the adult and continues to decrease over the first few months of life. The arterial blood pressure is lower in the infant, and increases to adult values by adolescence. The stroke volume increases with

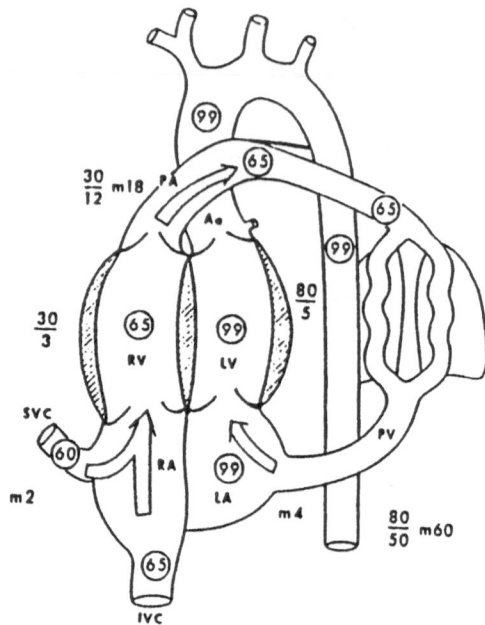

Figure 1.4. Mature circulation. Ao, aorta; LV, left ventricle; RV, right ventricle; RA, right atrium; LA, left atrium; PA, pulmonary artery; PV, pulmonary vein; SVC, superior vena cava; IVC, inferior vena cava; m, mean pressure. Circled numbers are oxygen saturation. (From Rudolph AM: Congenital Diseases of the Heart. Chicago, Year Book Medical, 1974, p. 19, with permission.)

age and cardiac output increases with body surface area, while heart rate decreases with age. The mature circulation must function to carry blood oxygenated by the lungs to all tissues of the body and return metabolic end products to the lungs and kidneys for removal.

Metabolic Change in the Cardiovascular System

It seems that the fetal cardiovascular system differs from the adult in terms of:

1. Thermoregulation
2. Oxygen consumption
3. Energy metabolism

Thermoregulation

Thermoregulation is the function of maintaining body temperature in the thermoneutral zone, by balancing heat production and heat loss. Shortly after birth, the infant's body temperature may drop 2 to 3°C, mostly due to evaporative loss and the high surface/body ratio. Peripheral vasoconstriction is the main mechanism by which the newborn can reduce heat loss. Infants are able to produce heat through nonshivering thermogenesis. This is a process whereby a catecholamine-activated lipase breaks down brown adipose tissue. The heat is produced by the oxidation of free fatty acid liberated from triglicerides. The cardiovascular effects of temperature regulation in the infant are similar to those in the adult. An increase in temperature causes a decrease in systemic vascular resistance and an increase in heart rate and cardiac output. A decrease in temperature causes vasoconstriction and a slight decrease in heart rate and cardiac output.

Oxygen Consumption

A full-term infant weighing approximately 3.5 kg and in a neutral thermal environment has an oxygen consumption of about 4.6 ml/kg/min. Studies have shown oxygen consumption increases to 7 ml/kg/min at 10 days and 8 ml/kg/min at 4 weeks. Theoretical reasons for this increase in basal oxygen consumption have

been an increase in the level of sympathetic activity, increase in arterial pO_2, and increase in muscular tone. Compared to adults, newborns seem to be able to increase oxygen consumption on exposure to cold. Myocardial oxygen consumption also is increased by inotropic agents, catecholamines, and exercise in the newborn and adult.

Energy Metabolism

The heart is primarily dependent on anaerobic metabolism. Myocardial adenosine 5'-triphosphate (ATP) is stored in the mitochondria. In fetal and newborn infants there is no age-related difference in the presence or absence of oxygen consumption per milligram of protein in the presence of adenosine 5'-diphosphate (ADP). Oxygen consumption in mitochondria, uncoupled by 2,4-dinitrophenol, was also higher in the fetus and newborn than in the adult. This suggests there may be increased electron transport in young animals. In addition, a great cytochrome c oxidase activity is found in fetal and newborn mitochondria when compared to the adult. Thus, there seems to be an increased aerobic capacity of the fetal and newborn mitochondria.

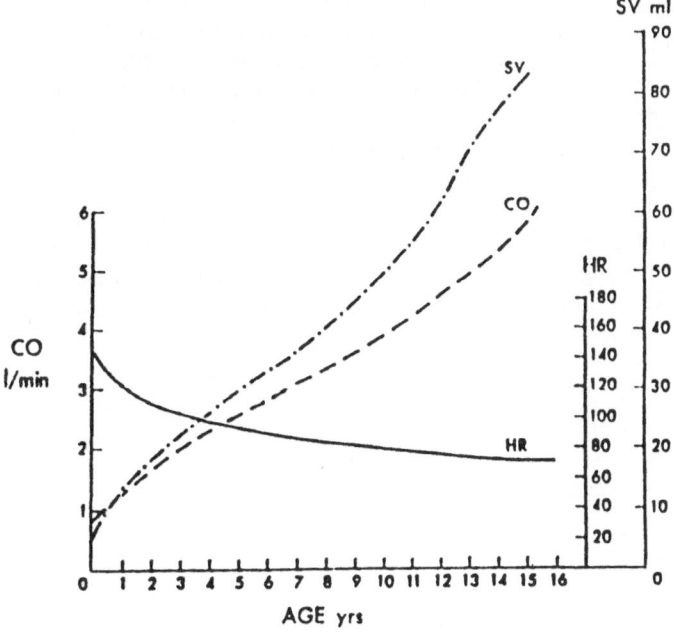

Figure 1.5. Changes in cardiac output (CO), stroke volume (SV), and heart rate (HR) with age. (From Rudolph AM: Congenital Diseases of the Heart, Chicago, Year Book Medical, 1974, p. 27, with permission.)

Changes with Postnatal Growth

After the adaptations that occur in the cardiocirculatory system in the perinatal period, several other changes occur during growth. There are gradual changes in heart rate, cardiac output, and blood pressure during infancy (Fig. 1.5). Resting heart rate decreases with age. Cardiac output, expressed as per meter of body height, decreases, while cardiac output per square meter of body surface area is constant. This difference could be explained as a change in body configuration. In fact, with growth, there is an increase in limb size and skeletal muscle, with a relative decrease in vital organ weight. Since blood flow to the muscle and in general to the extremities is quite low per unit of tissue mass, the total blood flow could be quite low in relation to body weight. Associated with body growth, there is an increase in stroke volume, which is due to the fact that heart rate decreases with age. Systemic arterial blood flow and systemic vascular resistance also increase.

Conclusion

In conclusion, several cardiocirculatory changes occur during the perinatal and postnatal period. In this chapter we report the major alterations that are known; but many other changes occur, and further investigations are necessary.

References

1. Rudolph AM, Heyman MA: The circulation of the fetus in utero. Circ Res 21:163–184, 1967.
2. Rudolph AM, Heyman MA: Circulatory changes with growth in the fetal lambs. Circ Res 26:289–299, 1970.
3. Rudolph AM, Heyman MA: Control of the fetal circulation. In: Proceedings of the Sir Barcroft Centenary Symposium: Fetal and Neonatal Physiology. Cambridge University Press, Cambridge, 1976, pp. 89–11.
4. Edelstone DI, Rudolph AM, Heyman MA: Liver and ductus venosus blood flows in fetal lambs in utero. Circ Res 42:426–433, 1978.
5. Edelstone DI: Regulation of blood flow through the ductus venosus. J Devel Physiol 2:219–238, 1980.
6 Walsh SZ, Meyer WW, Lind J (eds.). The Human and Neonatal Circulation. Springfield, 1974, pp. 129–137.
7. Lee JC, Dowing SE: Coronary flow and myocardial oxygen metabolism in fetal and newborn lamb. Yale J Biol Med 46:233–248, 1973.
8. Rudolph AM, Heyman MA: Cardiac output in the fetal lamb: the effect of spontaneous and induced changes of fetal heart on right and left ventricular output. Am J Obstet Gynecol 124:183–192, 1976.
9. Gilbert RD: Control of fetal cardiac output during changes in blood volume. Am J Physiol 238:H80–H86, 1980.
10. Friedman, WF: The intrinsic properties of the developing heart. In: Friedman WF, Lesch M, Sonnenblick EH (eds.). Neonatal Heart Disease. Grune & Stratton, New York, 1973, pp. 21–49.
11. Kirkpatrick SE, Pitlick PT, Friedman WF; Frank–Starling relationship as an important determination of fetal cardiac output. Am J Physiol 231:495–500, 1976.
12. Klopfentein HS, Rudolph AM: Postnatal changes in the circulation, and response to volume loading in sheep. Circ Res 42:839–845, 1978.
13. Williams LT, Lefkowitz RJ, Watanabe SM: Thyroid hormone regulation of β-adrenergic receptor number. *Biol Chem* 252:2787–2790, 1977.
14. Picardo S, Li C, Rudolph AM: Cardiovascular and metabolic responses to thyroid hormone in fetal lambs. In: XIII Conference of the Society for the Study of Fetal Physiology. Vancouver, 1986, p. 39.

CHAPTER 2

Anatomy of Cerebral Vessels in Infants and Children

Anthony J. Raimondi

The form, caliber, distribution, and pairing of arterial and venous structures in the newborn, infant, and child are distinctly different from what one observes in the adult, though the naming of the vessels is identical. Consequently, it is assumed that the reader is conversant with standard neuroradiological nomenclature. Within broad limits one may safely generalize that the younger the child the wider the caliber and the greater the redundancy of intracisternal and intrafissural vessels (such as the internal carotid, sylvian complex, basilar and posterior cerebrals). This may be related to the relatively greater size of the basal cisterns and the fissures. Also, the frontal lobes in the newborn and infant are extremely small. This latter anatomic characteristic is responsible for the central sulcus being closer to the coronal suture.

Cortical venous structures are much better visualized in infants and children than in adults. Other than this, the same generalities apply to the venous as to the arterial structures.

Internal Carotid Artery, Primary Branches, and Perforating Vessels

In Figure 2.1, the siphon (S) is tight in appearance; one should note the high and posteriorly located bifurcation of the internal carotid artery (1), with the A1 segment of the anterior cerebral artery coursing directly anteriorly and the M1 segment of the middle cerebral artery looping inferiorly to it before entering the sylvian fissure. The redundancy of these vessels is obvious. The ophthalmic (O) takes origin from the internal carotid artery immediately beneath

the origin of the ophthalmic nerve, and the bifurcation of the internal carotid allows the reader to evaluate the size of the supraclinoid cistern in which the internal carotid is located. Of particular interest is the size of the lingual artery (L) in the newborn. Indeed, judging from cerebral angiography, the majority of blood flow to the head in the newborn is to the tongue and thalamus. The sylvian complex stands out clearly in this illustration since there is no filling of the anterior or posterior cerebral systems.

In Figure 2.2, the anterior choroidal artery (1) is quite large, as are the perforating vessels going to the basal ganglia and thalami. Note the prominence of the medial anterior inferior temporal artery (2), which courses within the sylvian fissure and over the medial surface of the temporal lobe to the corpus amygdaloideum. This vessel is the route of anastomosis for collateral flow between the anterior and middle cerebral systems, since it may anastomose with Heubner's artery, to which it establishes branches on occasion. The posterior bifurcation of the internal carotid artery (arrow) may be well appreciated, as may the distribution of the primary sylvian vessels over the insular cortex, curving outward at the circular sulcus of the insula (arrowheads) to run around the frontal (F) and parietal (P) opercula to gain access to the surface of the hemisphere.

In Figure 2.3, the posterior communicating artery (1) has the appearance of a so-called embryologic posterior communicator in that it is large in size and continues directly into the posterior cerebral proper (2), which embraces the brainstem within the ambient cistern. The posterior inferior temporal artery (3) and the

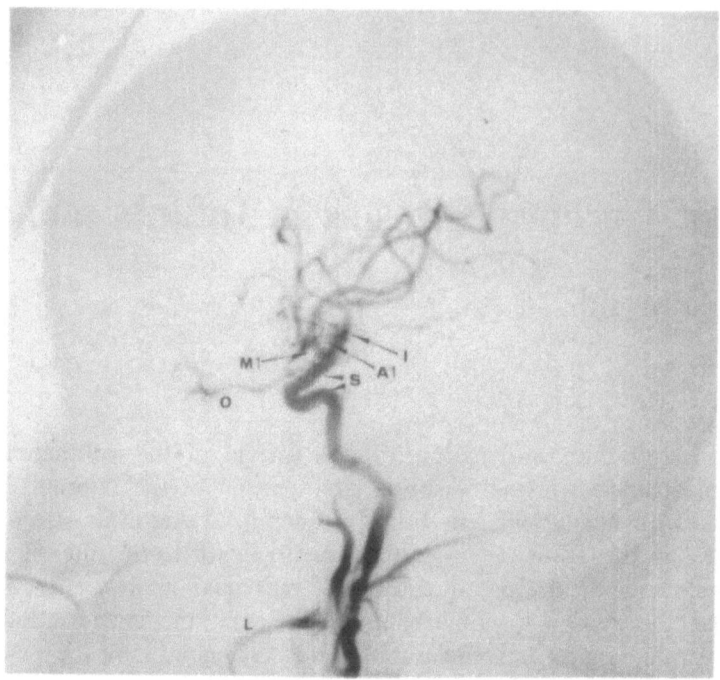

Figure 2.1.

internal occipital artery (4) nourish, respectively, the undersurface of the temporal lobe and the calcarine cortex on one hand, and the cuneate and parieto-occipital lobes on the other. One may appreciate the relative positions of the middle and posterior cerebral systems since there is only flash filling of the pericallosal system.

In Figure 2.4, the ophthalmic artery (1) allows one to appreciate both the course and length of the intracranial internal carotid artery, which has a high and lateral bifurcation (arrowhead).

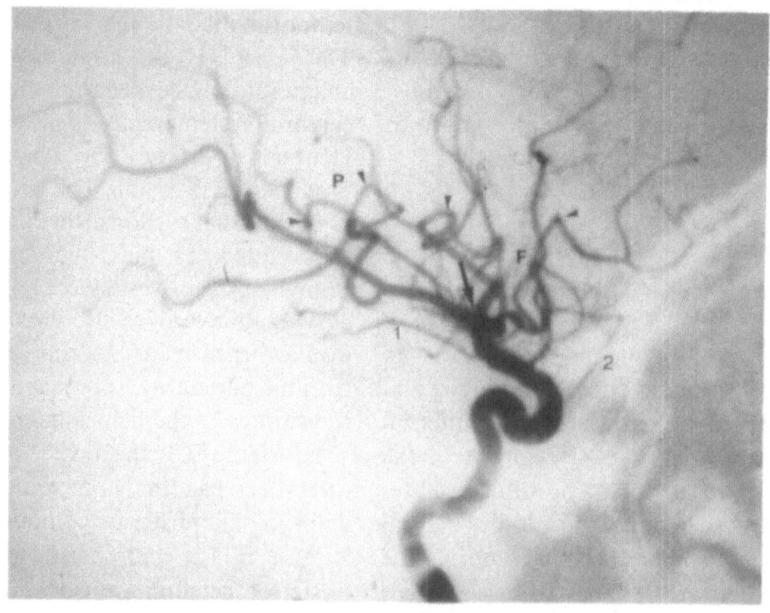

Figure 2.2.

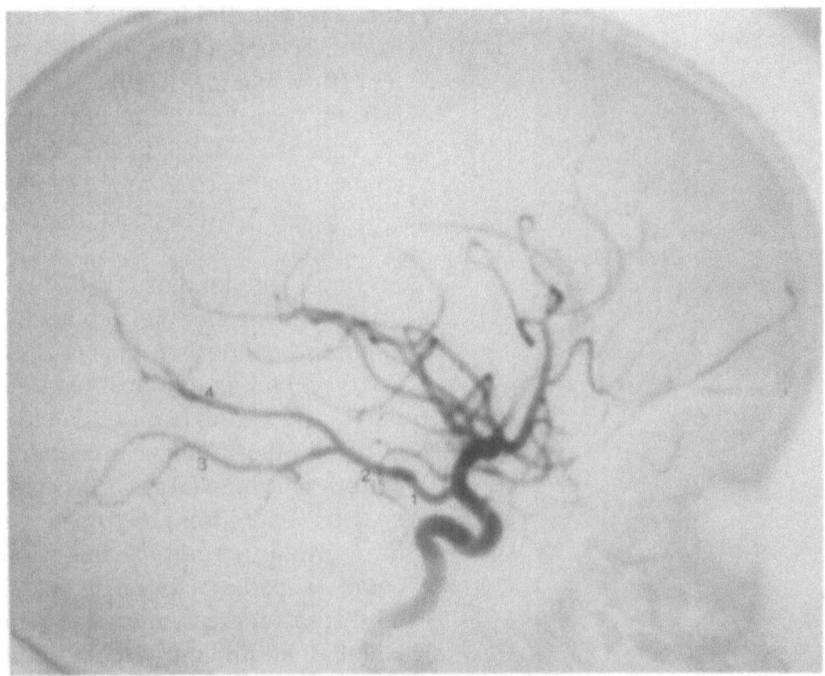

Figure 2.3.

The A1 portion of the anterior cerebral artery (2) also may be extremely redundant, though in premature infants it may be short and high, even following at times a superomedial course. The main trunk of the middle cerebral artery (3) generally is a mirror image of A1 in its course into or through the sylvian fissure before it curves over the insular cortex (4). The posterior communicating artery (5) courses through the interpeduncular cistern to join the posterior cerebral artery at the junction of its medial, mesencephalic (6), and lateral posterior cerebral

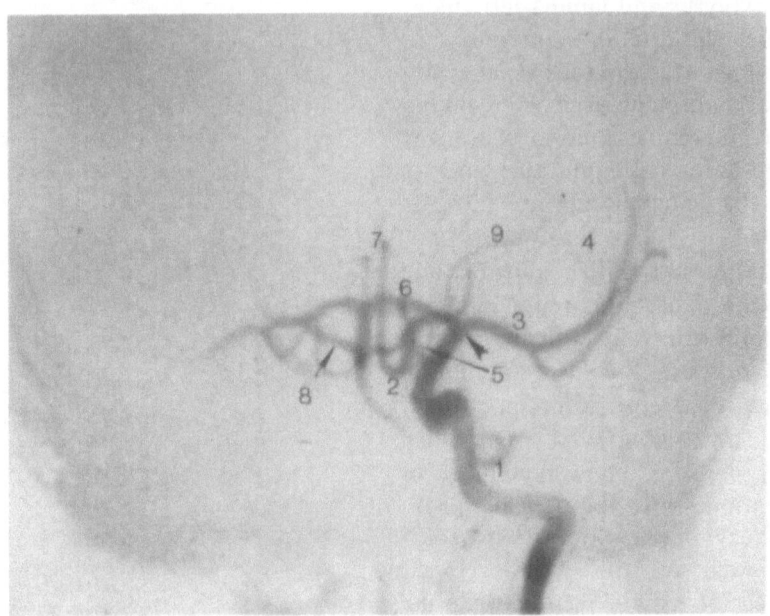

Figure 2.4.

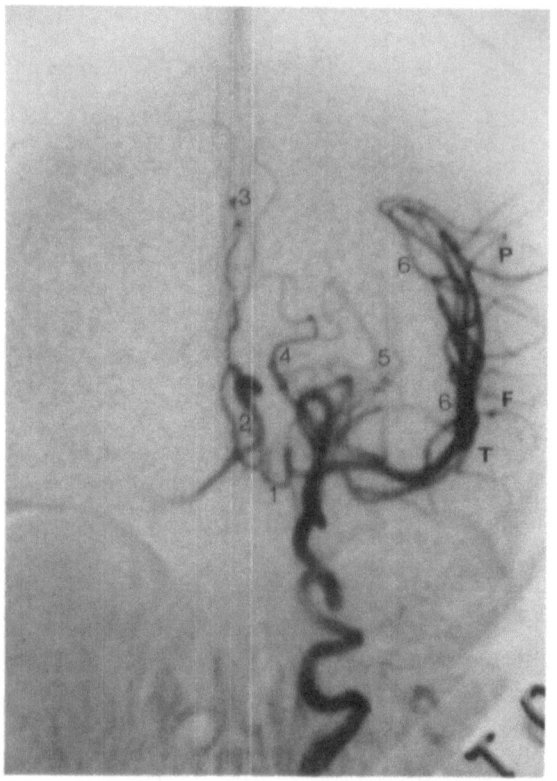

Figure 2.5.

complex with the temporal operculum (T), the frontal operculum (F), and the parietal operculum (P), being identifiable by the course of the sylvian branches from the opercular cortex through the sylvian fissure and sulci as they course to gain access to the cerebral convexity.

In Figure 2.6, the frontal basal branch (1) of the anterior cerebral system takes origin from the most inferior portion of the A2 segment, whereas the frontal polar branch (2) originates along the midportion of this vessel. Heubner's artery (H) originates most often from the body of A1 (arrowhead) and runs laterally toward the head of the caudate nucleus (arrow). The perforating branches of the middle cerebral system (3) arise from the superior surface of the intrasylvian portion of this vessel and then course superiorly through the anterior perforated substance to nourish the lentiform nuclei and the anterior limb of the internal capsule. The medial anterior temporal artery (4) curves over the medial surface of the temporal lobe and then generally gives origin to two branches: a superior branch (5) that courses superiorly and which, in the pathological condition, may establish anastomoses with Heubner's artery, and an inferior branch (6).

proper segments. The A2 portion of the anterior cerebral artery (7) swoops vertically in front of the para-olfactory gyrus and lamina terminalis. The superior cerebellar arteries (8) may be seen coming from the main trunk of the basilar artery and the anterior choroidal artery (9), taking origin from the internal carotid between the origin of the posterior communicator and its bifurcation and then coursing upward into the choroidal fissure.

In the half-axial projection in Figure 2.5, one may appreciate the remarkable redundancy of the internal carotid artery in both its cervical and intracranial portions. Similarly, the floppy course of the anterior cerebral artery in both its suprachiasmatic (1) and pre-III ventricular segments (2) may be seen. The wavy course of these vessels continues into the pericallosal (3) artery. Redundancy of the posterior cerebral artery (4), as well as the well-developed perforating vessels (5), may be seen between the anterior and middle cerebral systems. The insular cortex (6) has over its surface the sylvian

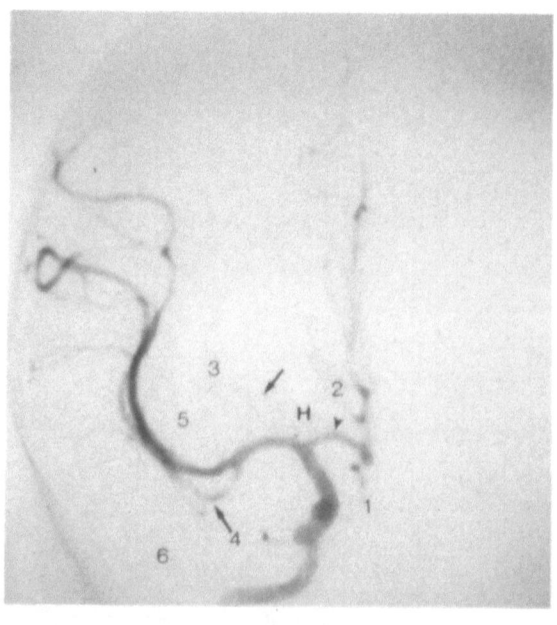

Figure 2.6.

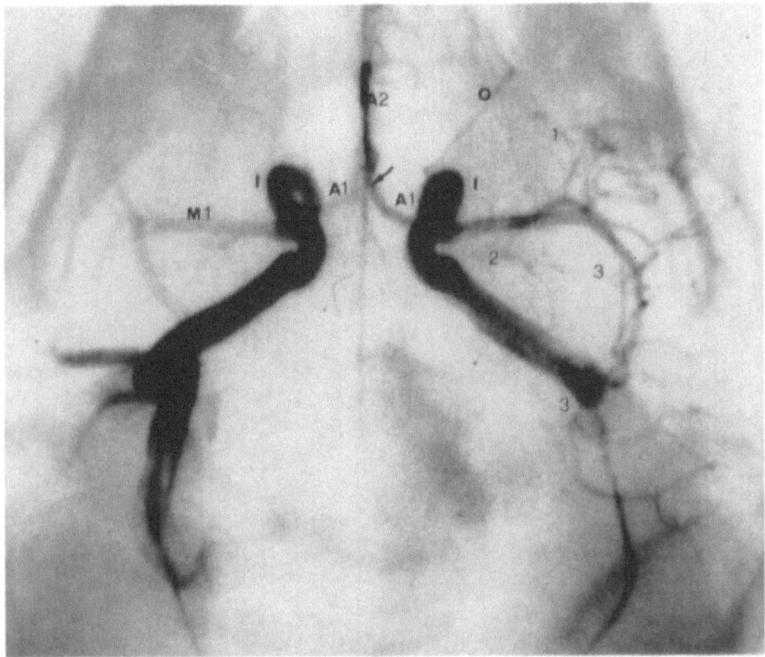

Figure 2.7.

The axial view shown in Figure 2.7 allows one to appreciate the circle of Willis and middle cerebral systems. The redundancy of the intracisternal internal carotid arteries (I) and the anteromedial course of the A-1 segments (A1) of the anterior cerebral arteries superior to the optic nerves and chiasm, to the region of the anterior communicating artery (arrow), is clearly shown. The anterior communicating artery almost invariably is not identifiable in normal angiography in childhood. The anterior course of the A2 segment of the anterior cerebral artery (A2) is best appreciated in the axial projection, as is the lateral course of the ophthalmic artery (O). The course of the middle cerebral artery through the sylvian fissure may be appreciated if one looks at the M1 portion (M1) of the middle cerebral artery on the left. The branches of the middle cerebral artery may be studied to advantage on the right. Here, one notices the anterior and medial course of the superior branch of the medial anterior temporal artery (1) and the initially medial and then lateral course of the perforating branches of the middle cerebral artery (2) as they penetrate the anterior perforated substance. The insular cortex (3) is covered by the main trunks of the sylvian system.

A variation in course of the posterior communicating artery (1), as well as the horizontal A1 portion of the anterior cerebral

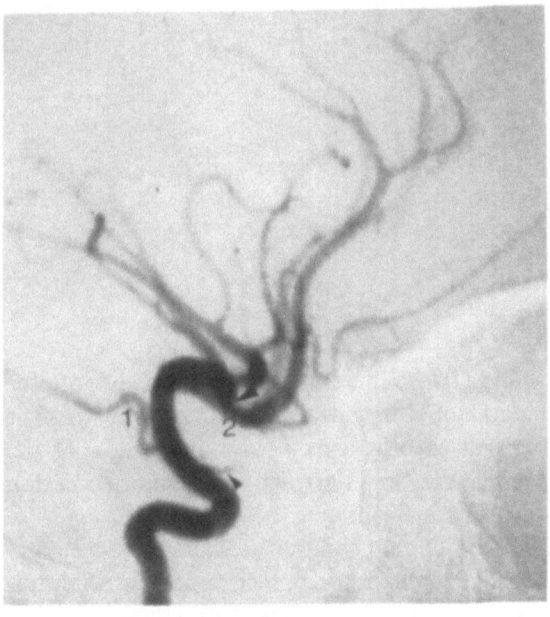

Figure 2.8.

Figure 2.9.

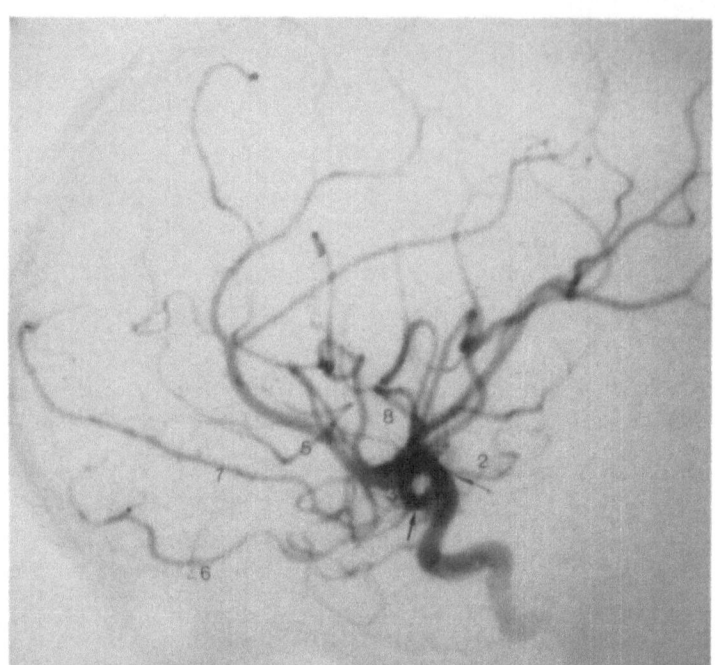

A

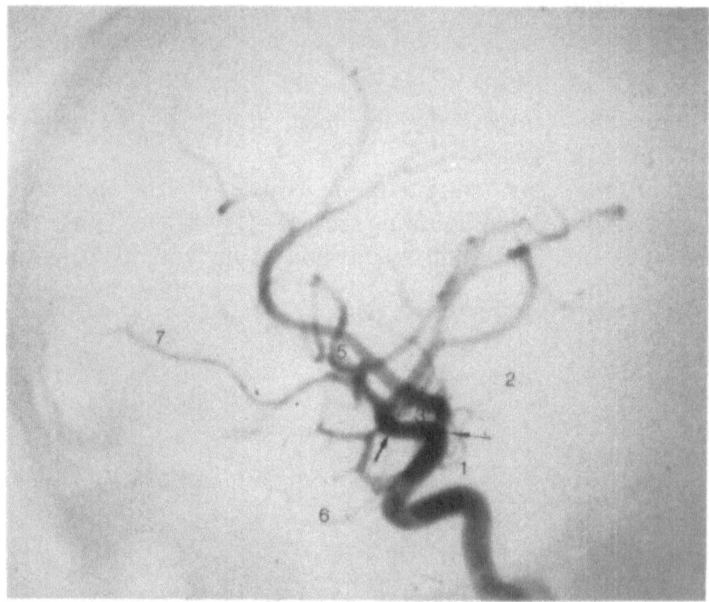

B

artery (2), are illustrated in Figure 2.8. Note the length of the intracisternal portion of the internal carotid artery from the origin of the ophthalmic (small arrowhead) to its bifurcation (large arrowhead).

Four different children are herein described to permit the reader to appreciate normal anatomical variations in the posterior communicating artery (1); anterior choroidal artery (2); bifurca-tion of internal carotid artery (thin arrow); the A-1 segment of the anterior cerebral artery (3): Heubner's artery (4) coming from the A-1 segment of the anterior cerebral artery; the varying types of A-2 of the anterior cerebral artery (3); the frontal basal artery (6); the frontal polar artery (7); the middle cerebral loop (bold arrow); the stain of the perforating branches of the middle cerebral system (8) (Fig. 2.9a–d).

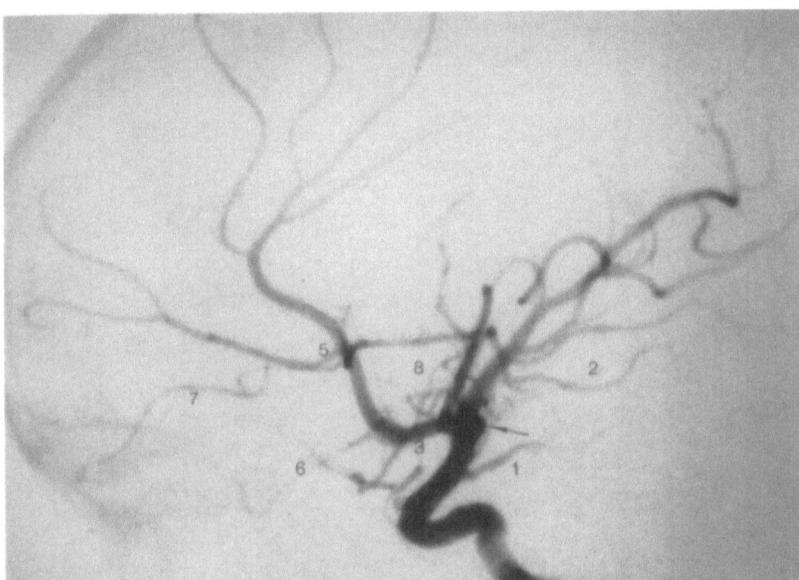

Figure 2.9. *Continued.*

C

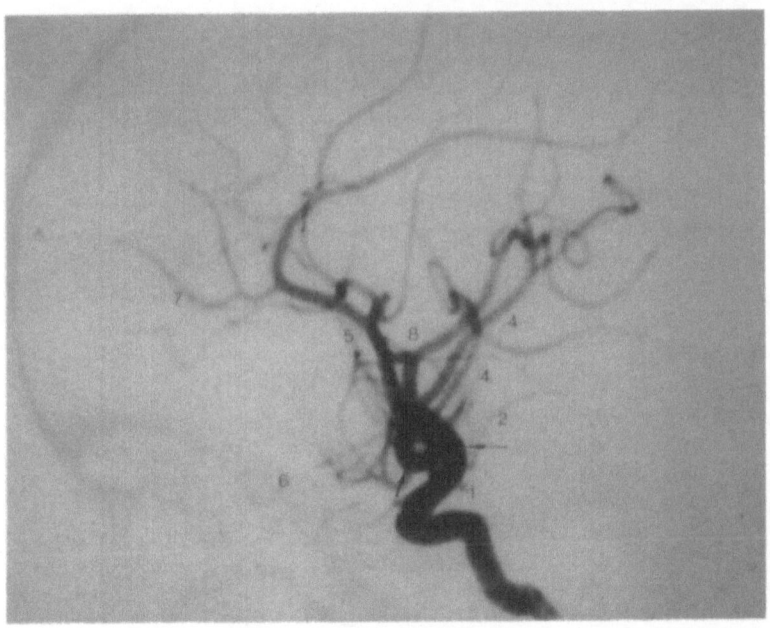

D

Secondary and Tertiary Branches of the Carotid System

In Figure 2.10, the lenticulostriate vessels stand out well between the intracisternal portion of the internal carotid artery and the anomalous origin of the anterior choroidal artery, which comes from the midportion of the posterior communi-cating artery. The early blush of the glomus of the choroid plexus within the trigone is well seen. The A2 portion of the anterior cerebral artery is located posterior to the middle cerebral trunk, a not uncommon observation in the newborn. The sylvian vessels are looping gently back onto themselves as they exit from the surface of the insular cortex through the sulci, indicating the marginal sulcus.

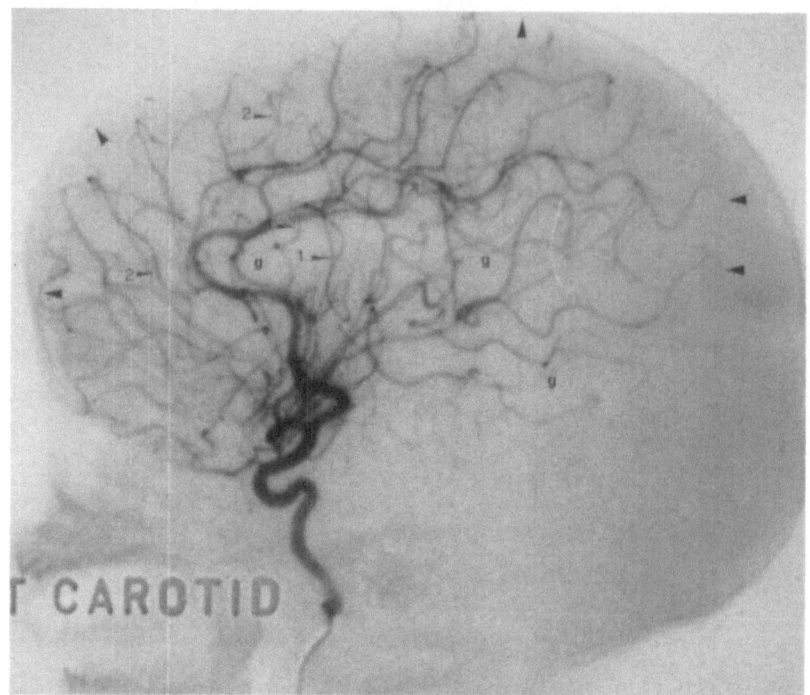

Figure 2.10.

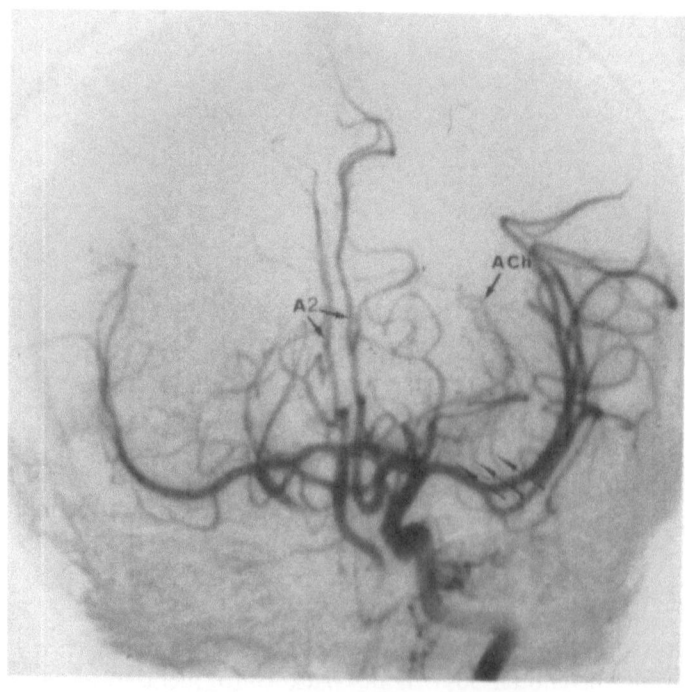

Figure 2.11.

Figure 2.12.

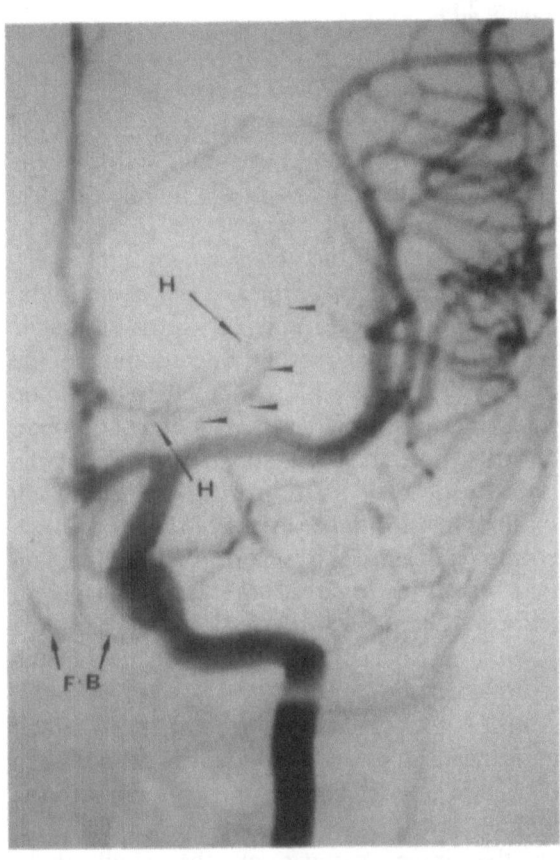

One notes that the gyri (g) are relatively uniform in width, separated by gently curving sulcal branches of the middle (1) and anterior (2) cerebral systems. This waviness of the sulcal arteries is most marked in the newborn. It is of interest to note that the terminal branches of the middle and anterior cerebral systems go out to the inner surface of the skull in the frontal and midparietal regions, but not in the posteroparietal and parieto-occipital regions (bold arrowheads).

In Figure 2.11, one notes a wide interval between the A2 segments of the anterior cerebral arteries (A2), staining of the choroid plexus as the anterior choroidal (A Ch) artery fills, and the many lenticulostriate branches of the intrasylvian portion of the middle cerebral artery (arrows).

In Figure 2.12, the initial rectilinear and then curvilinear courses of the frontobasal arteries (FB) provide one with information concerning the most inferomedial surfaces of each hemisphere. Heubner's artery (H) takes origin from

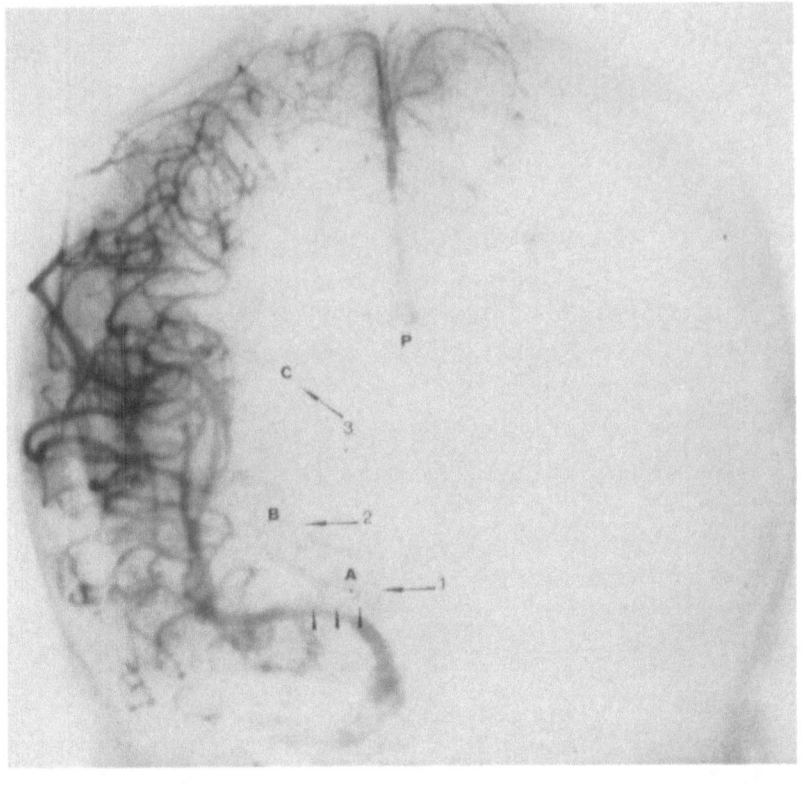

Figure 2.13.

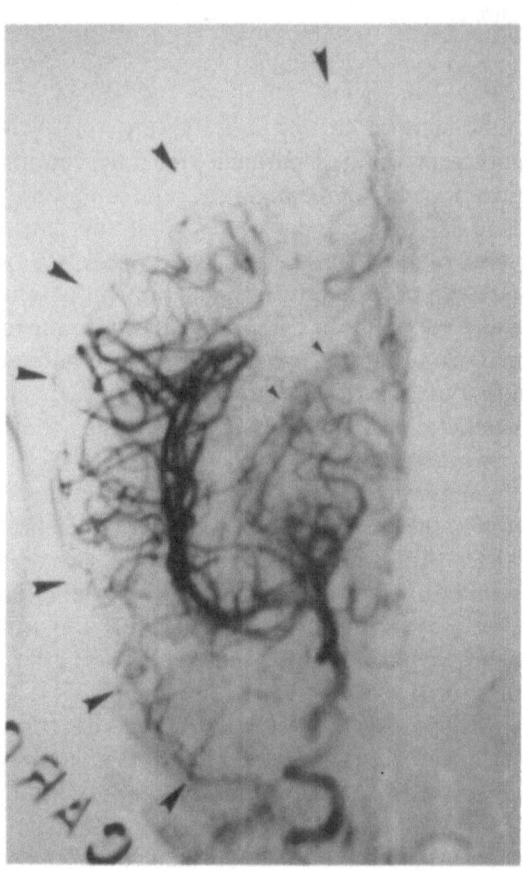

Figure 2.14.

A1 and then curves laterally toward the head of the caudate nucleus, where it crosses the lenticulostriate branches of the middle cerebral system (arrowheads).

In Figure 2.13, the anterior choroidal artery has an infracisternal portion (1), a choroidal fissure portion (2), and an intraventricular portion (3), which permit one to outline the uncus (A) where it is juxtaposed to the optic tract, the region of the lateral geniculate body and the optic tract (B), and the trigone of the lateral ventricle (C). The pericallosal plexus (P) outlines inferiorly the surface of the body of the corpus callosum and superiorly the cingulate gyri on either side of the interhemispheral fissure. The arrowheads indicate the anterior perforating substance at the bifurcation of the internal carotid artery.

In Figure 2.14, the choroidal blush (small arrowheads) allows one to identify precisely the choroidal fissure. The terminal branches of the middle cerebral system curve upon themselves at the inner surface of the skull (bold

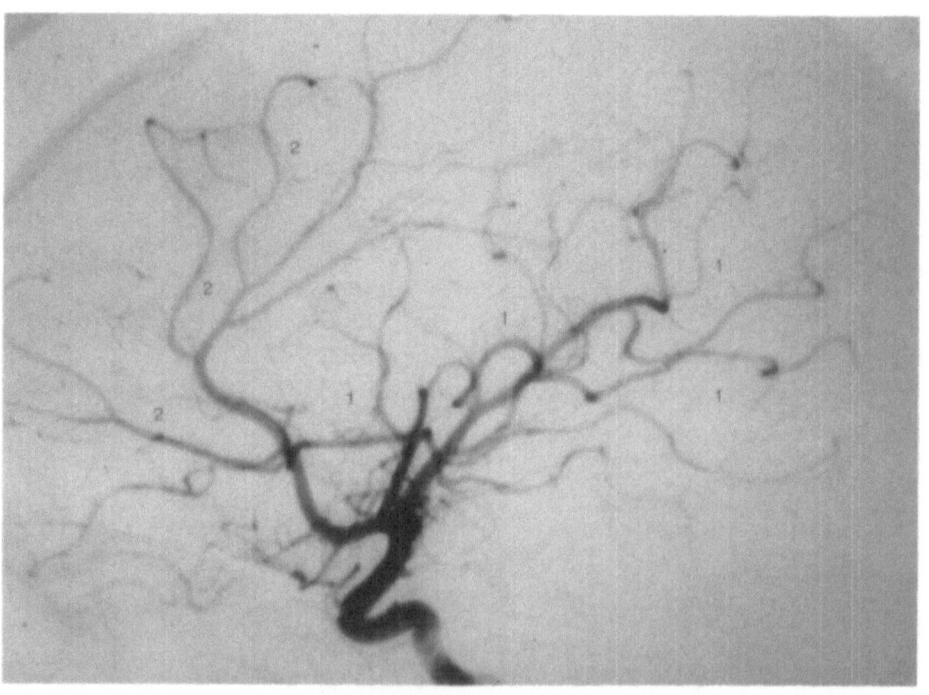

Figure 2.15.

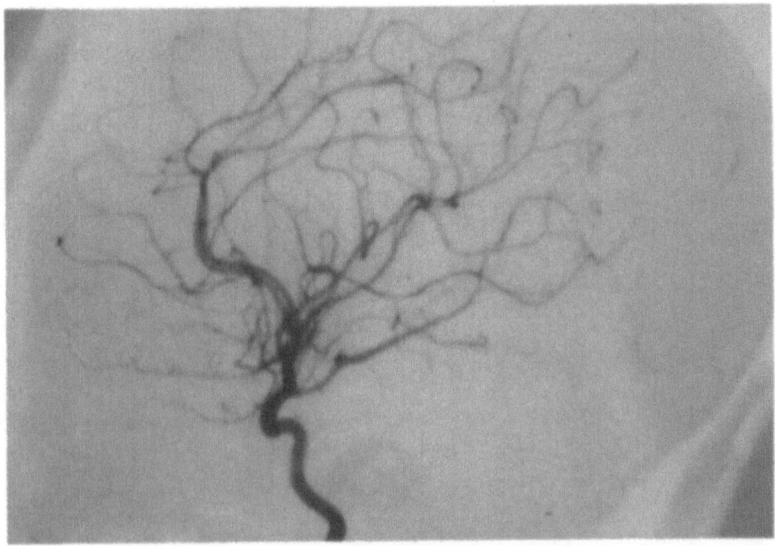

Figure 2.16.

arrowheads), from the inferior temporal area all the way to the vertex.

In Figure 2.15, the very delicate tertiary branches of the middle (1) and anterior (2) cerebral systems may be appreciated to advantage in this figure. Note that these vessels generally take origin at right angles to the major sulcal vessels, and that they course over the gyrus, is roughly parallel to one another. These vessels are extremely important in evaluating prognosis in infants with hydrocephalus, since if one is able to visualize them, irrespective of the ventricular size, he may predict that the child will attain normal psychomotor function, providing the shunting system is inserted in time and kept functioning.

The reader is urged to study Figure 2.16 carefully, to identify the exquisite tertiary branches of the sulcal arteries and appreciate the delicate, normal stain of the gyri (especially the

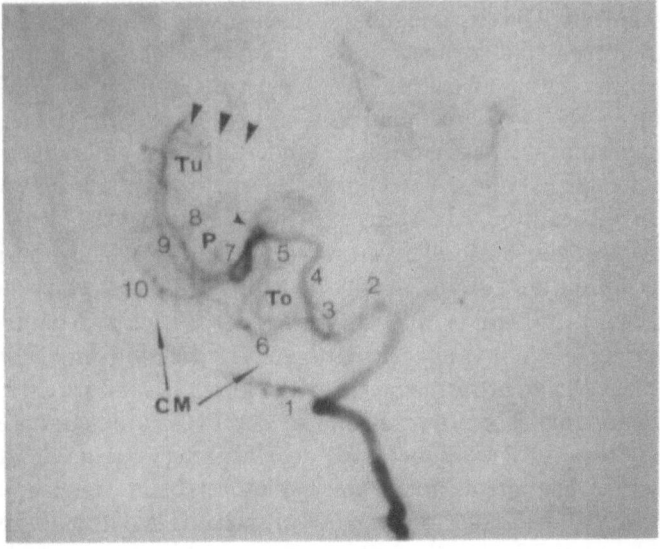

Figure 2.17.

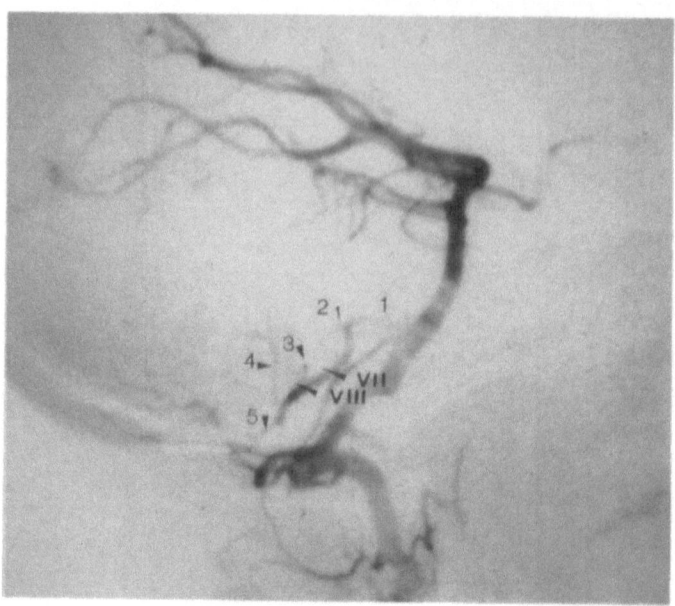

Figure 2.18.

gyrus rectus, the precentral gyrus, and the middle temporal gyrus).

In Figure 2.17, muscular branches (1) are quite prominent and establish anastomotic routes between the vertebral and occipital arteries. The posterior inferior cerebral artery (PICA) most often originates from the vertebral and courses around the medulla oblongata, where it may be divided into ventral (2), lateral (3), and dorsal or retromedullary (4) segments. The retromedullary segment follows a superomedial course along the inferior rim of the IV ventricle to the obex and then, within the vallecula, courses posteriorly as the supratonsillar segment (5) to the posterior tonsillar sulcus where the choroidal point (small arrowhead) may be seen, as may the prominent choroidal blush. The apex of the tonsil (6) rests within the cisterna magna. The retrotonsillar segment (7) curves inferiorly around the undersurface of the pyramis (P), at which point the vermian (9) and hemispheral (10) branches become identifiable. The artery of the superior pyramis (8) separates the tuber (Tu) from the pyramis (P). The great horizontal fissure (large arrowheads) separates the tuber below from the folium above, and is the line of demarcation between vascular supply to the

inferior portion of the cerebellum by the posterior inferior cerebellar artery and to the superior portion of the cerebellum by the superior cerebellar arteries. The tonsil (To) may be identified clearly, as may the cisterna magna (CM).

In Figure 2.18, the anterior inferior cerebellar artery (AICA) most often originates from the basilar artery, and generally has a caliber which is inversely proportional to that of the posterior inferior cerebellar artery. Within the pontine cistern (1), the anterior inferior cerebellar artery courses over the ventral surface of the pons inferiorly and laterally to enter the pontocerebellar cistern at the pontocerebellar angle. Before entering the cistern it gives off recurrent branches (2), which nourish the lateral surface of the pons and which are minute perforating vessels. Within the pontocerebellar cistern, the anterior inferior cerebellar artery gives origin to the internal auditory artery (3) at a point where it and PICA are juxtaposed to the seventh (VII) and eighth (VIII) nerves. As AICA exits from the pontocerebellar cistern, it terminates in two branches. The lateral branch, the major branch, runs within the ventral aspect of the great horizontal fissure, between the superior and

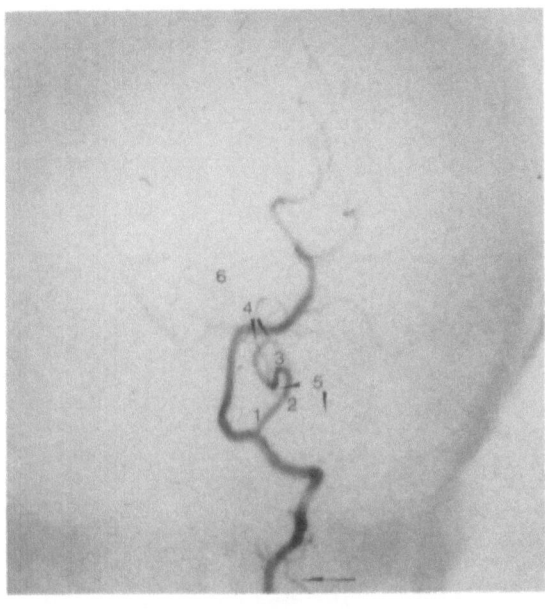

Figure 2.19.

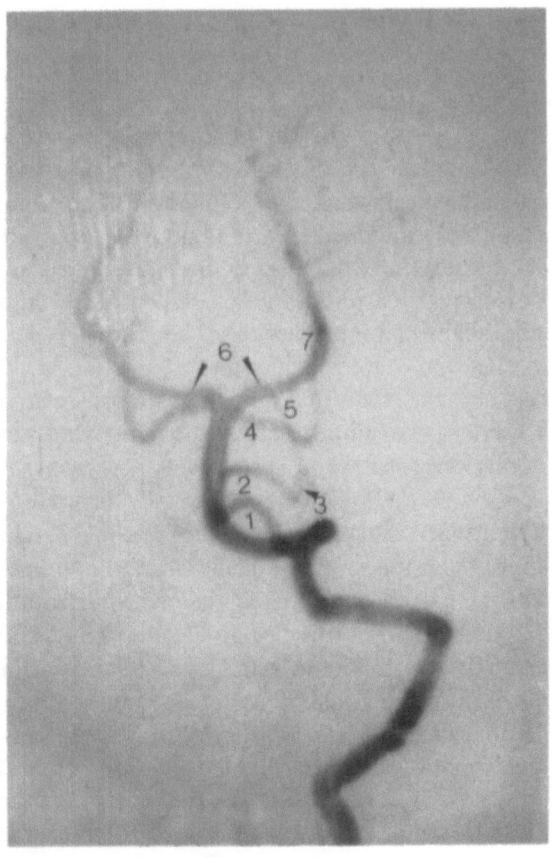

Figure 2.20.

inferior semilunar lobules (4). The medial branch (5) follows an inferior course toward the ventral lobule, where it anastomoses freely with the branches from PICA.

In Figure 2.19, one notes the course of the vertebral artery through the foramina transversaria of C2 and C1 with the muscular branches (arrow) at approximately the C2 level. The ventral medullary segment of PICA (1) courses laterally. The lateral medullary segment (2) has a wide curve onto the dorsal aspect of the medulla oblongata, where the dorsal medullary segment (3) may be seen. PICA proceeds more superiorly than longitudinally to the supratonsillar portion (4). The tonsillohemispheric branch (5) courses inferiorly and laterally. One notes to advantage the thalamoperforating branches of the mesencephalic portion of the posterior cerebral artery (6).

In the child shown in Figure 2.20, PICA (1) and AICA (2) are of approximately the same caliber, an exception to the rule that these vessels are inversely proportional to one another in caliber. At the pontocerebellar cistern (3), AICA is juxtaposed to the seventh and eighth cranial nerves. The superior cerebellar arteries (4) come off inferior to the posterior cerebral arteries. One notes the inferolateral direction of the posterior communicating artery (5), which goes to join the posterior cerebral artery. This point of junction is the line of demarcation between the mesencephalic portion of the posterior cerebral (6) and the posterior cerebral proper (7), which courses around the peduncles and into the ambient cistern.

In Figure 2.21, AICA courses along the ventral surface of the pons (1) to the point at which it gives origin to recurrent branches (2) that penetrate the lateral surface of the pons. Within the pontocerebellar cistern, AICA is juxtaposed to the seventh (VII) and eighth (VIII) cranial nerves. The exit of AICA from the pontocerebellar cistern is through the great horizontal fissure (GHF), at which point the superior terminal branch of AICA (3) courses upward between the superior semilunar lobule (SSL) and the inferior semilunar lobule (ISL). The superior cerebellar arteries (4) fill quite prominently in this phase.

In Figure 2.22, the muscular branches of the

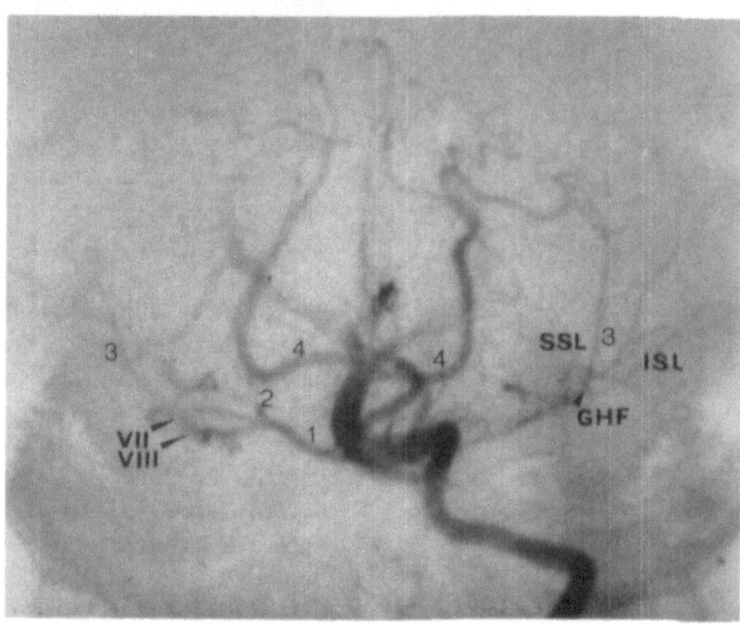

Figure 2.21.

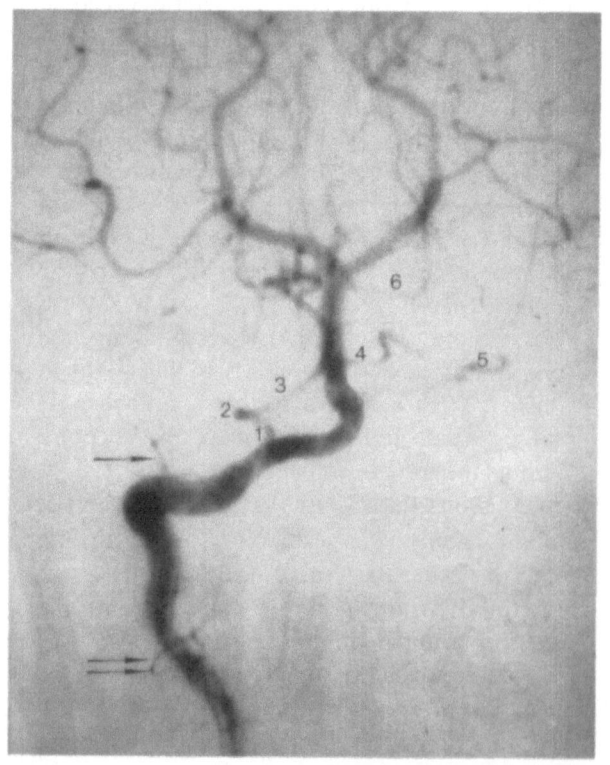

Figure 2.22.

vertebral artery are shown at the C2 level (double arrows) and the Cl level (single arrow). The ventral (1), lateral (2), and dorsal (3) medullary segments of PICA reveal it to be of the same caliber as AICA (4) on the opposite side. The loop of AICA upon itself (5) is the point at which this artery is juxtaposed to the seventh and eighth cranial nerves. The superior cerebellar artery (6) is well seen.

The axial view of Figure 2.23 affords one a superb opportunity to study the main branches of the vertebrobasilar system. AICA (1) may be seen coursing over the pons and then lateralward into the pontocerebellar system, where it loops (2) at the seventh and eighth cranial nerves and then goes on to exit at the great horizontal fissure, where it divides into lateral (3) and medial (4) terminal branches. The posterior portion of the circle of Willis also may be fully appreciated in the axial projection. The mesencephalic portions of the posterior cerebral arteries (5) are medial to the entry of the posterior communicating arteries (6) into the posterior cerebral system. The point at which the third cranial nerve passes between the

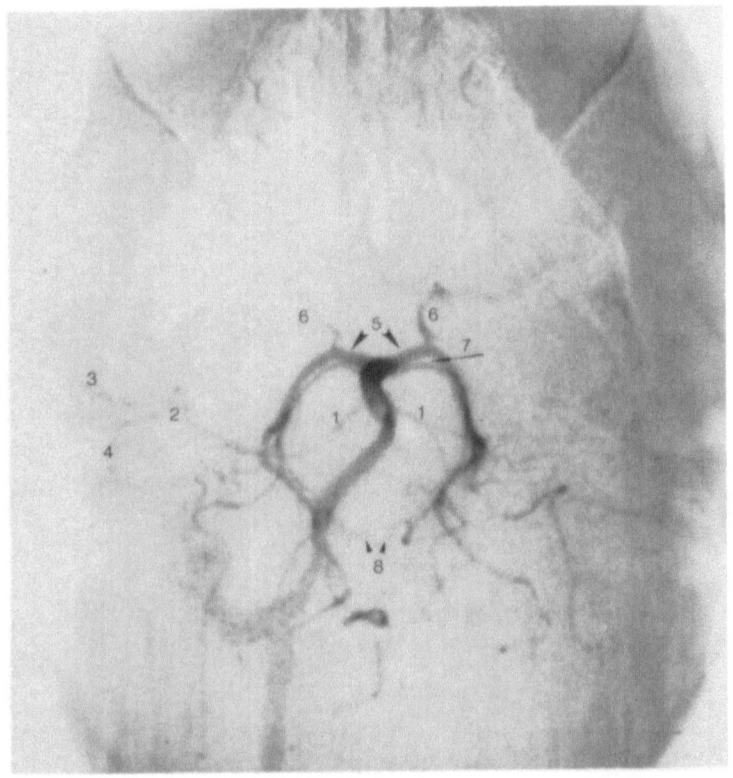

Figure 2.23.

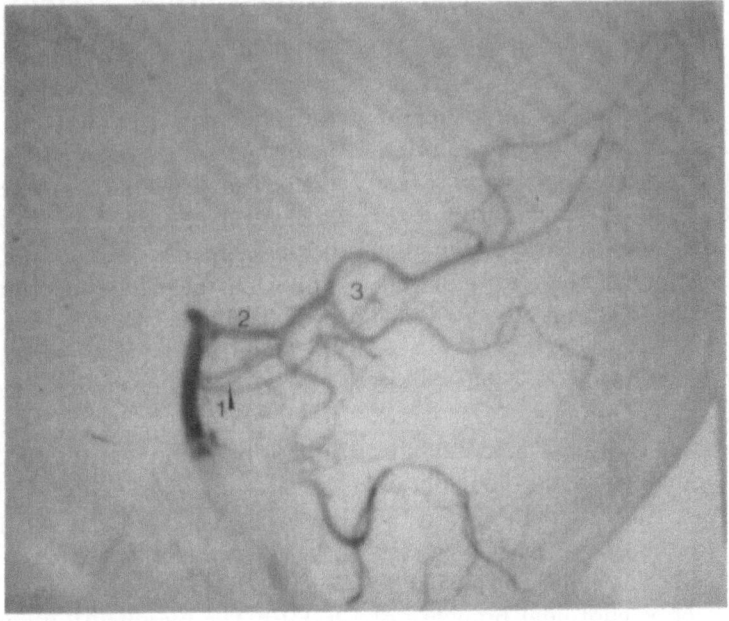

Figure 2.24.

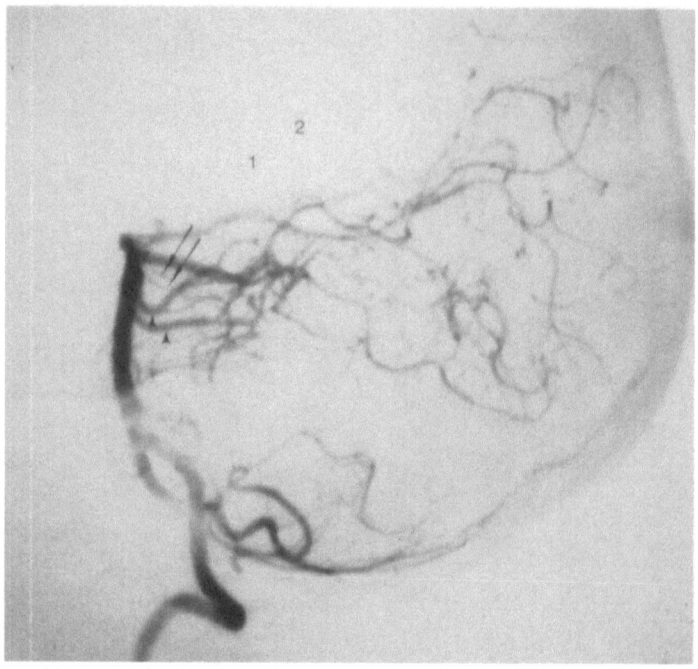

Figure 2.25.

posterior cerebral and superior cerebellar arteries is indicated (7). The collicular plate is outlined by the ramification of the collicular branches of the posterior cerebral system over its dorsal surface (8).

In Figure 2.24, there are at least three superior cerebellar branches coursing around the brainstem in the pontomesencephalic sulcus (1). The posterior cerebral artery (2) wraps around the peduncle within the ambient cistern and then courses over the tectum of the midbrain. The region of the collicular plate may be identified (3).

In Figure 2.25, the superior cerebellar vessels (arrowheads) are quite prominent. One notes very delicate circumferential mesencephalic arteries (arrows) wrapping around the midbrain from ventral to dorsal in their path, within the ambient cistern, to the dorsal surface of the midbrain and the collicular plate. The medial (1) and lateral (2) posterior choroidal branches of the posterior cerebral system are faintly visualized.

Secondary and Tertiary Branches of the Carotid System

Study of the superior and inferior cerebellar systems in Figure 2.26a allows one to identify the individual lobules of the vermis and hemispheres. The superior cerebellar artery divides into medial (1), intermediate (2), and lateral (3) branches, all of which nourish the dorsal superior surface of the cerebellum. Following the medial superior cerebellar arteries over the dome of the vermis, one may identify the culmen monticuli (CM) and then, posteroinferiorly, the culmen declive (CD) to the termination of the medial branches of the folium (Fo), which represent the superior border of the great horizontal fissure (GHF). The vermian branches of the posterior inferior cerebellar artery terminate at the tuber (Tu), which is the inferior border of the great horizontal fissure (GHF). The pyramis (Py) and uvula (Uv) may be identified by following the vermian branch of PICA.

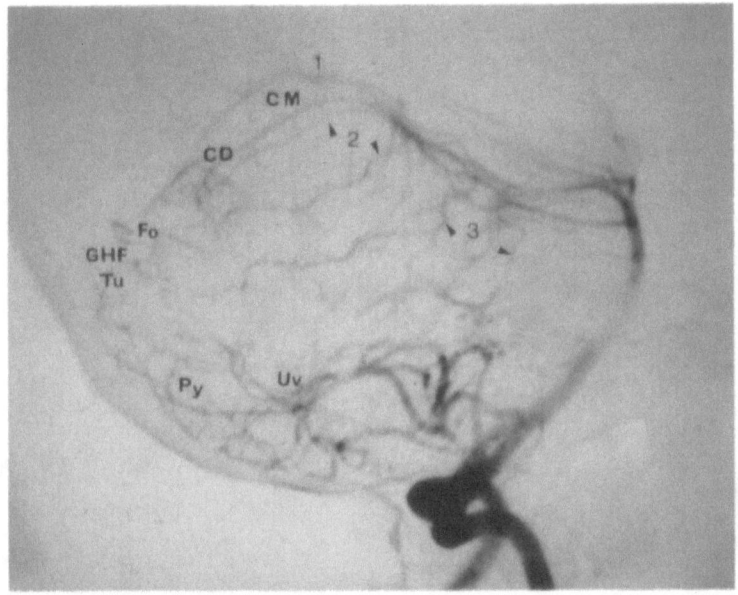

Figure 2.26.

In Figure 2.26b, the very delicate cerebellar sulcal arteries (arrowheads) originate from the secondary (medial, intermediate, lateral) superior cerebellar vessels. The cerebellar folia may be identified between the sulcal arteries. GHF, Great horizontal fissure.

In Figure 2.27, the hemispheral branch of PICA (1) may be seen coursing over the inferior

surface of the cerebellar hemisphere. One notes also the collicular branches of the posterior cerebral system (2) outlining the collicular plate.

In Figure 2.28, there is a rather prominent branch of PICA (1) that outlines the medial extension of the tonsil of the cerebellar hemisphere (To). The superior retrotonsillar segment (2) is quite prominent, as are the

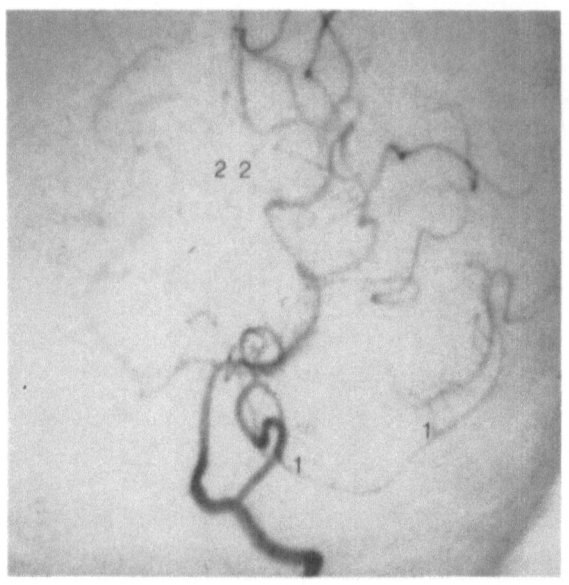

Figure 2.27.

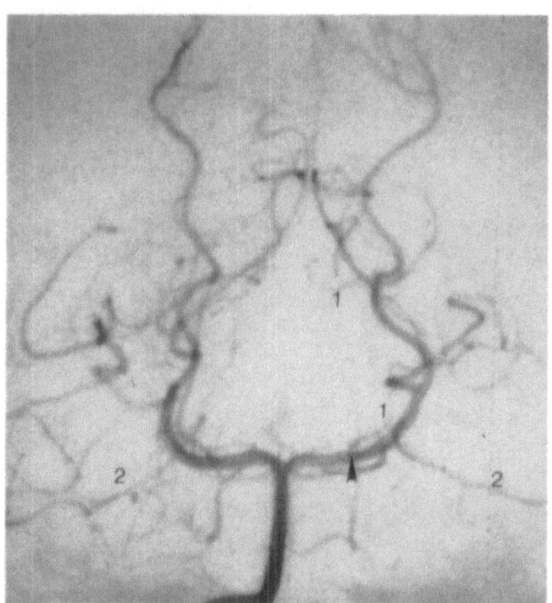

Figure 2.29.

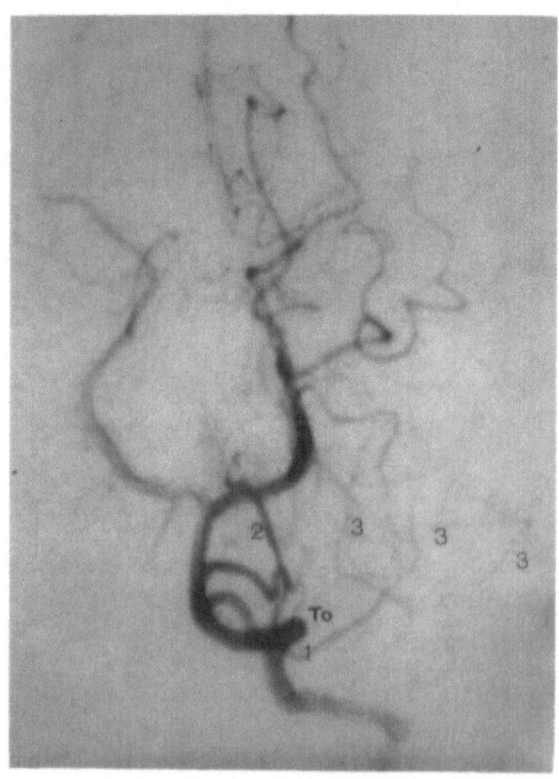

Figure 2.28.

terminal branches of the tonsillohemipheral artery (3).

In Figure 2.29, the medial posterior choroidal artery (1) may be seen to originate from the posterior cerebral artery at the mesencephalic segment (arrowhead) and to course around the midbrain, medial to the posterior cerebral artery within the ambient cistern. One notes two well-visualized posterior inferior temporal arteries (2) originating from the posterior cerebral artery and coursing along the tentorial surface of the temporal lobe.

In Figure 2.30, the thalamoperforating branches of the fundus of the basilar and mesencephalic portions of the posterior cerebral arteries (1) outline the more anterior portion of the thalamus. They penetrate the posterior perforating substance after coursing through the interpeduncular cistern. The medial (2) and lateral (3) posterior choroidal arteries are located, respectively, within the roof of the third ventricle and over the pulvinar of the thalamus. Thus, one may locate the anterior margin of the thalamus by identifying the anterior thalamoperforating vessel and the posterior surface of the thalamus by identifying the lateral posterior

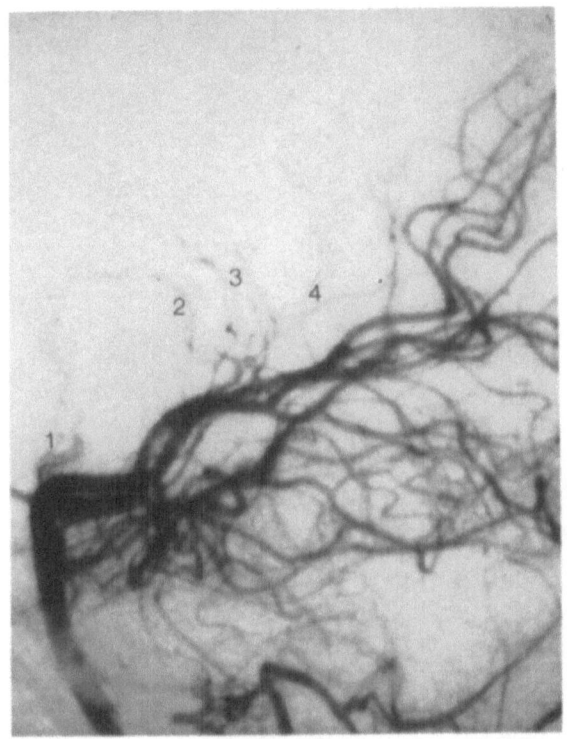

Figure 2.30.

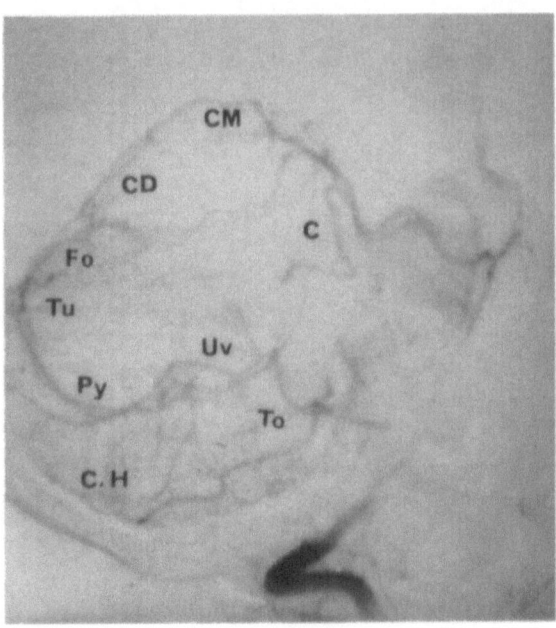

Figure 2.31.

choroidal artery. The inferior retrosplenial artery (4), another branch of the posterior cerebral, courses beneath the splenium of the corpus callosum and then within the pericallosal cistern. The posterior thalamoperforating vessels may be identified as a delicate cluster of branches of the posterior cerebral artery as they course superiorly between the anterior perforators and the lateral posterior choroidal artery, staining the thalamus.

The midarterial phase, shown in Figure 2.31, permits one to identify the secondary and tertiary branches of the superior and inferior cerebellar systems in order to visualize the cerebellar vermis and its lobules, as well as the inferior cerebellar hemisphere and the tonsil. C, lobulus centralis; CM, culmen monticuli; CD, culmen declive; Fo, folium; Tu, tuber; Py, pyramis; Uv, uvula; To, tonsil; CH, inferior cerebellar hemisphere.

Venous Studies

In Figure 2.32, the internal cerebral vein (IC), in fact, is the lesser vein of Galen. It and the basal vein of Rosenthal (BV) are the major tributaries to the great vein of Galen (G), which begins immediately posterior to the collicular plate and immediately inferior to the splenium of the corpus callosum. It then runs posterosuperiorly to enter the straight sinus (SS). The superficial middle cerebral vein (SMCv) rests within the sylvian fissure on the convex surface of the hemisphere. The deep middle cerebral vein (DMCv) rests within the sylvian fissure, coursing inferomedially to run along the floor of the middle fossa on the surface of the greater wing of the sphenoid. Th, Thalamic image.

In Figure 2.33, the vein of the septum pellucidum (s) runs within the septum pellucidum directly posteriorly, in the midline and its tributary to the internal cerebral vein (IC) at the foramen of Monro (arrowhead). The anterior caudate vein (ac) and the thalamostriate vein (ts) are both subependymal veins running, respectively, within the subependymal space over the surface of the head of the caudate nucleus and the thalamus. They are both tributary to the internal cerebral vein. Note the course of the

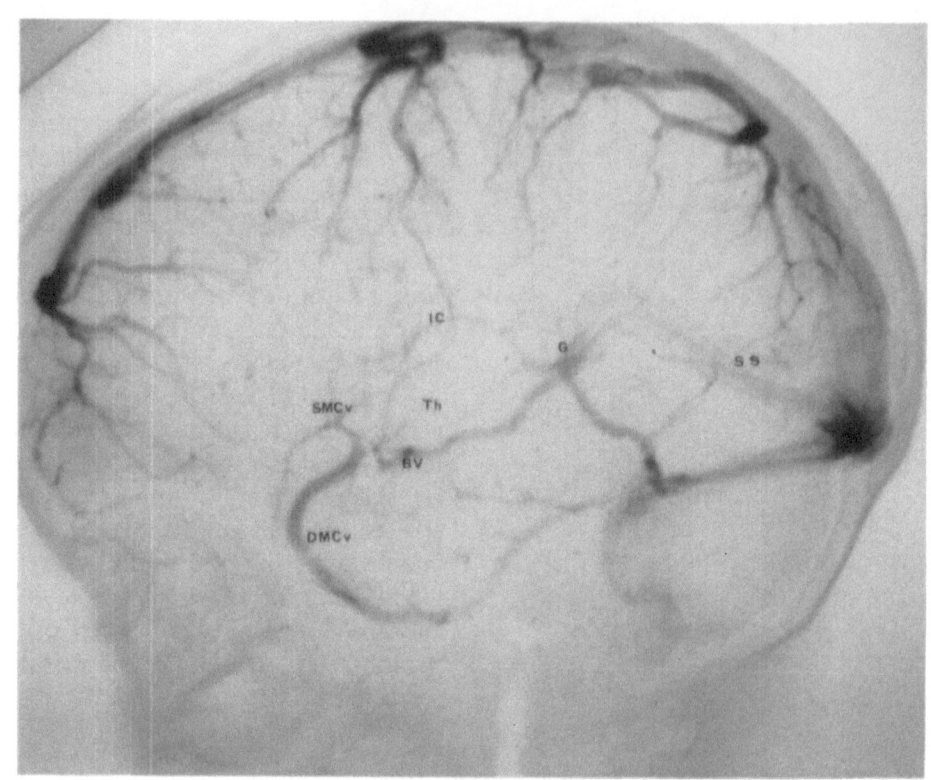

Figure 2.32.

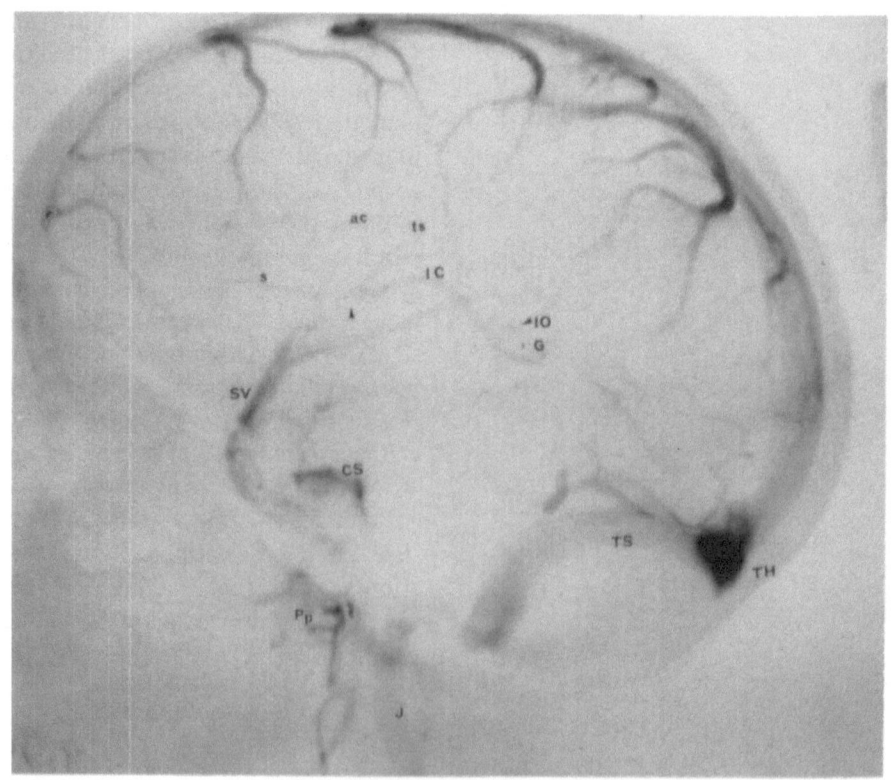

Figure 2.33.

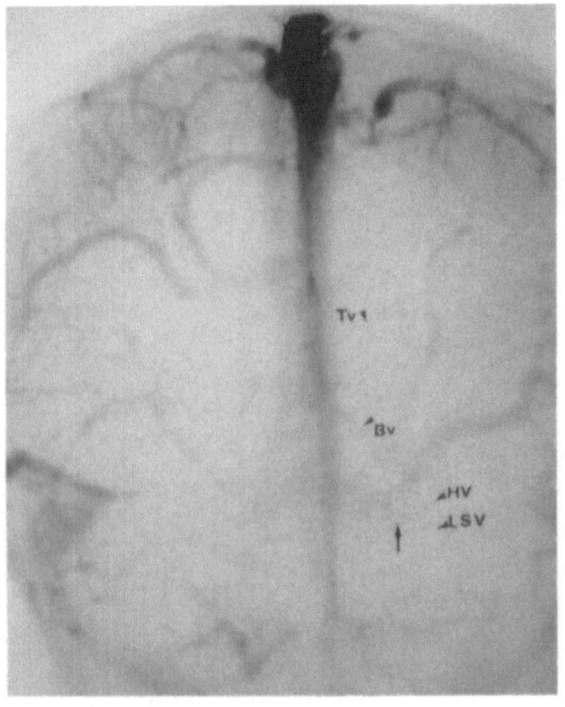

Figure 2.34.

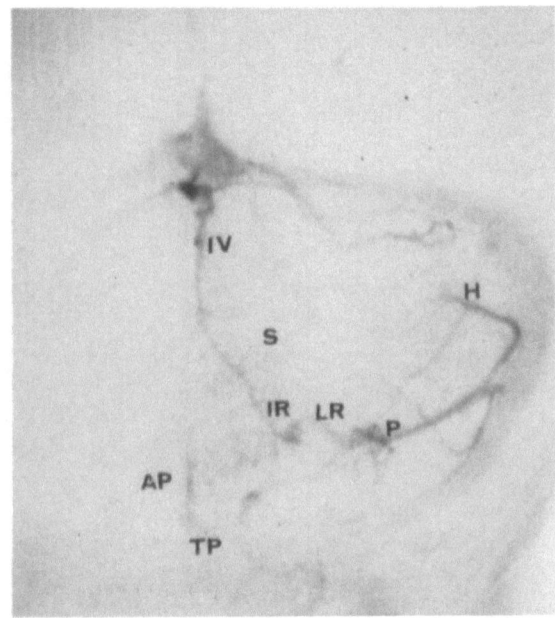

Figure 2.35.

great vein of Galen (G), outlining the inferior surface of the splenium of the corpus callosum. The internal occipital vein (IO) bridges from the medial surface of the most anterior portion of the occipital lobe into the great vein of Galen. In this illustration, the deep middle cerebral vein is labeled sylvian vein (SV) because both terms are used to describe this venous structure. The cavernous sinus (CS) is well visualized, with the relative space-filling defect in its inferior portion outlining the cluster of cranial nerves II, IV, VI, V1, V2. The torcular Herophili (TH) is completely filled, and the transverse sinus (TS) outlines the lateralmost insertion of the tentorium. Venous blood from the transverse sinus drains through the sigmoid sinus into the internal jugular vein (J). One also notes the pterygoid plexus (Pp).

In Figure 2.34, the thalamostriate vein (Tv) runs over the thalamus and caudate nucleus in the inferolateral surface of the lateral ventricle, and the basal vein (Bv) runs within the ambient cistern around the brainstem. The hippocampal (HV) and lenticulostriate (LSV) veins are

tributary to the vein of Rosenthal at the anterior perforating substance (arrow).

Some Veins of the Posterior Fossa (Figs. 2.35 and 2.36)

H, inferior hemispheral veins; P, petrosal vein; LR, vein of lateral recess; IR, inferior retrotonsillar vein; S, superior retrotonsillar vein; IV, inferior vermian vein; AP, anterior pontine vein; TP, transverse pontine vein. (Fig. 2.35)

SH, Superior hemispheral vein; SPS, superior petrosal sinus; P, petrosal vein; B, brachial vein; LR, vein of lateral recess; IV, inferior vermian vein (Fig. 2.36).

Sinuses and Cortical Draining Veins (Fig. 2.37)

SSS, Superior sagittal sinus; ISS, inferior sagittal sinus; SPS, superior petrosal sinus; IPS, inferior petrosal sinus; FA, ascending frontal vein; VL, vein of Labbé.

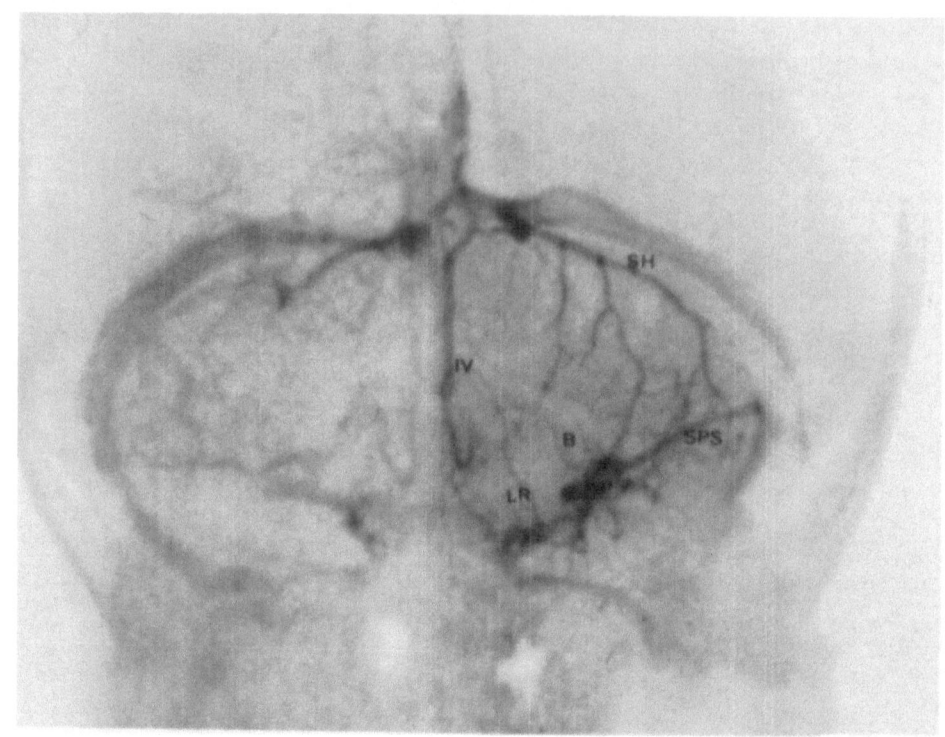

Figure 2.36.

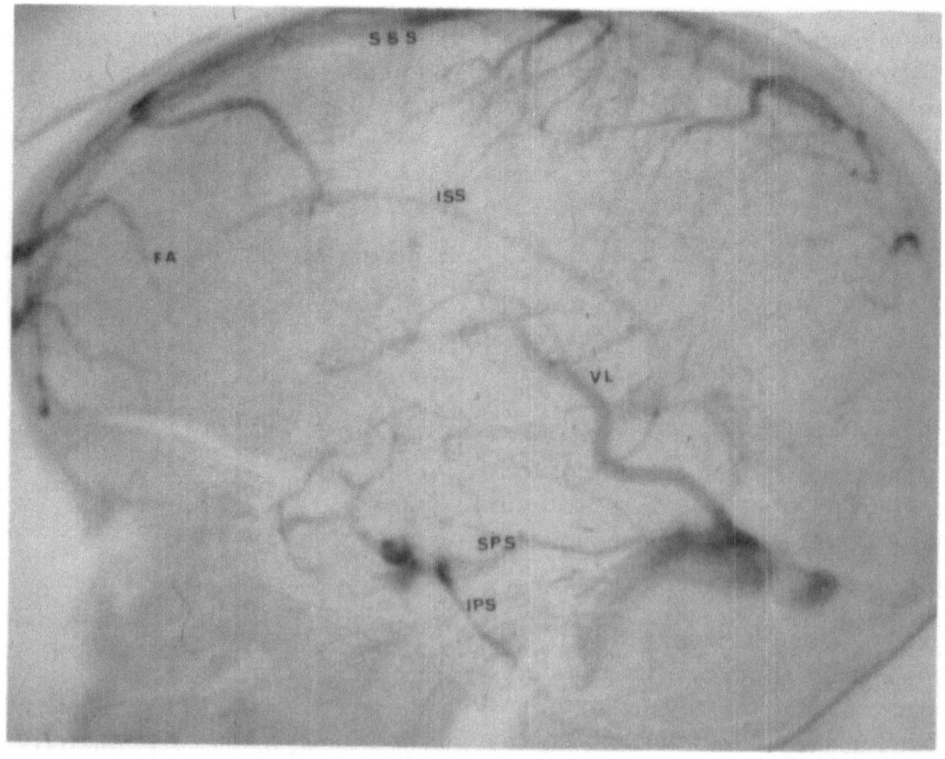

Figure 2.37.

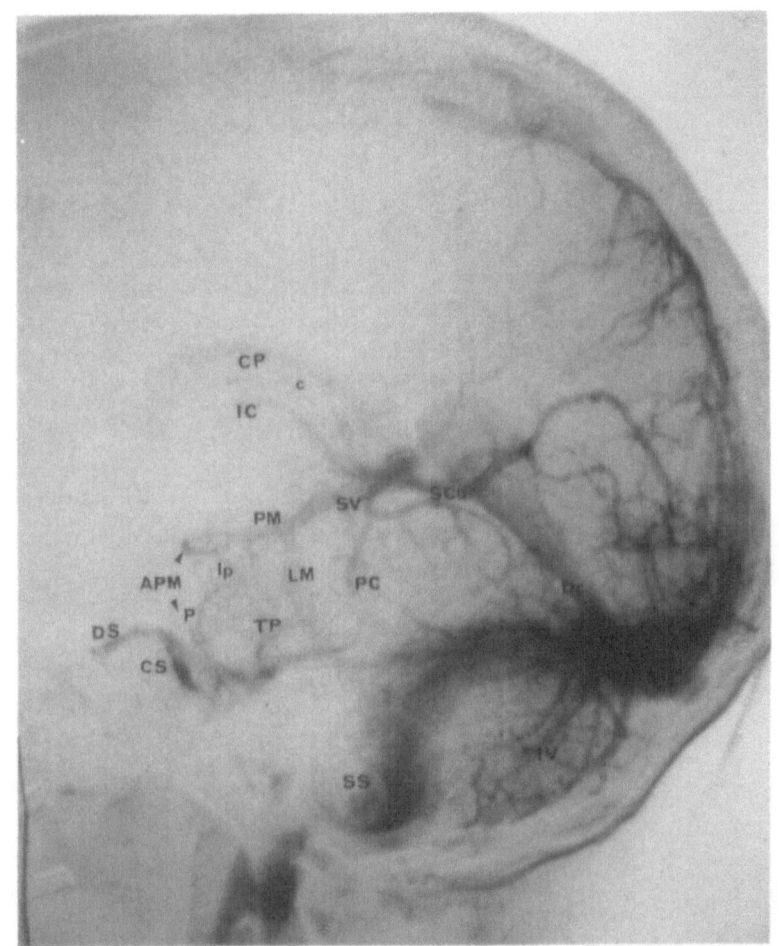

Figure 2.38.

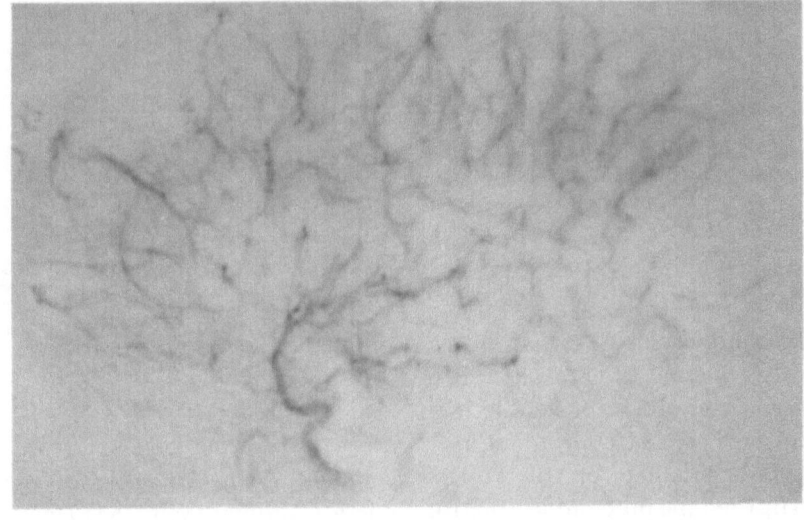

Figure 2.39.

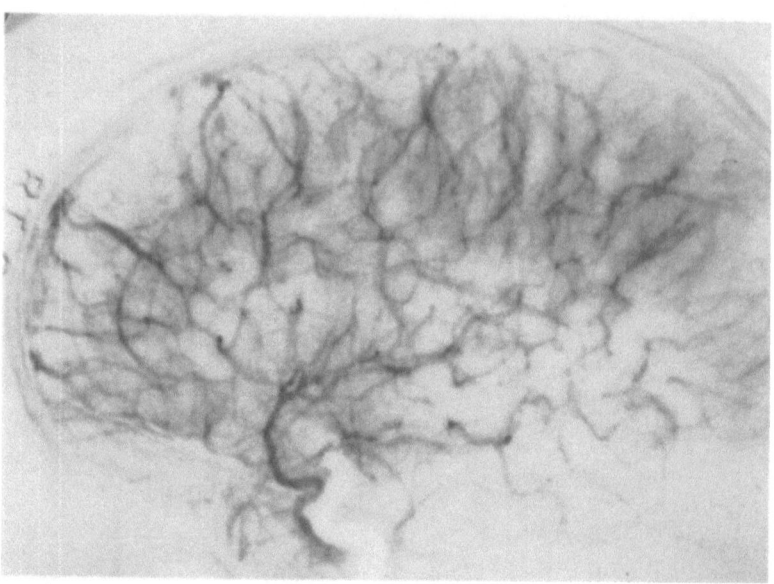

Figure 2.40.

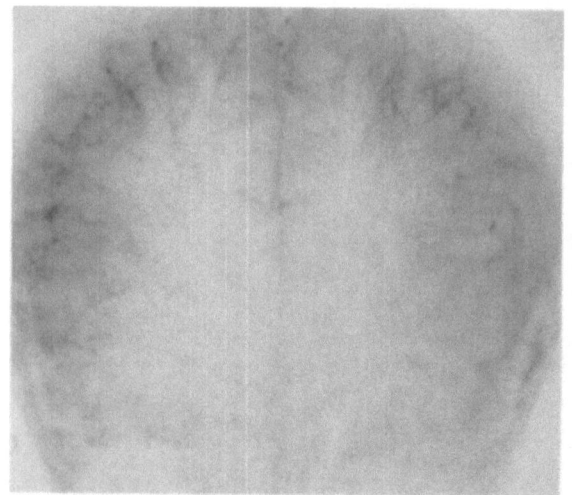

Figure 2.41.

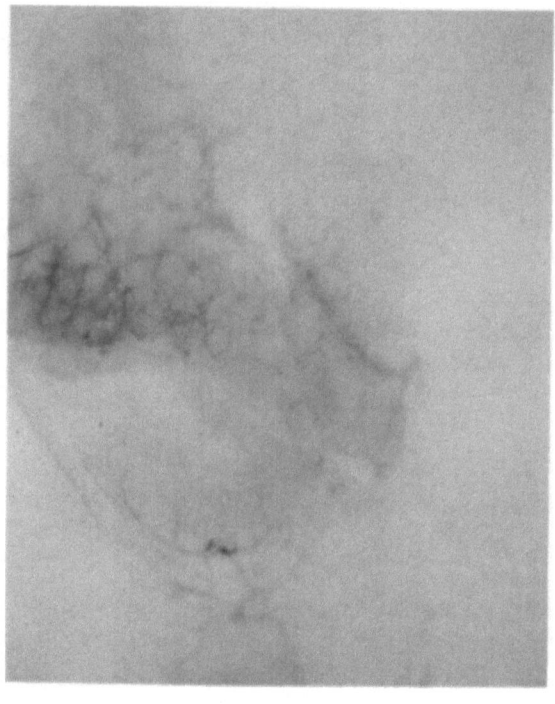

Figure 2.42.

Veins and Sinuses of the Midline (Fig. 2.38)

CP, Blush of the choroid plexus; c, vein of the choroid plexus; IC, internal cerebral vein; SV, superior vermian vein; PM, posterior mesencephalic vein; APM, anterior pontomesencephalic vein, consisting of the interpeduncular vein (lp) and the prepontine vein (P); LM, lateral mesencephalic vein; TP, transverse pontine vein; PC, precentral vein; SCu, supra- culminate vein; Dc, vein of the declive; IV, inferior vermian vein; SS, sigmoid sinus; CS, cavernous sinus; DS, diaphragma sellae sinus (Fig. 2.38).

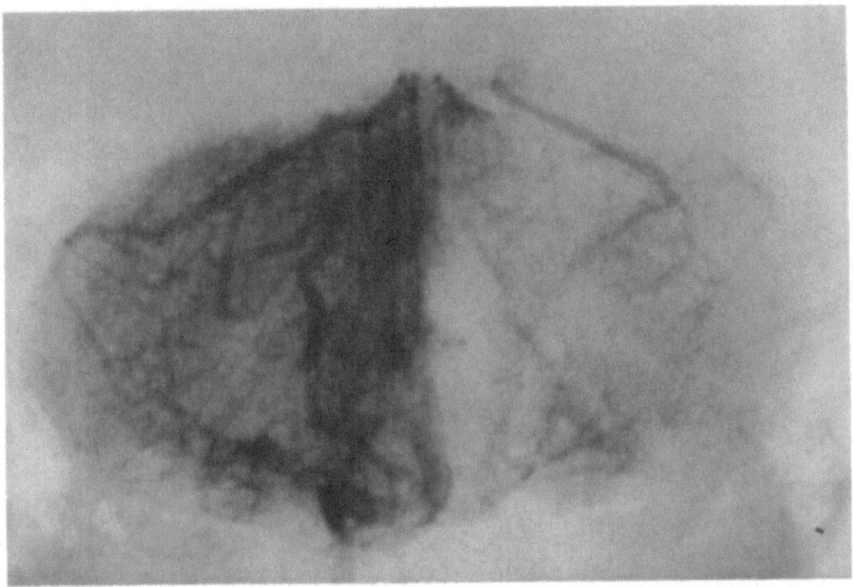

Figure 2.43.

Capillary Phases to Show Cerebrum and Cerebellum (Figs. 2.39 to 2.45)

Midcapillary phases to show gyral staining along sulcal borders (Fig. 2.39).

Midcapillary stain to show cortical stain in half-axial projection (Fig. 2.40).

Early capillary phase to show gyral staining of occipital and temporal lobes bordering upon lateral surface of tentorium (Fig. 2.41).

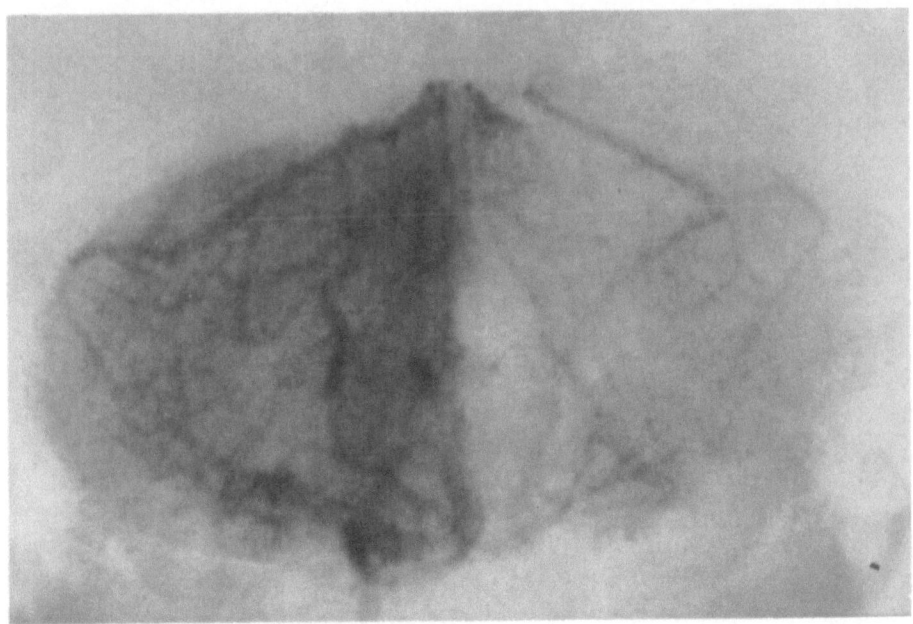

Figure 2.44.

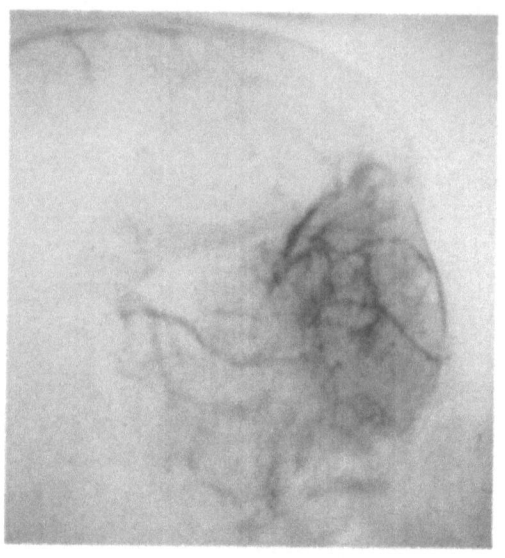

Figure 2.45.

show cerebellar hemispheres in half-axial projection (Fig. 2.43).

Late capillary stain to show inferior cerebellar hemisphere in lateral projection (Fig. 2.44).

Late capillary stain to show inferior cerebellar hemisphere in lateral projection (Fig. 2.45).

External Carotid Vessels

As can be seen in Figure 2.46, the retinal choroid (C) stains very well in infants. Meningeal vessels are indicated by the arrowheads and the occipital artery by the arrow.

In Figure 2.49, the lingual artery (L) and the internal maxillary artery (I) are well visualized, as is the anterior branch of the middle meningeal artery (arrowhead).

Figure 2.48 shows extracranial external carotid vessels. L, Lingual artery; F, facial artery; I, internal maxillary artery; S, superficial temporal artery; O, occipital artery.

Midcapillary stain to show the thalamus, midbrain, and cerebellar vermis and hemispheres (Fig. 2.42).

Late capillary phase with vermis filling to

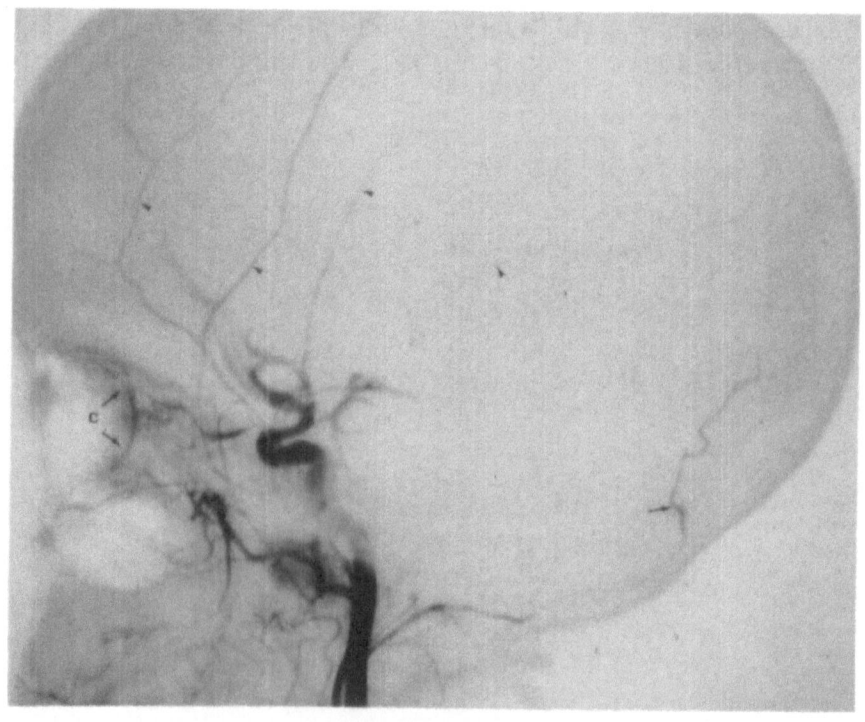

Figure 2.46.

Figure 2.47.

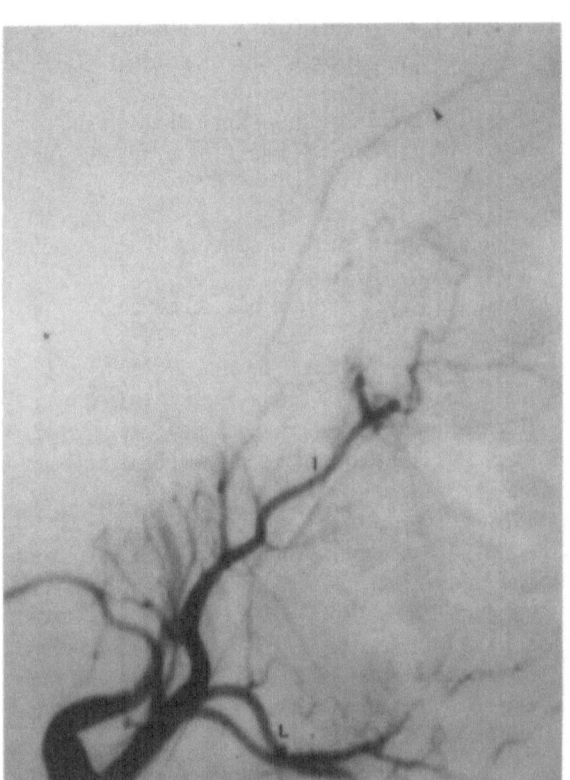

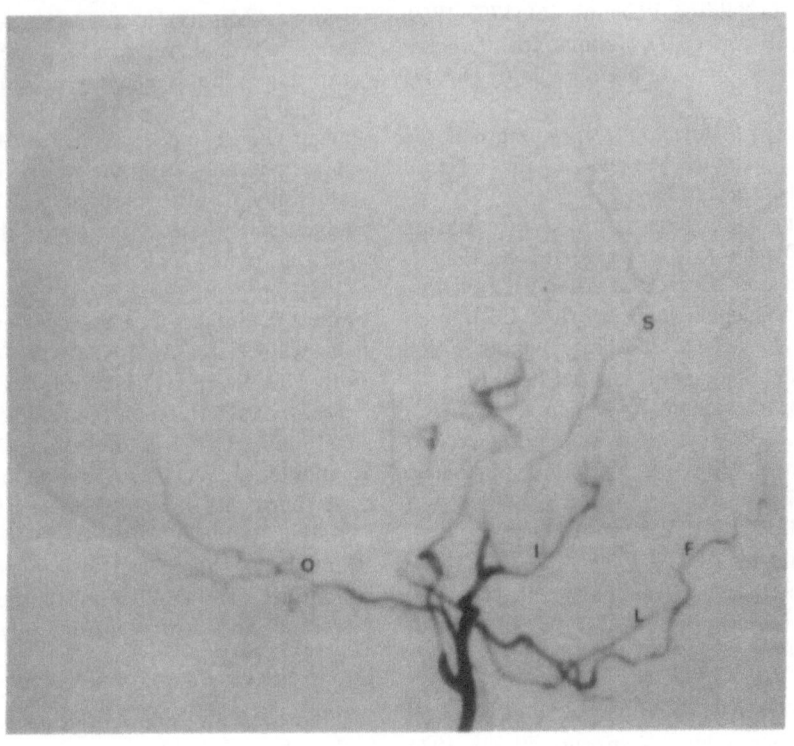

Figure 2.48.

Bibliography

Abbie AA: Blood supply of lateral geniculate body with note on morphology of choroidal arteries. J Anat 67:491, 1933.

Albertson KW, Doppman JL, Ramsey R: Spinal seizures induced by contrast media; a new method of comparing neurotoxicity of radio-opaque agents. Radiology 107:349, 1973.

Allen WE III, Kier EL, Rothman SLG: The maxillary artery: normal arteriographic anatomy. Am J Roentgenol Radium Ther Nucl Med 118:517, 1973.

Babin ES, Megret M: Variations in the drainage of the basal vein. Neuroradiology 6:154, 1973.

Ben-Amor M, Marion C, Heldt N: Normal and pathological radioanatomy of the superior choroid vein. Neuroradiology 3:16, 1971.

Billewicz O, Ben-Amor M: The posterior ventricular branches of the internal cerebral and basilar vein. Neuroradiology 2:37, 1971.

Boulos RS, Gilroy J, Meyer JS: Technique of cerebral angiography in children. Am J Roentgenol 101:121, 1967.

Carrea R: Angiography in children: preliminary report. Am Inst Med Exp 2:69, 1950.

Carrea R, Schuster G: Observations about retrograde brachial cerebral angiography in children. Acta Neurochir 9:456, 1961.

Castorina G, Fortuna A, Sollini A: Cerebral angiography in children. Policlinico 66:1797, 1959.

Desilets DT, Ruttenberg HD, Hoffman RB: Percutaneous catheterization in children. Radiology 87:119, 1966.

Eckstein A: Angioarchitectonics in young children; method of staining vessels. Z Ges Neurol Psychiatry 154:298, 1935.

Fischer PA: Angiographic picture of corpus callosum deficiency. Dtsch Z Nervenheilkd 180:40, 1959.

Fitz CR, Harwood-Nash DC: The Anterior Falx Artery Radiologicum. Punta del Este, 1974.

Fitz CR, Harwood-Nash DC: Early Venous Filling and Neuroradiologicum. Punta del Este, 1974.

Francisco CB, Davidson KC, Youngstrom KA, Schoolman A, Poser CM: Transfemoral cervicocephalic angiography in children. Pediatrics 33:119, 1964.

Harwood-Nash DC: Pediatric neuroradiology. Radiol Clin North Am 10:313, 1972.

Hassler O: Deep cerebral venous system in man; a microangiographic study on its areas of drainage and its anastomoses with the superficial cerebral veins. Neurology 16:505, 1965.

Horwitz NH, Wener L: Temporary cortical blindness following angiography. J Neurosurg 40:583, 1974.

Howieson J, Megison LC Jr: Complications of vertebral artery catheterization. Radiology 91:1109, 1968.

Huber P: Demonstration of impaired autoregulation in tumors and cerebral infarction by angiography. Acta Radiol Diagn 13:115, 1972.

Jensen HP: Unusual aspects in carotid artery angiography in early childhood hydrocephalus. Radiologie 6:465, 1966.

Lehmann R: The tolerance of cerebral angiography in children. Radiol. Diagn. 9:140, 1968.

LeMay M, Gooding CA: The clinical significance of the azygous anterior cerebral artery (ACA). Am J Roentgenol Radium Ther Nucl Med 98:602, 1966.

LePage JR: Transfemoral ascending lumbar catheterization of the epidural veins. III. Radiology 98:602, 1968.

Lie TA: Congenital Anomalies of the Carotid Arteries. Excerpta Medica Foundation, Amsterdam, 1968.

MacRae, DL, Castorina G: Variations in corpus callosum, septum pellucidum and fornix, and their effect on the encephalogram and cerebral angiogram. Acta Radiol Diagn 1:872, 1963.

Maki Y, Nakada Y, Watanabe O: Cerebral angiograms in children; the diameter of the main branches of the carotid system. Clin Neurol Tokyo Rinsho Sinkeigaku 9:308, 1969.

Marchese GS: Radiologia pediatrica: patologia cranica. Minerva Med 57:929, 1966.

Mingrino S, et al.: Agenesis of the septum pellucidum: an angiographic sign. Neurochirurgia (Stuttgart) 7:1, 1964.

Padget DG: The development of the cranial venous system in man, from the viewpoint of comparative anatomy. Contrib Embryol 32:212, 1948.

Padget DH: The development of the cranial arteries in the human embryo. Contrib Embryol 32:205, 1948.

Paraicz E, Szenasy J: Uber die Carotisangiographie im Kindesalter. Acta Neurochir 7:350, 1959.

Potts DG, Svare GT, Bergeron RT: The developing brain; correlation between radiologic and anatomical findings. Acta Radiol Diagn 9:430, 1969.

Raimondi AJ, White H: Cerebral angiography in the newborn and infants. I. General principles. Ann Radiol 10:146, 1967.

Raimondi AJ, Samuelson G, Yarzagaray L: Positive contrast (Conray 60) serial ventriculography in the normal and hydrocephalic infant. Ann Radiol 12:377, 1969.

Sangruchi V, Hitchcock E, Donaldson AA: Postangiography vertebral arteriovenous fistulae. Br J Surg 59:627, 1972.

Schelsinger B: The venous drainage of the brain, with special reference to the galenic system. Brain 62:274, 1939.

Stopford JSB: The functional significance of the arrangement of the cerebral and cerebellar veins. J Anat 64:257, 1930.

Takahashi M: Percutaneous catheterization in infants and children. In: Gyepes MT (ed.), Angiography in Infants and Children. Grune & Stratton, New York, 1974.

Takaku A., Suzuki J: Cerebral angiography in children and adults with mental retardation. I. Control series. Dev Med Child Neurol 14:756, 1972.

Taveras JM: Neuroradiology in children. In: Decker K (ed.), Clinical Neuroradiology. McGraw-Hill, New York, 1966, pp. 359–399.

Torkildsen A, Koppang K: Percutaneous carotid angiography in children. J Bras Neurol 2:xx, 1950.

Vermess M, Stein SC, Ajmone-Marsan C, DiChiro G: Angiography in "idiopathic" focal epilepsy. Am J Roentgenol Radium Ther Nucl Med 115:120, 1972.

Vigouroux R, Boudouresques J, Piganiol G, Vigouroux M: Valeur respective de la penumographie, de l'angiographie et de l'electroencephalographie au course des encephalopathies infantiles. Rev Neurol 90:662, 1954.

Vitek JJ: Microaneurysms of the carotid artery after "nontraumatic" percutaneous puncture. Radiology 106:101, 1973.

Vlahovitch, B: Insular guidemarks, carotid angiography of infants and children. Neurochirurgia 12:817, 1966.

Vogel FS, McClenahan JL: Anomalies of major cerebral arteries associated with congenital malformations of brain. Trans Am Neurol Assoc 77:132, 1952.

Vogelsang H, Bauer B: Current angiographic methods in cerebral diagnosis in infancy and childhood: report of 170 brachial angiographies. Fortschr Geb Roentgenstr 108:329, 1968.

Vogelsang H: Cerebral angiography through the brachial artery in infancy and childhood. Radiologie 6:461, 1966.

Wallace S, Anderson JH, Gianturco C: Thrombus formation during direct puncture cerebral angiography. Am J Roentgenol Radium Ther Nucl Med 119:613, 1973.

Wilson GH: Pediatric neuroarteriography. In: Gyepes MT (ed.), Angiography in Infants and Children. Grune & Stratton, New York, 1974.

Wilson GH: Technique in cerebral angiography in child. Wien Med Wochenschr 107:xx, 1957.

CHAPTER 3

Clinical Pictures of Vascular Pathology in Children

Ignacio Pascual-Castroviejo

Introduction

The incidence of both hemorrhagic and ischemic stroke in children under 14 years has been found to be 2.51[1] to 2.52[2] cases per 100,000 per year, although in these studies strokes related to perinatal causes, infection, and trauma were excluded.

Between 25 and 41% of the strokes are ischemic.[2,3] It has been described that only 1% of the thromboses and 5% of emboli occur in people under 35 years old.[4] We think, however, that the real incidence is somewhat higher. Most of the strokes affect the carotid artery and its principal or/and secondary branches. Obstruction of the vertebrobasilar arterial system and thrombosis of veins and venous sinuses are very infrequent, and even more rarely diagnosed. Males are moderately more affected than females.[5]

Ischemia

The term *ischemia* is used to describe the pathological situation caused by a transitory or permanent decrease in blood flow secondary to any mechanism. Ischemia may be *total* or *nonocclusive*, as is observed in cardiac arrest or in hypotensive shock, with cerebral lesions preferentially located in occipital zones. Regional or zonal ischemia describes cases of partial or total obstruction of a cerebral artery. It is necessary to differentiate ischemia from hypoxia (e.g., decreased arterial oxygen level, the blood flow being normal). Infarct is then a cerebral lesion, caused by ischemia (Fig. 3.1). It occurs primarily in a cerebral zone irrigated by a large- or middle-sized artery. In adults, atheromas or diffuse arteriosclerosis is almost the only cause of strokes by ischemia; however, arterial obstructions in children have numerous etiologies. Congenital heart disease has been the main cause of stroke in our series (31% of cases[5]), an observation that has been confirmed in other series.[6–9] The list of causes for ischemic stroke in children is extensive (Table 3.1) and unknown etiology is also high.

Until a few years ago, it was thought that persistence of signs and symptoms of ischemia for more than a few minutes could lead to irreversible brain damage. Experimental works[10–14] carried out in recent years in several mammalian species demonstrated that brain cells may resist ischemia more than had previously been suspected. Total cerebral ischemia for as long as 1 hr can be followed by at least partial recovery of metabolic and physiological tissue function.[15] Loss of consciousness and of electrical activity appear within 10 and 20 sec, respectively, of ischemia.[16] These events, however, do not have such significance in cell survival as does abnormal intracellular ion homeostasis, which can be detected within a few minutes. Impairment of the sodium pump leads to a marked increase of extracellular potassium concentration, and a fall in sodium and calcium concentrations, which are followed by the movement of both ions into the cell. Moreover, there is a release of calcium from mitochondria and endoplasmic reticulum. Astroglial swelling with cerebral edema is related to raised extracellular potassium concentration. High intracellular calcium con-

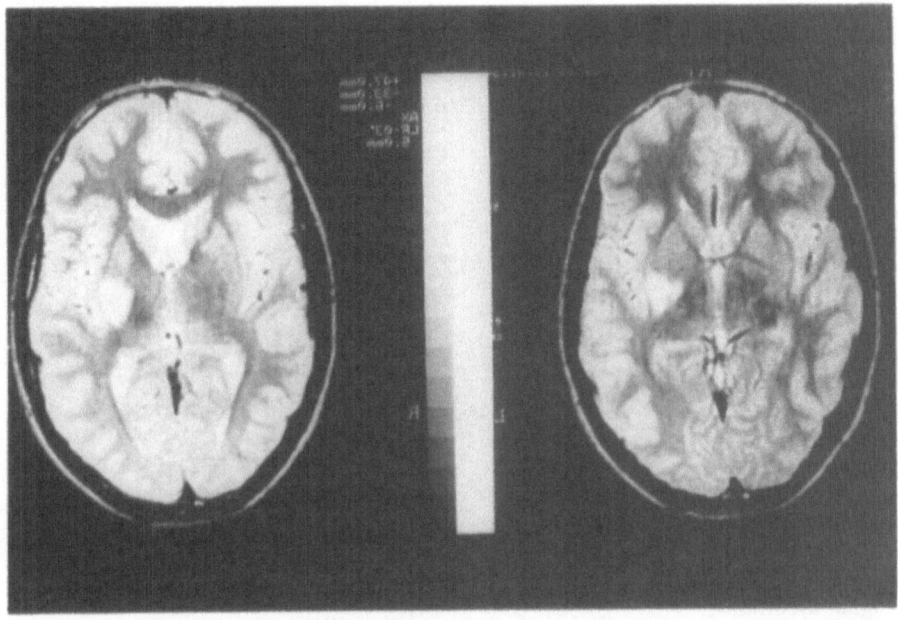

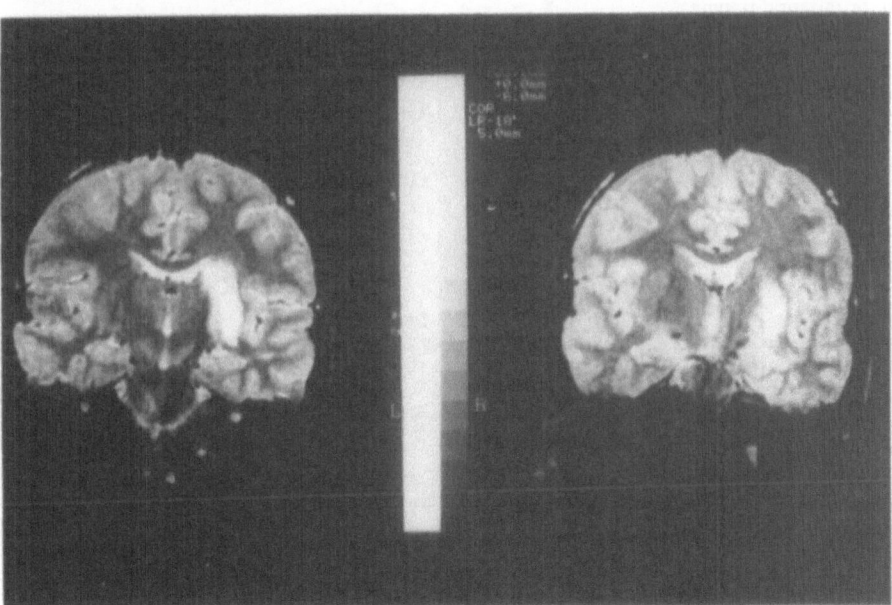

Figure 3.1. Magnetic resonance (MR) images showing hypersignal in a case of ischemic infarct secondary to one branch of the middle cerebral artery obstruction in axial (**A**) and frontal (**B**) views.

centration seems to play an important role in inducing ischemic cell lesion[17] and may be closely related both to deterioration of brain function during ischemia and to poor recovery during the perfusion period.[18,19]

Ischemia is accompanied by an increase in tissue lactate concentration because, in this event, glucose undergoes anaerobic metabolism, and there is a fall in tissue pH. It has been observed that acidosis and the concentration of lactic acid produce more severe harmful effects when ischemia is incomplete than in cases with

Table 3.1. Etiopathogenic factors of stroke in children

Idiopathic: 30 to 50% of the cases

Congenital heart disease

    Valvular disorders
    Congestive heart failure
    Septal defects
    Complex heart defects
    Emboli or hypertension of any origin
    Intracardiac tumor in relationship with tuberous
       esclerosis
    Surgical problems
    Polycynthemia or dehydration
    Problems caused by angiography

Acquired heart disease

    Rheumatic disease
    Endocarditis, myocarditis
    Myxoma
    Arrhythmias
    Surgical or angiographic problems
    Acute cardiogenic hypotension

Trauma

    Direct neck or intraoral trauma
    Closed head trauma
    Fat, air, or amniotic fluid embolization
    Strenuous exercise

Structural changes of the cerebrovascular system

    Vasculitis of unknown etiology
    Moyamoya syndrome
    Fibromuscular dysplasia
    Arteriovenous malformations
    Aneurysms
    Takayasu's syndrome
    Collagen disease [systemic lupus erythema tosus (SLE),
       polyarteritis nodosa (PAN)]
    Necrotizing angiitis
    Kinking or coiling
    Neurocutaneous syndromes
    Extrinsic compression (tumors)

Infections: local

    Tonsillitis
    Cavernous sinus thrombophlebitis
    Lymphadenitis
    Herpes ophthalmicus
    Malaria, paragonimiasis (Far East)
    Mucormycosis
    Meningitis

Infections: systemic

    Neonatal sepsis
    Pulmonary infections
    Viral infectious diseases
    Tuberculosis
    Mycoplasma pneumoniae

Hematological

    Intravascular coagulopathy
    Polycythemia
    Thrombocytosis
    Sickle cell disease

Metabolic disease

    Homocystinuria
    Fabry's disease
    Diabetes
    Dehydration
    Hyperlipidemia

Drug abuse

    Necrotizing angiitis (almost all types of drugs)
    Arterial spasms (LSD, cocaine and its free-base form or
       "crack")

Iatrogenic

    Umbilical vein catheters
    Radiotherapy (juxtasellar tumors)
    Intravascular use (diagnostic, therapeutic)

Data from refs. 1, 2, and 8.

complete interruption of blood flow.[20] This is in accordance with worsening of brain injury when glucose is administered, which is interpreted to be caused by the increased concentration of lactate. Other experimental works, on the contrary, have reported better tolerance, in terms of neurological recovery, of less severe incomplete ischemia than of complete ischemia.[21]

Carotid Obstructions

Infarctions in any zone of the supratentorial brain manifest the clinical symptomatology in the form of localized neurological alterations, which together are commonly known as ischemic stroke. The two main causes are arterial thrombosis and embolism. Although the disease can be observed in one or both carotid

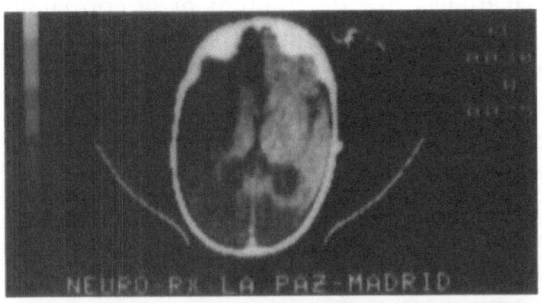

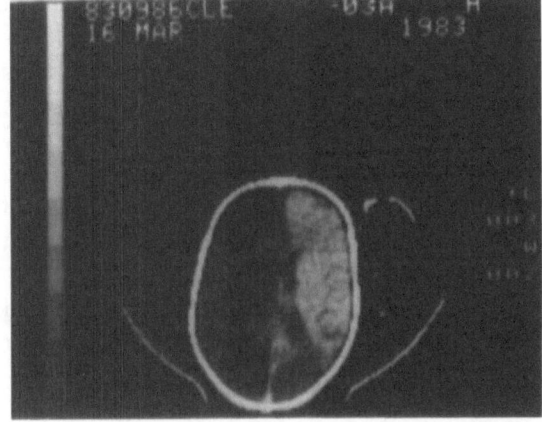

Figure 3.2. Complete obstruction of the left internal carotid artery in a child with congenital cardiopathy. The computerized tomography (CT) shows hypodensity of the left cerebral hemisphere and the occipital zone of the right hemisphere.

arteries (Fig. 3.2), or in any of their primary or secondary branches, obstruction of the territory of the middle cerebral artery is seen more frequently than any other,[5] especially in cases of congenital cardiopathy. Cerebral air embolism is very rare in children and can affect any vessel. Vascular insufficiency in the territory of the occipital branches of both posterior cerebral arteries is very frequently found after cardiac arrest.

Complete stroke is followed by focal neurological deficits. These clinical alterations are related to the affected zone of the brain, the origin being arterial thrombosis, emboli, hemorrhage, or venous occlusion. Neurological deficits in our series[5] were hemiplegia (85%; bilateral in 11%), generalized seizures (26%), focal seizures (18.5%), aphasia or disphasia (9.2%), and other symptoms (ataxia, transient dizziness, dysarthria) (27.7%). Headache, vomit-

ing, and loss of consciousness have been reported frequently.[9] Factors precipitating ischemic attacks are trauma, cardiac failure, deep breathing, crying, changes in body temperature, upper respiratory infection, severe changes of the cardiac rhythm such as in supraventricular tachycardia,[22] etc. (Table 3.1).

Bilateral obstruction of the carotids or any of their principal branches may occur.[23] According to our experience the prognosis of patients who present thrombosis of both middle cerebral arteries is bad.[23] Treatment depends upon the etiology of the obstruction, general care, and calcium antagonists in correct dosage.

Transient Ischemic Attacks

The term *transient ischemic attack* is used when the neurological deficits disappear within some minutes, although episodes having a duration of 24 hr or less may be called transient cerebral ischemic attacks (TCIAs). This disease is occasionally seen in children. It can be caused by problems of the carotid or the vertebrobasilar arteries. Transient episodes suggesting vertebrobasilar TCIAs are diplopia, ataxia, dizziness, dysphagia, and bilateral motor and/or sensory symptoms. Symptoms and signs suggesting carotid TCIAs are motor, sensory, speech, and visual disorders, in isolated or associated form. Distribution of motor and sensory problems may affect a part of or the entire arm, leg, face, or all the zones at the same time. Visual disease may present as monocular blindness having an onset with immediately completed deficit, or with upward, downward, or lateral progression. If a secondary vessel is affected, monocular field involvement may begin as partial blindness (superior or inferior half, peripheral field, blindness to different colors, etc.).

Conditions associated with TCIAs are mainly abnormalities of blood vessels, such as fibromuscular dysplasia, Moya–Moya syndrome, arteritis, arterial dissection, arterial stenosis, aneurysm or ectasia. Atherosclerosis is rarely the origin of TCIAs in children. Other miscellaneous conditions, such as migraine, hypotension, endocarditis, and hematological abnormalities may also be the cause of TCIAs.

Risk factors for TCIAs are any of the above-mentioned disorders, diabetes mellitus, and/or chronically elevated blood pressure, history of rheumatic heart disease, hypercholesterolemia, paroxysmal atrial tachycardia, and most of the severe cardiac diseases. Smoking rarely is a risk factor for children, although it is for adults.

Cerebral arteriography usually reveals the affected vessel. Computerized tomography (CT) and especially magnetic resonance (MR) images constitute the appropriate diagnostic studies to determine the damaged area of the brain.

Platelet antiaggregation agents are often used, although optimal dosage remains unknown, and calcium antagonists now constitute the most widely used drugs and those that give the best results, especially with regard to preventing future attacks.

Cerebral Hemorrhage

Intracrebral hematomas, if neonatal hemorrhages are excluded, are uncommon in children. Intracerebral hemorrhage secondary to ischemic infarctions, on the contrary, is very often seen. The most frequent causes of spontaneous hematomas are the rupture of arteriovenous malformations or aneurysms, bleeding diatheses, hypovitaminosis K (Fig. 3.3), hemophilia, trauma, bleeding into neoplasms, and rarely diabetic vasculopathies[24] or malignant hypertension. However, a low percentage of primitive hemorrhages of unknown etiology are reported in all series. Massive fatal hemorrhages are usually due to the rupture of vascular malformations (aneurysm or angioma).

Hemorrhagic infarction is usually associated with thrombotic or embolic stroke, the latter event documented in as many as 31% of patients with cerebral embolism.[25] This association is secondary to the use of anticoagulant therapy to prevent recurrent emboli not only in adults but also in children,[26] even though the use of anticoagulant therapy in pediatric patients with acute embolic stroke is not indicated.

The symptomatology is usually characterized by headache, vomiting, nuchal rigidity, focal or generalized seizures, and fever. Previous migraine-like headaches are quite common. Small and deep hematomas may be clinically silent. Voluminous intracerebral hemorrhages not only cause severe disturbances of motor, sensory, speech, language, and other cerebral functions

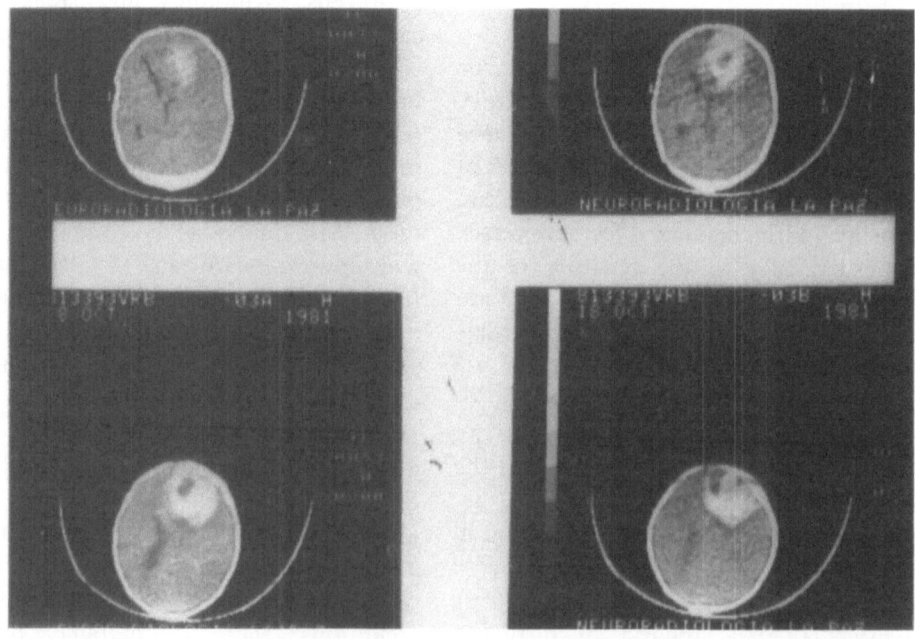

Figure 3.3. Intraparenchymatous hemorrhage in an infant with hypovitaminosis K; CT scan images.

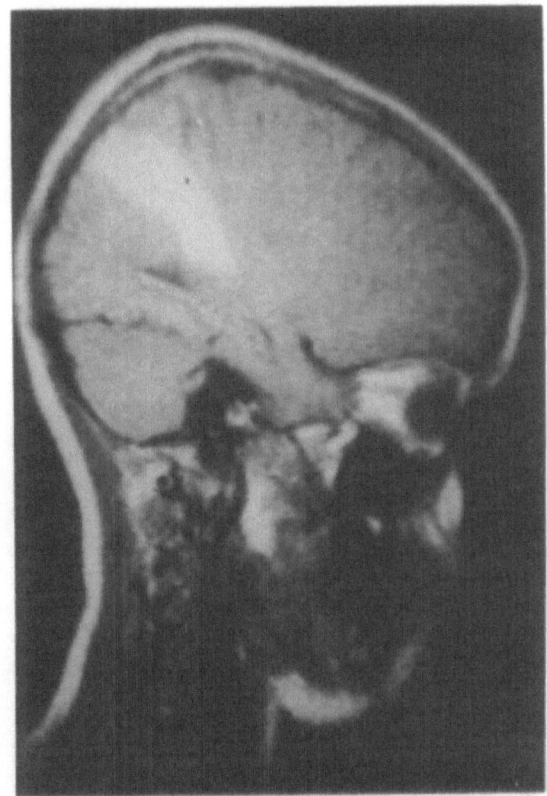

A

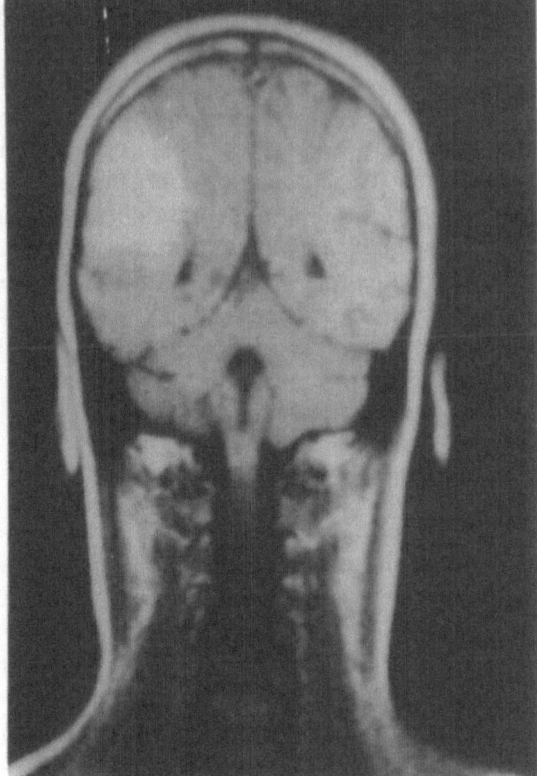

B

but also intracranial hypertension and hydrocephalus.

Computer tomography scans and MR images show very clearly the location (Fig. 3.4), size, aspect of the surrounding zones, and possible origin of the hemorrhage. Treatment is directed toward the cause of the hemorrhage, with surgery being indicated in cases of vascular malformation or in secondary hydrocephalus.

Vertebral Obstructions

Generalities and Clinical Findings

Occlusion of the vertebrobasilar arterial system is relatively rare in children. Approximately 40 cases affecting the entire vertebrobasilar system have been reported.[27] The most common clinical signs are vomiting, nausea, dizziness, ataxia, coughing, diplopia or other visual disorders, dysarthria, oculomotor or other cranial nerve deficit, nystagmus, headache, lethargy or irritability, staggering, dysphagia, nasal voice, hemiparesis or hemiplegia, and seizures. Tetraplegia, lethargy, or coma are more common in basilar artery occlusion whereas hemiparesis or hemiplegia of the contralateral side are more commonly seen in vertebral artery occlusion. Hypalgesia in some areas of the face, tongue, nose, or palate, Honner's syndrome, and cerebellar disorder on the same side of the arterial occlusion are usually seen in Wallenberg's syndrome [occlusion of the posterior inferior cerebellar artery (PICA)]. The basilar artery and one of the vertebral arteries are occluded with similar frequency. Complete or almost complete obstruction of one vertebral artery and incomplete occlusion of the other,[28,29] or complete occlusion of both vertebral arteries,[30] have been reported. Posterior circulation stroke in children occurs in males five times more often than in females.

Survival in cerebellar stroke results in 75% of cases, and complete recovery in only 20%. Severe mental, motor, and speech sequelae are found in 35% and minimal or discrete cerebellar, cranial nerve, or motor sequelae in 45%.[31]

←

Figure 3.4. A, B. Lateral and frontal views of MR images, showing hypersignal in a case of spontaneous intracerebral hemorrhage.

Although occlusion of the basilar artery seems to cause more severe clinical ictal alterations, sequelae are similar in basilar or vertebral occlusion. Adequate flow through collateral branches is indicative of a favorable outcome.[30]

Etiology

No clear origin may be found in more than 50% of cases. Mechanical injury to the C1–C2 vertebral artery segment has been reported as the most common cause,[31–35] especially in cervical spine manipulation, due to atlantoaxial instability in congenital odontoid aplasia. Other causes include Klippel–Feil[35] syndrome, direct trauma with or without fracture, vascular hypoplasia, cardiac abnormalities, arteritis, sepsis, hypercoagulable states, and migraine.[36] The vertebral arteries may suffer considerable stretching or kinking as they pass from the transverse foramen of C2 to C1. Any traumatism at this level increases the risk of lesion of the vessels, with consequent intimal injury that promotes platelet aggregation and formation of a thrombus at the site of the injured intima. This may lead to a vertebral occlusion.[37,38] Occasionally, this injured arterial region can be a source of recurrent emboli that obstruct the circulation of the vertebrobasilar system.[35]

Radiology

Computerized tomography and MR usually provide images that, in conjunction with clinical findings, help in the recognition of the arterial territory involved. In basilar artery occlusion, it is possible to observe bilateral pontine infarction or extensive brainstem ischemia, associated with cerebellar and posterior cerebral vascular damage.[39]

Occlusion of the PICA usually shows a wide ischemic zone in the cerebellum and vermis. Precise delineation of vertebrobasilar ischemia, however, appears difficult due to the numerous variations in distribution of the posterior fossa arterial supply. In spite of the images provided by the new, nonaggressive studies [CT, MR, and positron-emission tomography (PET)], the performance of vertebral arteriography is necessary if one wants to know the level and characteristics of the occluded artery, the morphology of vessels, and the collateral circulation (Fig. 3.5).

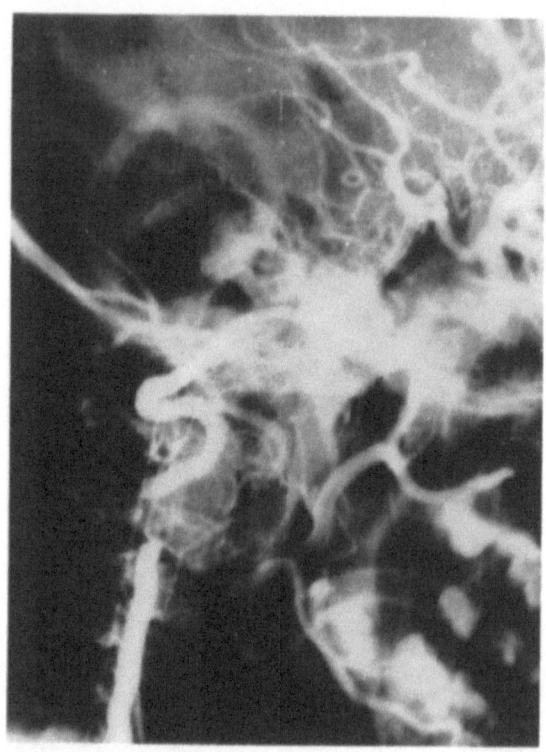

Figure 3.5. Lateral view of vertebral artery obstruction at the level of C2. The collateral vascularization makes possible the recanalization of the occluded artery at a higher level.

Treatment

The treatment of vertebrobasilar occlusion is conditioned to the etiology of the disease. General care, and administration of calcium antagonists may contribute to shorter recuperation and better prognosis. Aspirin is another drug to be used, if necessary, because it alters the aggregation–release reaction of blood platelets. Heparin-type anticoagulants are becoming less recommended.

Cerebellar Infarction

Isolated cerebellar infarction is rarely observed in children and young people, and its pathoetiology is variable.[40] According to our experience, however, it is more frequent than has been reported.[41] The clinical picture usually appears as intermittent dizziness and nausea, headache, vomiting, and difficulty in walking and talking. Cerebellar signs and symptoms, such as ataxia, nystagmus, slurred speech, and decomposition of movement on one or both sides, are commonly found. In cases with a large infarcted zone of the cerebellum, usually concomitant with an important edematous component, obstruction of the aqueduct or fourth ventricle causing obstructive hydrocephalus and intracranial hypertension may be observed. The brainstem may also be compressed by these voluminous infarcts, and diminution of consciousness or even coma can appear. The disease has been reported in infants, without any vascular disease, secondary to dehydration.[42] Our three cases presented without any known pathology.

Computerized tomography and MR images reveal nonspecific infarcted zones. These pathological images may persist for long periods of time, even several months, as a result of the necrosis.

Cerebellar infarction in children presents a clinical disease similar to other cerebellar disorders. Differential diagnosis with acute cerebellar ataxia, cerebellar tumors, drug intoxication, or acute labyrinthitis is always necessary.

Evolution of the disease, when no therapeutic solution is available, depends upon the volume of the infarction and the edema in the surrounding tissue, which can lead to stupor, coma, intracranial hypertension, or even death. General care, antiedematous treatment, and removal of the infarcted parenchyma when necessary are the therapeutic alternatives. Implanting of an intraventricular shunt before removing the necrotic tissue may be necessary in order to resolve the obstructive hydrocephalus. In two of our three patients we had to remove the infarcted zone. Complete recovery was achieved in all three cases.

Brainstem Hemorrhage

Primary brainstem hemorrhage is very frequent in adults, but very rare in children. Prevalence of this disease, however, is now greater than before, because of greater ease in diagnosis provided by CT and MR studies. Vertebrobasilar arteriography usually shows normal images. At autopsy small angiomas have been found in children with brainstem hemorrhage.[43]

Clinical presentations are very different between adults and children. Sudden onset of coma, quadriplegia, constricted pupils, and respiratory arrest in patients having systemic hypertension, followed by death within a short time, maybe minutes or hours after onset, or survival with considerable deficits, is the most usual clinical picture observed in adults. The survival rate, however, has increased in recent years.[44,45] Children, on the contrary, present a subacute disease, usually without systemic hypertension, although they show cranial nerve paralysis, vomiting, hemilateral or bilateral paresis or paralysis, sphincter problems, hypotonic extremities, and loss of consciousness that can reach a semicomatose or comatose state. This picture may be preceded by a history of headache, fever, and general malaise over a few days or hours. The disease can be seen in children of all ages. Computerized tomography and MR images reveal the hemorrhage to be an area of high density and hypersignal, respectively. Extent and regression of the hemorrhage can be clearly identified by these studies. Complete recovery, or only minimal sequelae, such as paresis of some of the cranial nerves, mild hypo- or hyperesthesia and hyperreflexia, is mostly seen in children.[46]

Venous Thrombosis

Cerebral venous thrombosis has been considered a relatively uncommon disease. It can be found in all veins and venous sinuses, that is to say, cortical deep veins; sagittal, transverse, straight, petrosal, and cavernous sinuses, torcula, and jugular veins. However, sagittal and lateral sinuses are the most frequently affected because of the proximity of the auditory system and its many infections. With the introduction of new antibiotics, thrombosis of the cavernous sinus is rare. Thrombosis of the superior sagittal sinus is one of the best known, because of the possibility of identifying it by CT, MR, or cerebral angiography.

In the past, most venous thromboses in children were the result of a complication of infection, principally meningitis, or of a septic focus arising from adjacent areas, as a complication of mastoiditis or infection of the paranasal sinuses, or as a result of dehydration. Presently, venous thrombosis is more frequently seen in neonates delivered with asphyxia,[47] as a manifestation of hypercoagulable states such as polycythemia in children with congenital heart malformations who show blood hyperviscosity,[48] and in patients with postraumatic or postsurgical complications. Invasion of the sinus by local neoplasms, use of oral contraceptives, and pregnancy are very seldom the cause of venous thrombosis in children and young people, although they are frequently seen in adults.

Clinical symptoms usually appear with acute or subacute onset. They are mostly nonspecific, although a certain relationship with the original illness may commonly be established. Headaches, seizures, lethargy and/or stupor or coma, fever, nausea or vomiting, drowsiness, hemiparesis, aphasia, or dysphasia are commonly observed. A bulging anterior fontanelle is usually seen in infants. The high mortality and morbidity reported in the past and attributed to complications of trauma, intracranial infections, or surgery now constitute a less important problem. Deep cerebral venous thrombosis, however, can have a high mortality with presentation of a comatous state very early on.[49]

Diagnosis of cerebral sinus and venous thrombosis must be established by angiography that shows in the venous phase nonfilling of the thrombosed sinus or vein. Other neuroradiological studies, however, may help in the diagnosis of these disorders. Computerized tomography can reveal normal or small ventricles, hemorrhages, low-density areas, and increased density of dural sinuses and the tentorium.[50] Magnetic resonance imaging has been reported lately as a positive complementary study in the diagnosis of dural sinus thrombosis.[51–53] Thoracic vertebra 1(T1)-weighted images show an absence of normal flow void within the sinuses, while the thrombus appears hyperintense in both T1 and T2 images during the first few days after thrombosis. In partial thrombosis, it is possible to distinguish the central hyperintense signal belonging to the thrombus, which is surrounded by a peripheral halo of a signal void that corresponds to flowing blood.

Treatment in the acute phase is mainly limited to general care. Anti-inflammatory and antiepileptic drugs are most often administered. Anticoagulant use has been considered ill-advised.[54] Experimental repair of the sagittal sinus by bypass has been performed with very positive results.[55]

Alternating Hemiplegia

Alternating hemiplegia is a very rare disorder, one first described by Verret and Steele.[56] The onset of the disease is before 18 months of age and more frequently between 3 and 9 months of age.[57,58] The disorder is usually marked by episodes of hemiplegia, tonic fits, acute dystonia, or a combination of these. The hemiplegic attacks may involve either side, and their duration ranges from some minutes to several days. Their intensity may also be variable. These attacks can affect both sides of the body, either alternatively or simultaneously, and are often accompanied by predominantly unilateral nystagmus and/or autonomic nervous system phenomena such as respiratory disturbances, vasomotor changes, or autonomic spells. The tonic fits can be unilateral or bilateral and are very often accompanied by a brief loss of consciousness, screaming, and irritability. Dystonic postures, choreoathetoid movements, dystonic head turning or tilting toward the side more affected, are also frequently noted. Psychomotor retardation is often seen and appears more evident with the passing of time. Motor sequelae (spasticity, ataxia, or choreoathetosis) may be observed in some children, especially in those who have had more severe and frequent attacks.

The nosology of the syndrome includes a relationship with migraine, something that has been suggested by the clinical signs. The possibility that the attacks of alternating hemiplegia represent atypical manifestations of epilepsy has also been discussed, and may also be related to paroxysmal dyskinesias and the common types of hemiplegia. The exact nature of alternating hemiplegia, however, still remains unknown. The pathophysiology seems to be at least partly related to intermittent dysfunction of the brainstem.

Electroencephalograms (EEGs) show ictal and interictal normalities, although an excess of slow wave activity is observed in some cases.[56,57] Neuroradiological studies (CT, MR, and cerebral arteriographies) fail to reveal marked abnormalities.

Anticonvulsant and conventional antimigraine drugs are ineffective, but calcium antagonists seem to be effective. Beneficial effects on the interictal condition are noted in most patients. An important reduction in frequency and/or duration and severity of attacks, an interictal decrease, and improvement in mental development seem to result from treatment with flunarizine.[58] The recommended dose is 5 mg on alternate days for children with a body weight below 20 kg, and 5 mg/day for children weighing 20 kg or more. A daily dose of 5 mg/day or more for children of all weights as well as the administration of other calcium-entry blockers may have a positive effect as well.

References

1. Raybaud CA, Livet MO, Jiddane M, Pinsard N: Radiology of ischemic strokes in children. Neuroradiology 27:567–578, 1985.
2. Schoenberg BS, Mellinger JF, Schoenberg DG. Cerebrovascular disease in infants and children: a study of incidence, clinical features, and survival. Neurology 28:763–768, 1978.
3. Egg-Olofsson O, Ringheim Y: Stroke in Children. Clinical characteristics and prognosis. Acta Paediatr. Scand 72: 391–395, 1983.
4. Matsumoto N, Whisnant JP, Kurland LT, Okazaki H: Natural history of stroke in Rochester, Minnesota, 1955 through 1969: an extension of a previous study 1945 through 1954. Stroke 4:20–29, 1973.
5. Pascual-Pascual SI, Pascual-Castroviejo I, Velez A: Accidentes cerebrovasculares isquémicos en la infancia. In: Yaya Huaman R, Sancho Rieger J, Lainez Andres JM. (eds.). Accidentes Cerebrovasculares Isquémicos en Adultos Jóvenes. MCR, Barcelona, 1987, 141–153.
6. Gold AP, Challenor YB, Gilles SH: Strokes in Children (part 1). Stroke 4:835–94, 1973.
7. Terplan KL: Patterns of brain damage in infants and children with congenital heart disease. Am J Dis Child 125:175–185, 1973.
8. Adams HP, Butler MJ, Biller J, Toffol GJ: Nonhemorrhagic cerebral infarction in young adults. Arch Neurol 43:793–796, 1986.
9. Kurokawa T, Chen YJ, Tomita S, Kishiwara T, Kitamura K: Cerebrovascular occlusive disease with and without the Moyamoya vascular network in children. Neuropediatrics 16:29–32, 1985.
10. Hossmann KA, Sato K: Recovery of neuronal function after prolonged cerebral ischemia. Science 168:375–376, 1970.
11. Hossmann KA, Kleinhues R: Reversibility of ischemic brain damage. Arch Neurol 19:375–384, 1973.
12. Garcia JH, Kamijyo Y: Cerebral infarction. Evaluation of histopathological changes after occlusion of a middle cerebral artery in primates. J Neuropathol Exp Neurol 33:408–421, 1974.
13. Garcia JH, Mitchem HL, Briggs L, Morawetz R, Hudetz AG, Hazebrig JB, Halsey JH, Conger KA: Transient focal ischemia in subhuman primates. Neuronal injury as a function of local cerebral blood flow. J Neuropathol Exp Neurol 42:44–60, 1983.
14. Plum F: What causes infarction in ischemic brain? The Robert Wartenberg Lecture. Neurology 33:222–233, 1983.
15. Hossmann KA, Zimmerman V: Resuscitation of brain after one hour of complete ischemia. I. Physiological and morphological observations. Brain Res 81:59–74, 1974.
16. Astrup J, Siesjo BK, Symon L: Thresholds in cerebral ischemia. The ischemic penumbra. Stroke 12:723–725, 1981.
17. Faber JL, Chien KR, Mittnacht S Jr: The pathogenesis of irreversible cell injury in ischemia. Am J Pathol 102:271–281, 1981.
18. Uematsu D, Greemberg JH, Reivich M, Karp A: In vivo measurement of cytosolic free calcium during cerebral ischemia and reperfusion. Ann Neurol 24:420–428, 1988.
19. Uematsu D, Grenberg JH, Reivich M, Hickey F: Direct evidence for calcium induced ischemic and reperfusion injury. Ann Neurol 26:280–283, 1989.
20. Rechncrona S, Rosen I, Siesjo BK: Excessive cellular acidosis: an important mechanism of neuronal damage in the brain. Acta Physiol Scand 110:435–437, 1980.
21. Steen PA, Michenfelder JD, Milde JH: Incomplete versus complete cerebral ischemia: Improved outcome with a minimal blood flow. Ann Neurol 6:389–398, 1979.

22. Atluru VL, Epstein LG, Gootman N: Childhood stroke and supraventricular tachycardia. Pediat Neurol 1:54–56, 1985.

23. Pascual-Castroviejo I, Larrauri J: Bilateral thrombosis of the middle cerebral artery in a child aged 14 months. Dev Med Child Neurol 13:613–620, 1971.

24. Atluru VL: Spontaneous intracerebral hematomas in juvenile diabetic ketoacidosis. Pediatr Neurol 2:167–169, 1986.

25. Weisberg LA: Nonseptic cardiogenic cerebral embolic stroke: clinical CT correlations. Neurology 35:896–899, 1985.

26. Kelley RE: Hemorrhagic cerebral infarction in pediatric patients. Pediatr Neurol 2:111–114, 1986.

27. Phillips PC, Lorentsen KJ, Shropshire LC, Ahn HS: Congenital odontoid aplasia and posterior circulation stroke in childhood. Ann Neurol 23:410–413, 1988.

28. Ouvrier RA, Hopkins IJ: Occlusive diseases of the vertebrobasilar arterial system in childhood. Dev Med Child Neurol 12:186–192, 1970.

29. De Vivo DC, Farrell FW: Vertebrobasilar occlusive disease in children. A recognizable clinical entity. Arch Neurol 26:278–281, 1972.

30. Pascual-Castroviejo I, Pascual-Pascual JI, Mulas F, Roche MC, Tendero A: Bilateral obstruction of the vertebral arteries in a three-year-old child. Dev Med Child Neurol 19:232–238, 1977.

31. Pascual-Pascual JI, Pascual-Castroviejo I, Tendero A, Roche MC: Oclusiones del territorio vertebrobasilar en la infancia. Presentación de un caso y revisión de la literatura. Ann Esp Pediatr 10:665–672, 1977.

32. Latchaw RE, Seeger JF, Gabrielsen TO: Vertebrobasilar arterial occlusion in children. Neuroradiology 8:141–147, 1974.

33. Jain S, Maheshwari MC, Tandon PN, Goulatia RK: Idiopathic basilar artery occlusion in childhood. Stroke 15:563–565, 1984.

34. Singer WD, Haller JS, Wolpert SM: Occlusive vertebrobasilar artery disease associated with cervical spine anomaly. Am J Dis Child 129:492–495, 1975.

35. Ross CA, Curnes JT, Greenwood RS: Recurrent vertebrobasilar embolism in an infant with Klippel–Feil anomaly. Pediatr Neurol 3:181–183, 1987.

36. Dunn DW: Vertebrobasilar occlusive disease and childhood migrain. Pediatr Neurol 1:252–254, 1985.

37. Ford FR, Clark D: Thrombosis of the basilar artery with softening in the cerebellum and brainstem due to manipulation of the neck. Bull Johns Hopkins Hosp 98:37–42, 1956.

38. Bell HS: Basilar artery insufficiency due to atlanto-axial instability. Am Surg 35:695–700, 1969.

39. Bonafe A, Manelfe C, Scotto, B, Pradere MY, Rascol A: Role of computed tomography in vertebrobasilar ischemia. Neuroradiology 27:484–493, 1985.

40. Bergen BJ, Batnitzky S, Norantz RA, Erice HI: Cerebellar infarction with associated hydrocephalus due to vertebral artery occlusion in a child. Neurosurgery 8:383–387, 1981.

41. Aoki N, Toyofuku T, Komiya K: Cerebellar infarction. Neuropediatrics 17:124–128, 1986.

42. Fischer EG, Strand RD, Gilles FH: Cerebellar necrosis simulating tumor in infancy. J Pediatr 81:98–100, 1972.

43. Zeller RS, Chutorian AM: Vascular malformations of the pons in children. Neurology 25:776–780, 1975.

44. Burns J, Lisak R, Shut L, Silberberg D: Recovery following brainstem hemorrhage. Ann Neurol 7:183–184, 1980.

45. Lavy E, Rothman S, Reches A: Primary pontine hemorrhage with complete recovery. Arch Neurol 38:320, 1981.

46. Minami T, Kurokawa T, Inoue T, Takaki S, Goya N, Yoshida M, Kishikawa T: Primary brainstem hemorrhage in a child: usefulness of auditory brainstem response (ABR). Neuropediatrics 15:99–101, 1984.

47. Konishi Y, Kuriyama M, Sudo M, Konishi K, Hayakawa K, Ishii Y: Superior sagittal sinus thrombosis in neonates. Pediatr Neurol 3:222–225, 1987.

48. Schubiger G, Schubiger D, Tonz O: Thrombose des sinus saggital superior beim Neugeborenen—Diagnoses durch computer tomographie. Helv Paediatr Acta 37:193–199, 1982.

49. Elck JJ, Miller KD, Bell KA, Tutton RH: Computed tomography of deep cerebral venous thrombosis in children. Radiology 37:399–402, 1981.

50. Rao KCG, Knipp HC, Wagner EJ: Computed tomographic findings in cerebral sinus and venous thrombosis. Radiology 140:391–398, 1981.

51. Macchi PJ, Grossman RI, Gomori JM, Goldberg HI, Zimmerman RA, Bilaniuk LT: High field MR imaging of cerebral venous thrombosis. J Comput Assist Tomogr 10:10–15, 1986.

52. McArdle CB, Mirfakhraee M, Amparo EG, Kulkarni MV: MR imaging of transverse/sigmoid

dural sinus and jugular vein thrombosis. J Comput Assist Tomogr 11:831–838, 1987.

53. Baram TZ, Butler IJ, Nelson MD, McArdle CB: Transverse sinus thrombosis in newborns: clinical and magnetic resonance imaging findings. Ann Neurol 24:792–794, 1988.

54. Gettelfinger DM, Kokment E: Superior sagittal sinus thrombosis. Arch Neurol 34:2–6, 1977.

55. Sindou M, Mazoyer JF, Fischer G, Pialat J, Fourcade C: Experimental bypass for sagittal sinus repair. Preliminary report. J Neurosurg 44:325–330, 1976.

56. Verret S, Steele J: Alternating hemiplegia in childhood: a report of eight patients with complicated migraine beginning in infancy. Paediatrics 47:675–680, 1971.

57. Krägeloh I, Aicardi J: Alternating hemiplegia in infants: report of five cases. Dev Med Child Neurol 22:784–791, 1980.

58. Casaer P, Aicardi J, Curatolo P, Dias K, Maia M, Matte J, Pineda M, Peuplard F, Preney-Cramatte S, Stephenson J, Szliwowski H: Flunarizine in alternating hemiplegia in childhood. An international study in 12 children. Neuropediatrics 18:191–195, 1987.

CHAPTER 4

Agenesis and Prenatal Occlusion of the Cerebral Vessels

Shizuo Oi

Introduction

The concept of cerebrovascular accident in the embryonal and fetal periods remains obscure. The normal developmental status of the vascular system must be further analyzed not only from the morphological but also the physiological points of view. The pathophysiology and outcomes of these disorders are complicated mainly by developmental factors.

This chapter deals with the concept of a genesis and prenatal occlusion of the fetal vessels of the central nervous system (CNS), analyzing vascular development along with the neuronal maturation processes. Also emphasized in this concept are the vascular developmental anomalies and their close relationship to the dysgenetic states of the fetal brain. Developmental etiopathophysiology of the encephalodysplasic and encephaloclastic malformations are given particular attention.

Neuronal Maturation and Vascular Development*

In Streeter's classification,[1] the blood vessels of the human brain develop in the following stages: first stage (primordial endothelial vascular plexus: mesenchymal tissue hemangioblast endothelial cells, primitive vasculogenic cells, endothelial vascular meshwork); second stage (primordial endothelial vascular plexus of the head arteries, capillaries, and veins); third stage (three separate vascular systems: superficial vessels of the head, meningeal vessels, and

cerebral vessels); fourth stage (vascular adaptations to the growing brain); and fifth stage (late histologic changes in the walls of the vessels). Subsequently, the basic structures of the major blood vessels of the brain are completed within 7 weeks of gestational age, so that the vascular development of the brain occurs between neurulation and the beginning of neuronal differentiation.

Transition from the prevascular to the vascular period is accomplished during the fourth gestational week. In the prevascular period, the conceptus receives nourishment from the cytoplasm of the ovum, the yolk sac, and possibly uterine secretion. During this period of transition, diffusion is the major mechanism for nutrient delivery (Fig. 4.1A).

The first aortic arch appears at 3 weeks of gestational age. During the stages when the first and second aortic arches develop, the primitive internal carotid and trigeminal arteries occur as branches of the first aortic arch. Then the first two aortic arches begin to involute, and the primitive internal carotid arteries appear as extensions of the third aortic arch (at the end of the week).[2] The exact manner by which the basilar artery is formed remains unclear, but certainly it develops at a later stage, at about 4 weeks of gestational age. A single median artery is formed from a primitive double-basilar artery in the rostral region, but the caudal end remains plexiform. This caudal region is replaced in the mature stage with the inferior cerebellar arteries (6 weeks of gestational age). This fact may suggest the later development of the cerebellar hemispheres. The vertebral arteries are formed as longitudinal anastomoses between the upper segmental branches of the dorsal aorta at 5

---

* See Marcelletti and Picardo, Chapter 1, in this volume.

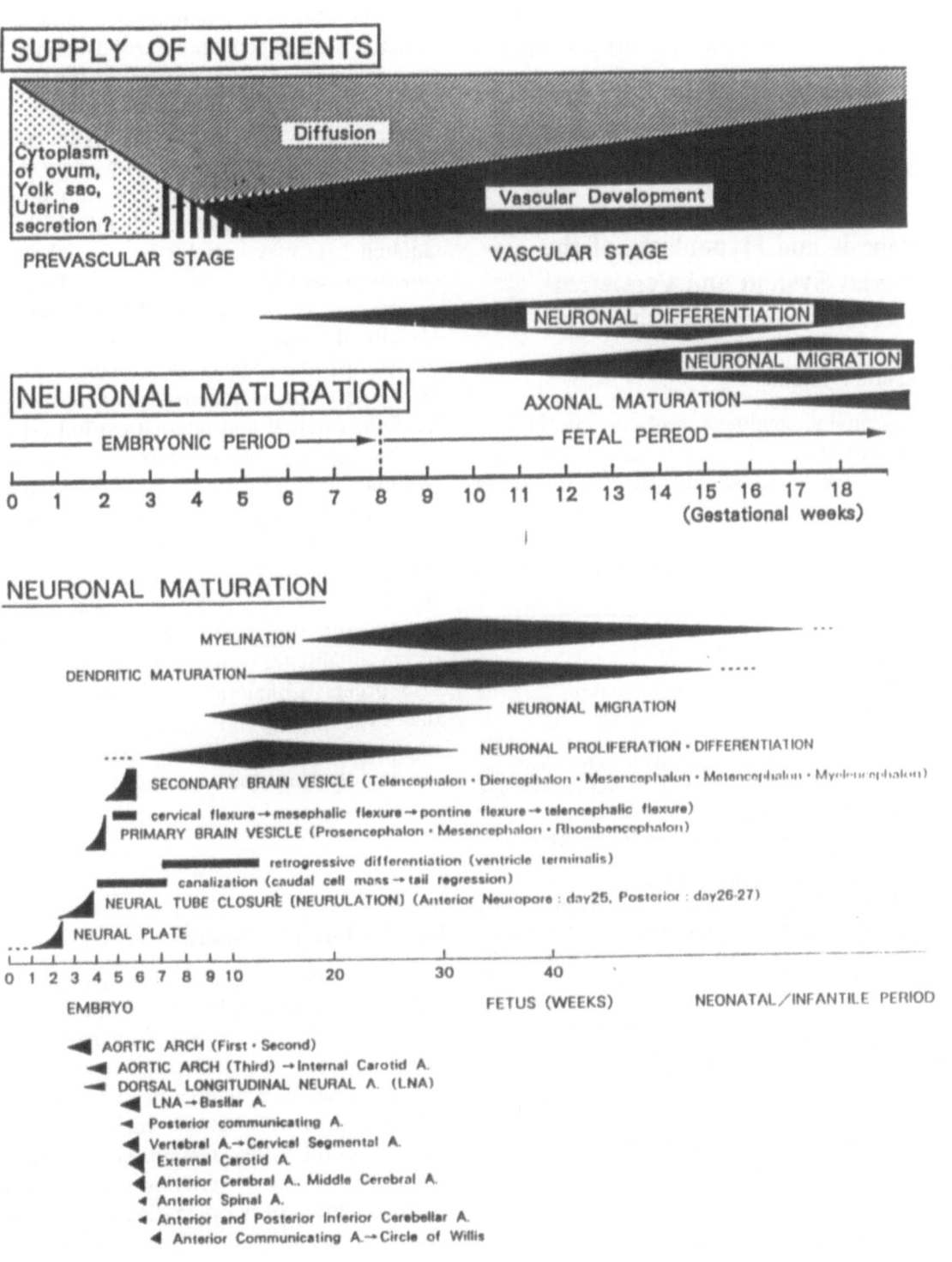

Figure 4.1. Neuronal maturation and vascular development in the normal embryo and fetus. (**A**) Neuronal maturation and supply of nutrients. (**B**) Neuronal maturation and vascular development.

weeks of gestational age. The anterior cerebral and middle cerebral arteries appear at 5 weeks of gestational age. By 7 weeks of gestational age, the anterior communicating artery develops and the circle of Willis is formed. Consequently, the essential structures of the cerebral vascular system are completed in the embryonic period (Fig. 4.1B).

Agenesis and Hypoplasia of the Arterial System and Persistent Arteries

Carotid System

Congenital anomalous vasculatures in the head and neck are listed in Table 4.1. In the carotid system, there are various sites of abnormal

Table 4.1. Congenital anomalous vasculatures in the head and neck.

Carotid system
1. Bicarotid trunk
2. Variation in common carotid bifurcation
3. Abnormal origins of common carotid
4. Absence of common carotid (right side: internal and external carotids aris separately from the innominate artery; left side: internal and external carotids arise independently from the aortic arch)
5. Tortuosity of the internal carotid (S-, C-shaped curves or kinking and looping)
6. Hypoplasia and aplasia of the internal carotid
7. Partial absence of one segment of the internal carotid (anterior and posterior communicating arteries are well developed, giving origin to the major branches of the carotid arterial system)

Vertebral–basilar system
1. Hypoplasia and aplasia of vertebral arteries
2. Partial absence of vertebral arteries
3. Duplications of vertebral arteries
4. Translocations and common trunks of vertebral arteries
5. Abnormal origins of vertebral arteries

Carotid–basilar anastomosis
1. Persistent primitive trigeminal artery
2. Peristent primitive acoustic (or ortic) artery
3. Peristent primitive hyperglossal artery

Other remnant arteries
1. Stapedial
2. Persistent primitive ophthalmic
3. Heubner's
4. Peristent first cervical intersegmental

origin of the common carotid artery. The bicarotid trunk is a common trunk, shared by the right and left common carotid arteries. Sometimes, the left common carotid artery arises abnormally close to the base of the innominate artery. Rarely, both carotid arteries arise independently, but directly, from the aorta.[2] Bifurcation of the common carotid artery should be at the level of the fourth cervical (vertebra) level in adults; the level is slightly higher in children. It may rarely be, in abnormal conditions, as high as the first cervical vertebra or as low as the second thoracic vertebra. Usually, this anomalous position is recognized bilaterally.[1] Absence of the common carotid artery develops as independent vessel origins from the external and internal carotid arteries, and there may be various forms of abnormally tortuous internal carotid arteries. S- or C-shaped curves (Vollmar type I) may not be significant clinically, but coiling or looping (Vollmar type II) (Fig. 4.2A) or kinking (Vollmar type III) may cause ischemic insults, requiring patch grafting or graft interposition. Complete or partial absence of the internal carotid artery also occurs. Collateral circulations, including the external carotid artery or the anterior/posterior communicating arteries, are usually well developed in such cases.

Vertebral–Basilar System

In the vertebral–basilar system, hypoplasia or aplasia of the vertebral artery on one side is not rarely recognized. There may be partial absence of the vertebral artery (Fig. 4.2B and C). In a case presented here, there was a well-developed collateral circulation between each of the patient vessels, but the patient remained asymptomatic. Abnormal origins of vertebral arteries include right vertebral artery originating from the right common carotid artery, right vertebral artery originating from the right internal carotid artery, right vertebral artery from the aortic arch, left vertebral artery from the aortic arch, and the left vertebral artery from the left internal carotid artery.

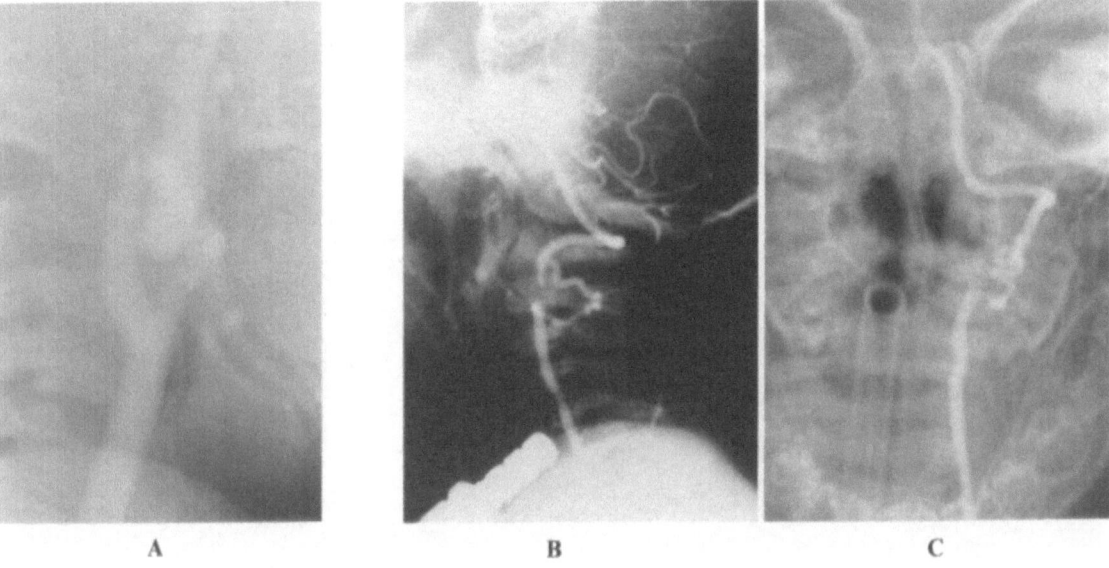

Figure 4.2. A. Coiling of the internal carotid artery (Vollmer type II). **B,C.** Partial absence of vertebral artery.

Carotid–Basilar Anastomosis

By 7 weeks of gestational age, there are numerous numbers of vascular networks, plexuses, and anastomoses in the embryo head and neck. These anastomotic channels disappear in the fourth stage of vascular development (rearrangement). Sometimes, however, some of them remain as a remnant (rudimental) artery (Table 4.1). These are commonly seen as carotid–basilar anastomoses and include the primitive trigeminal artery, primitive acoustic (otic) artery, and primitive hypoglossal artery.[3] The clinical significance of these remnant arteries with carotid–basilar anastomoses is that these (1) are sometimes associated with aneurysm of arteriovenous malformation, (2) may cause irritation of the adjacent cranial nerves (i.e., trigeminal neuralgia by primitive trigeminal artery), and (3) may be a causative factor of ischemic insults in the cerebrum when the patient's cerebral circulation is unsteady, such as in seizure, hypotension, etc., The main mechanism is in the "steal phenomenon" via the anastomotic channel (Fig. 4.3).

Prenatal Arterial Occlusion in the Fetal Brain

Cerebrovascular accident is a rare clinical entity in the fetal period, but recently such specific pathophysiology has been disclosed both in hemorrhagic and ischemic lesions. The most common hemorrhagic lesion involving the fetal brain is intrauterine intraventricular hemorrhage.[4] Intraventricular hemorrhage is a well-described clinical entity, as a specific form of cerebrovascular accident occurring in premature neonates. However, it still may not be well known that intraventricular hemorrhage is not a rare in utero event: 6% of stillborns have been observed to have this evidence at autopsy.[5,6] The ischemic insult, on the other hand, seems to be much less common in the fetal period.

Vascular disruptive lesions occurring in monozygotic twins include various forms of ischemic insults in the brain, renal defects, gastrointestinal defects, aplasia cutis congenita, hemifacial microsomia, and limb defects.[7] One specific feature known at the present time is

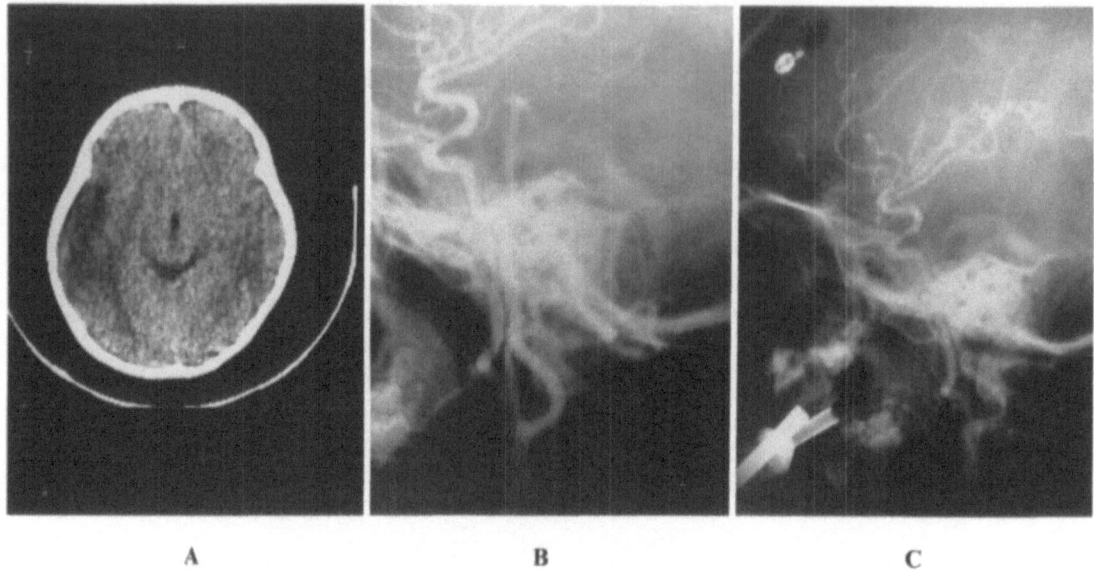

A   B   C

Figure 4.3. A 5-year-old male with generalized convulsions followed by prolonged coma. **A.** Computerized tomography demonstrated bilateral, diffuse, low-density changes in the cerebral hemisphere, more markedly in the temporal lobes. **B.** The carotid angiogram revealed a persistent hypoglossal artery. C. Increased intracranial pressure was controlled under continuous pressure monitoring, and the persistent artery was ligated to prevent the "steal phenomenon". (The vertebral angiogram showed normal vasculature.) The patient improved gradually and returned to a normal status.

cerebral infarction occurring in a single twin fetus. The mechanism of this unique condition is that thromboplastic materials pass through the placenta from the dead twin to the circulation of the living twin via vein-to-vein and artery-to-artery anastomoses, causing disseminated intravascular coagulation, followed by cerebral infarction[8-10] (Fig. 4.4). In the central nervous system, vascular disruption may result in encephalodysplasia or encephaloclastic insults such as porencephaly of the developing brain. Jung et al.[11] reviewed their series of 56 cases of congenital hydroanencephaly and porencephaly, observing that 6 cases (11%) were documented to be associated with monozygotic twins. They also reported the data involving 24 cases of congenital hydroanencephaly and porencephaly associated with twinning. In these cases, the finding of a preponderance of monozygotic twins, and the common association of a deceased cotwin, support the hypothesis of a vascular disruptive etiology.[11]

Primary Versus Secondary Vascular Maldevelopment in the Fetal Brain

It has been well established that a specific maldevelopment or morphological change of the embryonic central nervous system appears with a certain teratogen in a certain period of gestational life (critical period and stage specificity). This concept is well established, especially in the field of experimental teratology.[12] However, little is known concerning the relation between malformations of the central nervous system and vascular maldevelopment. It seems to be an extremely important concept that the development of the vascular system is seen in the late stage of the embryonic period and the vascular involvement in developing such morphological changes of the brain is limited to a certain period. Therefore, vascular hypoplasia may be either the cause or the result of the various CNS anomalies.

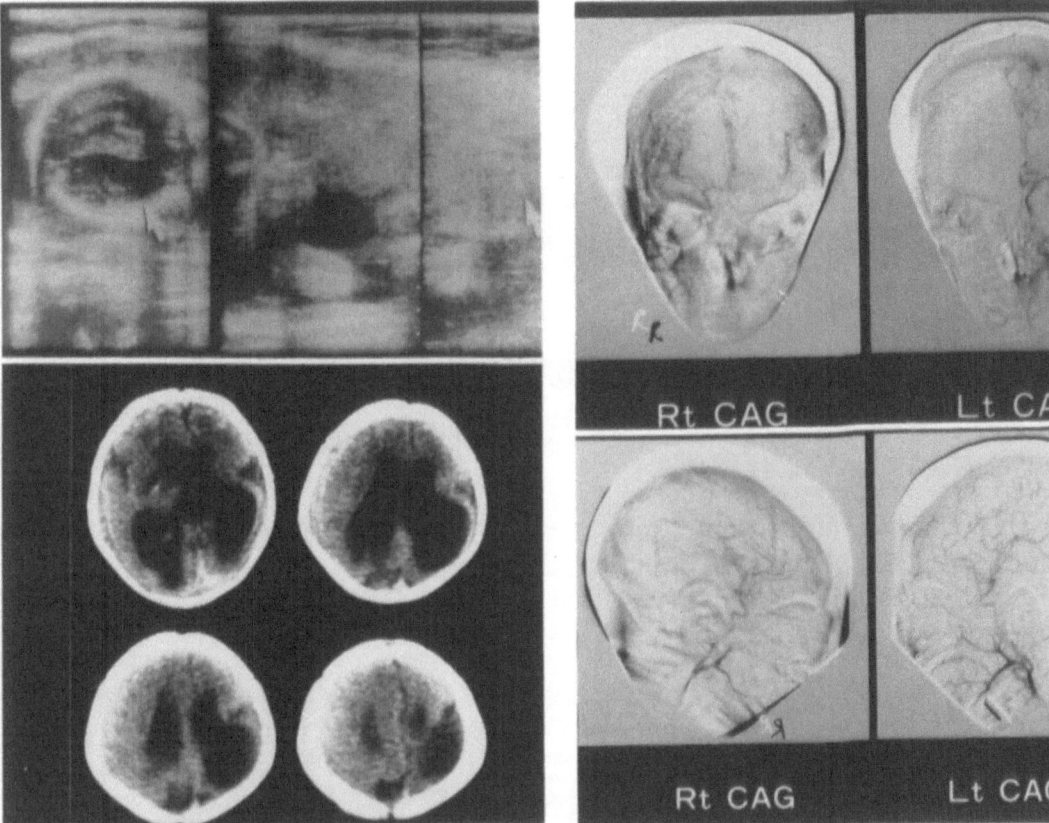

Figure 4.4. Cerebral infarction in an infant associated with a macerated cotwin. A twin pregnancy was diagnosed at 16 weeks of gestation. **A**. At 29 weeks of gestational age, ultrasonography demonstrated in utero death of twin 1 and dilated ventricles in twin 2 (left arrow). A calcified spot was also recognized in the placenta (right arrow). **B**. Computerized tomo-graphy obtained at birth revealed asymmetrically dilated ventricle and dysgenetic or encephaloclastic right cerebral hemisphere. **C**. Carotid angiogram (CAG) disclosed occlusion of major branches of the right middle cerebral artery. (From Shimoji, T. with permission.)

The supply of nutrients for the development of embryonic tissue differs depending on the stage. During the initial weeks of embryonal life, the cytoplasm of the ovum, the yolk sac, and possibly uterine secretions are the sources of nourishment to the conceptus. Transition from this primitive form of nourishment to the mature form (with the vascular supply) occurs in the fourth week of gestational age. During the transition period between this primitive pre-vascular stage and the time of vascular development, diffusion may play an important role in nourishment. Thus, if malnourishment may be a cause for development of CNS anomalies, it may involve brain development,

resulting in encephalodysplasia in the early embryonic period, prior to or during the prevascular stage. At that time, the later vascular development with the expected brain growth is suppressed, and vascular hypoplasia develops as a secondary change (encephalodysplasic mal-formation). Or, it may exist also as an associated lesion in brain parenchymal and vascular development.

On the other hand, the malnourishment may develop as a result of a primary vascular lesion during the vascular stage, especially in the fetal period. Neuronal maturation may already be completed either with neuronal differentiation or neuronal migration, after cell proliferation, in

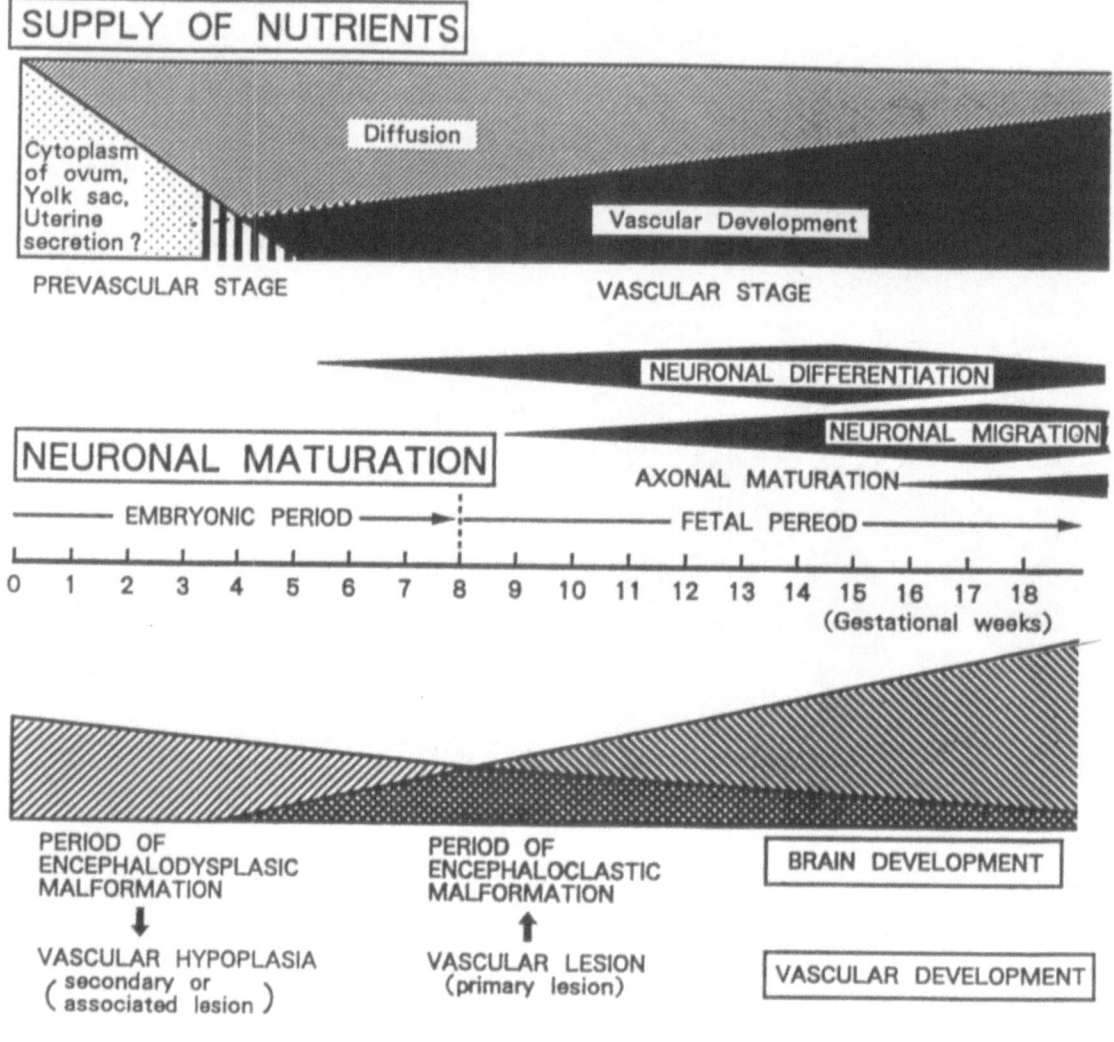

Figure 4.5. Encephalodysplasic malformation versus encephaloclastic malformation.

these cases. The morphological changes are mainly regressive in form, in which once-completed brain structure is destroyed and further maturation is stopped (encephaloclastic malformation) (Fig. 4.5).

Anencephaly and Vascular Structures

Anencephaly is one of the most severe forms of cephalic dysraphia, in which the telencephalon is poorly formed.[13] The common carotid arteries are intact and numerous prominent branches of the external carotid artery develop. The internal carotid arteries are small and subdivide into smaller vessels in the intracranial portion. In the posterior circulation, the major trunks are intact.

Cranium Bifidum Cysticum and Vascular Structures

Cranium bifidum cysticum, such as encephalocele, encephalomeningocele, encephalomeningocystocele, and so forth, is the product of a postneurulation disorder. The brain structure is completely formed, but some part of the normally developed brain herniates through the developmental defect of the meninges and skull with the major trunks of extra- and intracranial vasculature. The vascular structures are also deformed. The result is that the distorted brain and its corresponding vessels herniate into the sac maintaining the circulation from the intracranial parent arteries.[13]

Hydranencephaly and Vascular Structures

This form of malformation is the most severe type of encephaloclastic malformation, and the regression in the once-completed brain structure is the underlying condition; the secondary destructive processes are likely due to prenatal occlusion of the internal carotid artery. The cerebral hemispheres are absent, and it is often associated with hydrocephalus. The internal carotid artery may be hypoplastic. Some authors have reported that no carotid artery thrombosis or embolism may be present in the angiographic findings and that this fact is against the theory of vascular impairment.[14]

Holoprosencephaly and Vascular Structures

Holoprosencephaly is a malformative disorder that interferes with the development of the telencephalon. A single (azygos) anterior cerebral artery and bilateral middle cerebral arteries are present. Other variations of major vessels, such as persistent primitive trigeminal artery, abnormal origin of the anterior cerebral artery, a hypoplastic anterior cerebral artery, absence of the normal insular pattern, etc., have been reported.[14] The posterior circulation is intact.

Porencephaly and Vascular Structures

Porencephaly, a cerebral defect involving cortex and white matter through to the ventricular surface, may develop as a result of either vascular involvement or a primary dysgenic lesion. Yokovlev and Wadsworth[15] proposed a concept of "schizencephaly" as "encephalodysplastic porencephaly." It had been well recognized that the most common pathogenesis of the "encephaloclastic porencephaly" involved circulatory disturbances.

In the cases they reported, it was concluded that the symmetric congenital clefts in the cerebral mantle developed as a result of a failure of growth and differentiation of circumscribed areas of the cerebral mantle during the first 2 months of fetal life. The underlying condition may include a cell migration disorder. The thickness and the richly cellular structure of the plate of gray matter in the wall of the clefts and the persistence of the myelinated tangential fibers in the pia–ependymal layers seem to be incompatible with the essentially destructive effects of venous stasis and of a circulatory disturbance. However, the vascular structures may be affected secondarily, a result of these primary parenchymal morphological changes, differing from the encephaloclastic form of porencephaly (in which the prenatal occlusive vascular insult is the primary lesion).

Encephaloclastic porencephaly rarely develops as a result of local parenchymal destruction by intracerebral hemorrhage, such as periventricular hemorrhage in premature infants.[16] The porencephalic cavity may expand in the later, postnatal period and the extensive cerebral defects may cause neuronal degeneration of the subcortical nuclei and such chronological changes as retrograde cellular degeneration.[17] Hydrocephalus or further deterioration of vascular supply in the adjacent brain parenchyma associated with these lesions always remains a consideration.

Hypotheses on the Embryopathogenesis of Dysraphism, and a Vascular Basis Theory

Stevenson et al.[18] proposed an embryopathogenetic hypothesis of dysraphism: a vascular basis for neural tube defects. Closure of the neural tube, they proposed, is dependent upon vascularization of the neural system and its supporting tissues. According to this hypothesis, a disturbance in the timely development of vasculature may limit nutrients available to the neural tissue and thereby prevent closure. In their autopsy observations on six fetuses with spina bifida, abnormalities of the arterial supply to the region of the spine defect were demonstrated. Because embryologically these arteries develop prior to closure of the neural tube, it was suggested that the vascular disturbance limited nutrition to the developing neural tissue and supporting structures, preventing appropriate growth and closure.[18] There are reports supporting the hypothesis of a vascular basis of cephalic dysraphism in the literature.[19]

Acknowledgments. The author acknowledges the permission of Dr. Takeyoshi Shimoji, Chairman, Department of Neurosurgery, Okinawa Nambu Hospital to cite his valuable case in this chapter. The author also expresses sincere appreciation to Professors Satoshi Matsumoto and Professor Anthony J. Raimondi for kind suggestions on the concept dealt with in this chapter.

References

1. Kier EL: Development of cerebral vessels. In: Newton TH, Potts DG (eds.). Radiology of the Skull and Brain, Chapter 55, C. V. Mosby, Saint Louis, 1974, pp. 1089–1130.
2. Lemire RJ, Leaser JD, Leech RW, Alvord EC: Normal and Abnormal Development of the Human Nervous System. Harper & Row, New York, 1975.
3. Raimondi AJ: Pediatric Neuroradiology. Saunders, Philadelphia, 1972.
4. Oi S, Matsumoto S: Hydrocephalus in premature infants—characteristics and therapeutic problems. Child's Nerv Syst 5:76–82, 1989.
5. Leech RW, Kohnen P: Subependymal and intraventricular hemorrhages in the newborn. Am J Pathol 77:465–475, 1974.
6. Harcke HT, Naeye RL, Storch A: Perinatal cerebral intraventricular hemorrhage. J Pediatr 80:37–42, 1972.
7. Hoyme HE, Higginbottom MC, Jones KL: Vascular etiology of disruptive structural defects in monozygotic twins. Pediatrics 67:288–294, 1981.
8. Bulla M, von Lilen T, Goecke H, Roth B, Ortmann M, Heising J: Renal and cerebral

necrosis in survivors after in utero deth of co-twin. Arch Gynecol 240:119–124, 1987.
9. Benirschke K: Twin placenta in perinatal mortality. NY State J Med 61:1499–1507, 1961.
10. Moore CM, McAdams AJ, Sutherland J: Intrauterine disseminated intravascular coagulation: a syndrome of multiple pregnancy with a dead twin fetus. J Pediatr 74:523–528, 1969.
11. Jung JH, Graham JM Jr, Schultz N, Smith DW: Congenital hydranencephaly/porencephaly due to vascular disruption in monozygotic twins. Pediatrics 73:467–469, 1984.
12. Oi S, Kokunai T, Okuda Y, Sasaki M, Matsumono S: Identical embryopathogenesis for exencephaly and myeloschisis: an experimental study. J Neurosurg. 72:450–458, 1990.
13. Oi S, Matsumoto S: Morphological evaluation for neuronal maturation in anencephaly and encephalocele in human neonates: a proposal of reclassification of cephalic dysraphism. Child's Nerv Syst 6:350–355, 1990.
14. Wolpert SM: Vascular studies of congenital anomalies. In: Newton TH, Potts DG (eds.). Radiology of the Skull and Brain, chapter 87. C. V. Mosby, Saint Louis, 1974.
15. Yokovlev PL, Wadsworth RC: Schizencephalies —a study of the congenital clefts in the cerebral mantle. I. Clefts with fused lips. J Neuropathol Exp Neurol 5:116–130, 1946.
16. Pastermak JF, Mantovani JF, Volpe JJ: Porencephaly from periventricular intracerebral hemorrhage in a premature infant. Am J Dis Child 134:673–675, 1980.
17. Takada K, Shiota M, Ando M, Kimura M, Inoue K: Porencephaly and hydranencephaly— a neuropathological study of four autopsy cases. Brain Dev 11:51–56, 1989.
18. Stevenson RE, Kelly AC, Aylsworth AS, Phelan MC: Vascular basis for neural tube defects: a hypothesis. Pediatrics 80:102–106, 1987.
19. Vogal FS: The anatomic character of the vascular anomalies associated with anencephaly: with consideration of the role of abnormal angiogenesis in the pathogenesis of the cerebral malformation. Am J Pathol 39:163–169, 1961.

CHAPTER 5

Arteriovenous Malformations—Indications and Strategies for Surgery

Norihiko Tamaki and Kazumasa Ehara

Introduction

A vascular malformation is defined as a localized collection of metamorphic vessels, abnormal in number, in structure, and in function. This primary disease is sometimes referred to as *angioma*. However, this disorder is considered not to be a neoplasm, but rather a maldevelopment or a mal-production of cerebral vessels in early fetal life. However, the true pathogenesis is still unknown.

These may be classified into four types according to the histological finding of the composition of the vascular wall and intervening cerebral tissue: (1) arteriovenous malformation (AVM), (2) venous malformation, (3) cavernous angioma, and (4) capillary angioma.[1] Transitional forms exhibiting the histologic characteristics of more than one of the above-mentioned types are sometimes encountered within a malformation. Arteriovenous malformation has been defined as consisting of arteries, malformed veins with thin or thick walls, and veins. Usually, this type of malformation is surrounded by gliotic tissue. Features contributing to clinical and neuroradiological differential diagnosis of different types of vascular malformations are shown in Table 5.1.[2]

Incidence of Cerebral Arteriovenous Malformations

Arteriovenous malformations of the brain are uncommon. In the McCormick series,[1] 30 patients (0.52%) were found in 5850 consecutive autopsy cases; there were also 179 cases of venous malformations, 52 capillary angiomas, and 19 cavernous angiomas (Table 5.2). The majority of these cases were believed to be asymptomatic during life. However, in the clinical literature, approximately 8% of subarachnoid hemorrhages have been estimated to be due to an AVM, one-tenth the incidence of cerebral aneurysm.

In children, AVMs are the one of the most frequent causes of intracranial hemorrhage after the age of infancy (Table 5.3). According to a Japanese nationwide investigation, there were 168 patients with AVMs among 1251 patients (all children) with cerebrovascular disease.[3] There were 125 cases with subarachnoid hemorrhage (SAH) due to rupture of AVMs; their incidence was 4 times higher than SAH due to aneurysms (27 cases) in patients under 15 years old.

Clinical Manifestation

Arteriovenous malformations in children under 7 years old were found to be relatively rare, according to the nationwide investigation from 1986 to 1988 (Fig. 5.1). This figure also suggests that two-thirds of AVMs were found after an attack of intracranial bleeding, irrespective of age. Headache and seizures are the next most frequent symptoms (Table 5.4). Large AVMs (> 5 cm) make up about 10% of cases under 15 years old (Table 5.5), and posterior fossa AVMs represent approximately 16% of the cases of this age group (Table 5.6).

Table 5.1. Clinical features of different types of cerebrovascular malformations.

Feature	Arteriovenous malformation	Venous malformation	Cavernous angioma	Capillary angioma
Age	20–40 years (children seldom)	Middle age (children rarely)	Middle age	Middle or old age
Sex	Male > female (1,4:1)	?	?	?
Heredity	Seldom	?	Seldom	Rendu–Osler disease
Size	Occult to giant	Small to large strip	Ovoid, 2–5 cm	Very tiny (<1 cm)
Location	Every site	Cerebral, cerebellar	Everywhere, intrinsic or extrinsic	Pons
Shape	Spider, wedge shaped	Umbrella shaped	Honeycomed	Petechial
Multiple	Seldom	Solitary	Seldom	?
Aneurysm	10%	?	?	Rare
Clinical symptom	Silent to stormy	Usually silent	Silent to acute	Usually silent

From ref. 2.

Table 5.2. Histological type of 274 vascular malformations (in 5850) autopsy cases).

Histological type	Number of cases
Venous angioma (+varix)	175 (+4)
Capillary angioma	52
AVM[a]	30
Cavernous angioma	19
Total:	274

From ref. 1.
[a] AVM, Arteriovenous malformation.

Table 5.3. Etiology of cerebrovascular disease in children.

Etiology	Number of incidents of intracranial hemorrhage	Number of incidents of cerebrovascular disease
Neonatal intracranial hemorrhage	432	432
Cerebral occlusive disease	10	395
Intracranial vascular malformations	125	189
AVM	125	168
Malformation of vein of Galen	0	9
Cavernous angioma	0	8
Dural AVM	0	4
Idiopathic intracranial hemorrhage	101	101
Vitamin K deficiency	43	43
Aneurysm	27	37
Hemorrhagic disease	18	18
Tumor hemorrhage	13	13
Spinal AVM	0	9
Others	2	4
Total:	986	1251

From ref. 3.

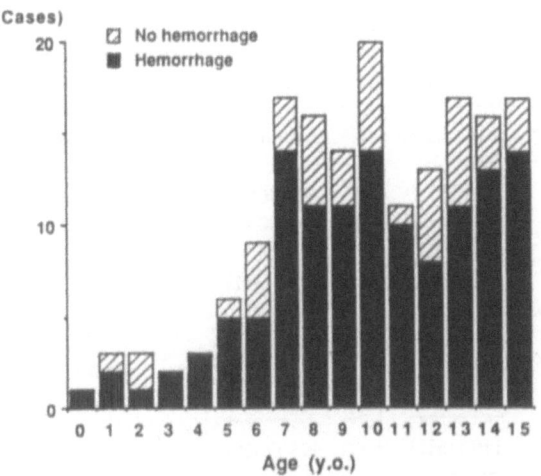

Figure 5.1. Age distribution of cerebral arteriovenous malformations from a Japanese nationwide investigation of cerebrovascular disease in children. (From ref. 3.)

Table 5.4. Clinical symptoms and signs in arteriovenous malformations in children.

Symptoms and signs	Number of cases
SAH symptoms[a]	125
Headache	38
Seizure	18
Loss of consciousness	6
Hemiparesis	2
Cranial nerve palsy	2

From ref. 3.
[a] SAH, subarachnoid hemorrhage.

Table 5.5. Size of arteriovenous malformations in children.

Size	Number of SAH cases	Total number of AVM
Small (<2.5 cm)	60 (77%)	78
Medium (<5 cm)	55 (71%)	78
Large (>5 cm)	10 (56%)	18

From ref. 3.

Table 5.6. Location of arteriovenous malformations in children.

Location	Number of SAH cases	Total number of AVM
Frontal	14 (47%)[a]	30
Temporal	25 (83%)	30
Parietal	22 (71%)	31
Occipital	18 (58%)	31
Paraventricular	21 (78%)	27
Thalamus	18 (90%)	20
Cerebellum	19 (90%)	21
Brainstem	4 (67%)	6

From ref. 3.
[a] Statistically significant ($p < 0.01$).

approximately 10 to 15%. According to our follow-up data of 151 cases, the 15-year survival rate for conservative treatment (27 cases) was 84% (Fig. 5.2). In contrast, the 15-year survival rate for patients with AVMs totally removed was 97%, and that with subtotal removal was

Natural Course of Untreated Arteriovenous Malformations

There are several reports bearing on the natural history of cerebral AVMs that suggest a yearly rate of hemorrhage ranging from 1 to 2.7% in patients with unruptured AVMs and 2 to 4% in those with ruptured AVMs.[4,5] If one-third of the patients were to die after the next hemorrhage, the mortality rate at 15 years would be

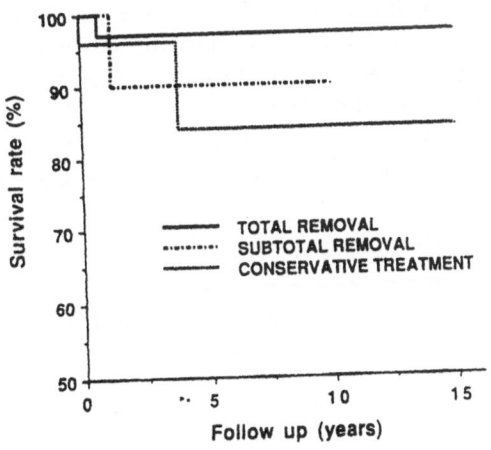

Figure 5.2. Relationship between treatment and survival rate at 15-year follow-up. (From ref. 6)

Table 5.7. Treatment and outcome at discharge and last follow-up.

| Treatment group | Number of cases | Satisfactory outcome[a] | | Number of deaths At follow-up |
		At discharge	At follow-up	
1. Total excision	81	67 (83%)	70 (86%)	1
2. Subtotal excision	15	10 (67%)	9 (60%)	1
3. Partial excision	5	3 (60%)	3 (60%)	1
4. Other procedures: Hematoma removal, craniotomy, ventricular shunt, embolization, feeder clipping, and radiation	21	10 (48%)	9 (43%)	3
5. Conservative treatment	29	24 (83%)	23 (79%)	2
Total:	151	119 (75%)	119 (75%)	8

From ref. 6.
[a] Excellent and good; satisfactory outcome.

90%.[6] The younger the patient, the more favorable the outcome, which may be expected to be a very long life if the AVM is surgically excised.

Indications for Surgery

Surgical treatment of an AVM is generally indicated if the risk of operation is less than the risk determined by conservative treatment. In terms of both the long-term survival rate and the rate of satisfactory outcome at final follow-up, total excision in general showed more favorable results than subtotal excision or conservative treatment (Table 5.7). However, the indication for total excision of AVMs should also be considered and decided upon the basis of surgical risks presented by individual AVMs. The surgical outcome was clearly related to the age of the patients in our series, as in those reported by others. In AVM patients under 19 years old, satisfactory outcome was expected in approximately 92% of the patients treated surgically either with total or subtotal excision, a rate which is definitely better than the surgical results of patients over 50 years old ($p < 0.05$) (Table 5.8). The preoperative clinical condition was also related to the surgical outcome. Morbidity was higher in patients with a disturbance of consciousness (Glasgow coma scale < 12 or Hunt's grade 3 to 5) before surgery.[6]

The size of the AVM has been considered to be one of the most important prognostic factors. Many authors categorized the AVMs by size into two to four groups. In our experience in 96 cases with total or subtotal excision, there was a good postoperative outcome if the size of the AVM was less than 4 cm. Patients with AVMs larger than 4 cm clearly showed a lower rate of satisfactory outcome. In addition, there was no postoperative symptomatic hemorrhage in cases of AVMs smaller than 4 cm in diameter.

Table 5.8. Age and surgical outcome.

Age (years)	Excellent	Good	Fair	Poor	Total	Satisfactory outcome
0–19	10	13	2	0	25	23 (92%)[a]
20–49	13	31	11	0	55	44 (80%)
50–	5	5	4	2	16	10 (63%)[a]

From ref. 6.
[a] Statistically significant ($P < 0.05$) at ages 0–19 years and over 50 years, by chi-square analysis.

Table 5.9. Lussenhop's angiographical grading.

Grading feature	Grade
One named artery	1
Two named arteries	2
Three named arteries	3
Four named arteries	4

From ref. 7.

Table 5.10. Spetzler's angiographical grading system.

Grading feature	Points assigned[a]
Size of AVM	1
Small (<3 cm)	2
Medium (3–6 cm)	3
Large (>6 cm)	
Eloquence of adjacent brain	
Non-eloquent	0
Eloquent	1
Pattern of venous drainage	
Superficial only	0
Deep	1

From ref. 8.

[a] Grade = (size) + (eloquence) + (veinous drainage); that is, (1, 2, 3) + (0 or 1) + (0 or 1).

Table 5.11. Our angiographical grading system.

Angiographical factors	Points[a]
Size of AVM	
Small (<4 cm)	0
Large (≥4 cm)	2
Location	
Superficial	0
Deep	1
Feeding artery	
One or two artery systems	0
Three or more artery systems	1

From ref. 6.

[a] Angiographical grade is calculated by summing these points.

widely used in practice (Table 5.10).[8] However, to our knowledge, until now there has been no correlation between grading system and outcome in children.

According to multiple regression analysis, using our angiographical data and surgical outcome of 96 surgical cases of AVMs, the expected Karnofsky scale may be given as follows when size, location, and the pattern of feeders are scored from 0 to 1, respectively:[6]

$$\text{Karnofsky scale} = 87.1 - 11.5(\text{size})$$
$$- 5.4(\text{location}) - 5.1(\text{feeder})$$

This formula means that size is the most important factor relating directly to surgical outcome ($p < 0.001$). Location ($p = 0.176$) and feeder ($p = 0.216$) also related well to the surgical outcome. On the basis of this formula, the angiographic grading system was simplified, as is shown in Table 5.11. Size was categorized into two groups, which were assigned 0 or 2 points. Location and feeders were categorized into two groups and were assigned 0 or 1 point. The grade of an AVM was determined by summing the points assigned for each category and then classifying from grade 0 to 4. In addition, the predicted Karnofsky scale was calculated using this grading system and the linear regression as follows:

$$\text{Predicted Karnofsky scale} = 87.2 - 5.6(\text{grade})$$

However, symptomatic hemorrhage occurred in 4 (18%) of 22 patients with AVMs larger than 4 cm. Thus, it appears reasonable to categorize the AVMs by size into two groups: small (< 4 cm), and large (< 4 cm).

It has been suggested that other factors, such as location of the AVM, pattern of the feeders, and the characteristics of venous drainage, are also important predictors of operative morbidity. Some grading systems have been proposed on the basis of these factors. Lussenhop proposed a grading system for determining the operability of AVMs mainly on the basis of the pattern and number of named feeding arteries (Table 5.9).[7] This grading system clearly related to the size of AVMs. The grading scale of Spetzler and Martin appeared to provide a better prediction of surgical outcome, and is

The 96 surgically treated AVMs were graded in order to evaluate the validity of this system in terms of the degree of surgical difficulty and the postoperative outcome. Correlation of this grading system to degree of surgical difficulty, represented by the rate of total excision, was also good ($p < 0.005$). The rate of total excisability decreases significantly as the grade of the lesion rises ($p < 0.05$). The percentage of satisfactory outcome after surgery also decreased significantly as the grade of the lesion increased ($p < 0.001$). There was also significant correlation between mean Karnofsky scale and this AVM grading.

This angiographical grading system, combined with the patient's age and the preoperative clinical condition, also facilitates the achievement of special strategies to prevent postoperative complications in treating high-grade or "difficult" AVMs.

Hemodynamic Aspects

Among various postoperative complications, the normal perfusion pressure breakthrough (NPPB) phenomenon appears to be closely associated with the postoperative outcome.[9] The overall incidence of the breakthrough phenomenon leading to postoperative morbidity appears variable, ranging from 1.4 to 18%, while its incidence in large AVMs > 4 or 5 cm is reported to be significantly higher, ranging from 19 to 37%.

It has been suggested that factors contributing to the development of NPPB include the following[9,10-12]:

1. Large arteriovenous shunt
2. Angiographical evidence of steal
3. Recruitment of the perforating vessels
4. Low cortical blood flow around AVMs
5. Impaired autoregulation of the vessels
6. Low cortical artery pressure before excision
7. Increased pressure of the cortical arteries after excision
8. A sudden and excessive increase in cortical blood flow after excision

There are many methods to measure the cerebral blood flow. However, if there exists a high-flow, large arteriovenous (AV) shunt, some

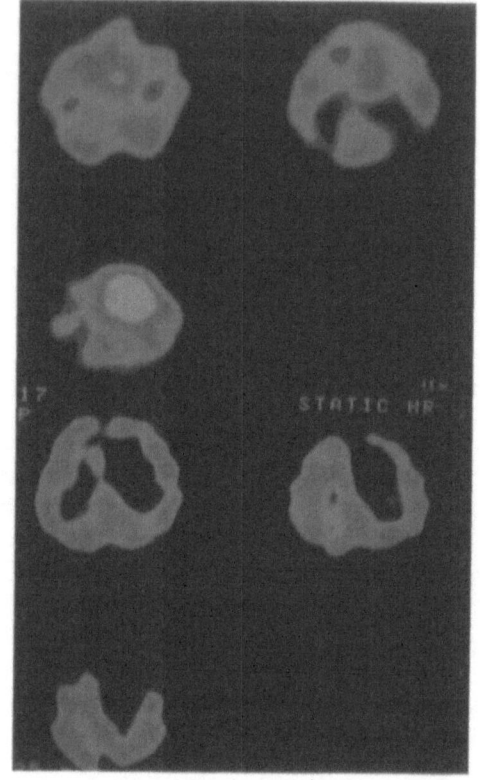

Figure 5.3. Upper three images are ^{133}Xe SPECT (single-photon emission tomography) blood-flow images in patient with an AVM in the left frontal lobe. Lower three images are [123]iodoamphetamine blood flow images of the same patient.

methods may be very sensitive to the shunt flow and others may not interfere with the AV shunt. The upper three images of Figure 5.3 are[133]Xe SPECT (single-photon emission tomography) images of a large, right frontal AVM in a child with a very high-flow region in the nidus. In contrast, the lower three images, [123]io-doamphetamine SPECT images of the same patient, show a completely cold lesion in the same area. Different findings depend on the sensitivity of the AV shunt. A better understanding of cerebral hemodynamics of intracranial shunt flow and in the surrounding brain has become possible by:

1. Estimation of intracranial shunt flow or resistance of shunt

a. Intraoperative measurement of mean arterial blood pressure and flow or velocity of feeding arteries
b. Measurement of velocity of flow in and diameter of the carotid artery using Doppler flowmetry
c. Measurement of flow in the middle cerebral artery using transcranial Doppler flowmetry
d. Measurement of the mean transit time using digital subtraction angiography or the dynamic computerized tomography (CT) scan
2. Estimation of perfusion pressure, autoregulation, and steal phenomenon in the surrounding cerebral tissue
a. Direct cortical blood-flow measurement, using either thermogradient or the laser–Doppler flowmeters
b. Measurement of autoregulation with increased blood pressure or CO_2 response using SPECT or positron-emission tomography (PET)

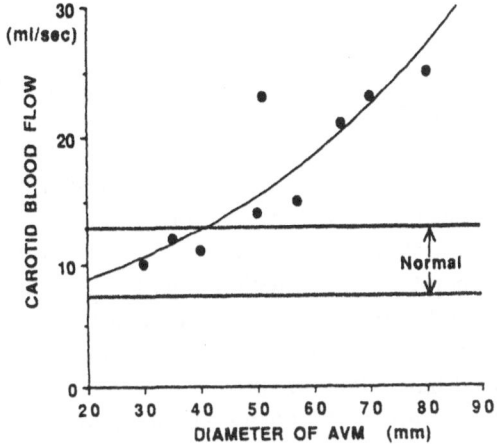

Figure 5.4. Relationship between the diameter of the AVMs and flow values with the carotid Doppler flowmeter.

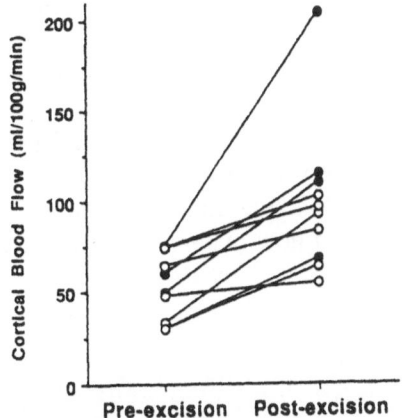

Figure 5.5. Intraoperative cortical blood-flow study with the thermogradient flowmeter. Closed circles are preexcision and postexcision flow values in the cases of the large AVMs (> 4 cm). Open circles are those of the small AVMs (> 4 cm).

For assessment of intracranial shunt flow, carotid Doppler flowmetry was done in nine cases of supratentorial AVMs of various size, using Doppler flowmetry (QFM 2000 XA; Hayashi Electric Co., Kawasaki City, Japan), as shown in Figure 5.4. Carotid blood flow in the AVM increased exponentially, approaching two times the normal common carotid flow when the longest diameter of the AVM exceeded 5 cm.

To predict the risk of the NPPB, intraoperative cortical blood flow surrounding the nidus of AVMs was measured in 10 cases of supratentorial AVMs using the thermogradient flowmeter (Nihon Electric Co., Tokyo, Japan) (Fig. 5.5). In the large AVMs, over 4 cm in size, postexcision cortical blood flow increased more than twice as much as that of the preexcision values. There were two cases of postoperative hemorrhage out of four large AVMs, probably due to NPPB. In contrast, the patients with small AVMs showed slightly increased cortical blood flow after excision, and had no postoperative hemorrhagic complications.

If the AVM is large and has a high flow as estimated by angiography and by the measurement described above, special strategies must be used to reduce the risk of NPPB syndrome.

Surgical Procedure

General Consideration

Arteriovenous malformations are among the most difficult neurosurgical procedures. The technical difficulties are usually compounded by the size and the location of the malformation.

The larger the AVM, the more difficult the excision. Even when it is small, great care is needed when it is deeply seated, especially if it is close to a critical area.

Intraarterial pressure and arterial blood gases should be monitored, induced hypotension should be used to reduce bleeding, and for large, high-flow shunt AVMs, various cortical blood-flow monitors are sometimes used. This latter study endeavors to help avoid ischemic complications or to detect postexcision increase in cortical blood flow of surrounding tissue so as to avoid an NPPB phenomenon. In order to reduce venous pressure, the head should be elevated above the level of the patient's heart.[13]

One of the most important decisions in AVM surgery is where and how to identify and occlude the main feeding arteries. If clipping of long large feeders is close to the nidus, large amounts of blood flow into the small, thin-walled arterioles adjacent to the AVM may cause postoperative hemorrhage. There are three types of feeding arteries: circumferential, terminal, and penetrating.[14] It is very important to understand the three-dimensional anatomical structure of brain and vessels and flow dynamics preoperatively.

The approach to the nidus is also an important point, especially in excising deep AVMs adjacent to an eloquent or vital area. Sometimes difficulties are encountered in finding the nidus of the AVM and the feeding arteries (which sometimes run through the cerebral tissue). In such cases, dissection is started from the subarachnoid spaces or cortical sulci, close to the drainer, so as to find the nidus.

After identification and temporary occlusion of the main feeding arteries, dissection of the nidus of the AVM is done between it and the surrounding gliotic tissue, coagulating small shunting arterioles and venules running into the AVM. When the color of the drainer changes from red to blue, after occlusion of major feeders, it is possible to occlude and cut some of the drainers. After dissection is completed, the largest drainer may be cut. Large AVMs may sometimes be separated into several compartments, and to avoid the risk of incomplete resection intraoperative digital subtraction angiography is quite useful (Fig. 5.6). Large-dose barbiturate therapy is sometimes effective to reduce brain swelling during excision[15].

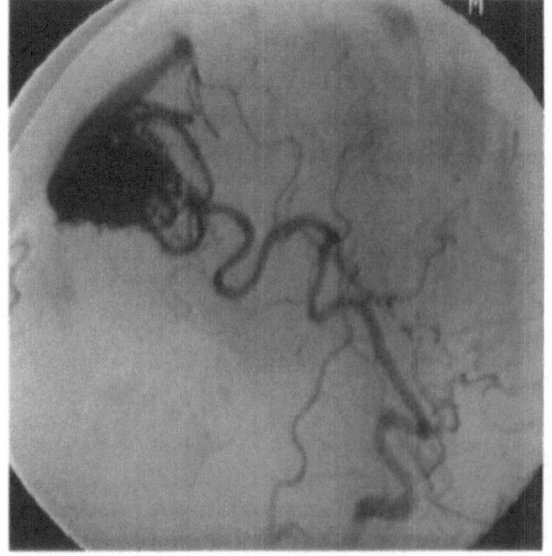

Figure 5.6. Intraoperative digital angiography clearly displays the feeding arteries and the nidus of the AVM.

Strategies for Excision of Large, High-Flow Arteriovenous Malformations

Prevention of NPPB is important for successful surgery on high-flow AVMs, so the following strategy has been tried in an effort to prevent the NPPB phenomenon:

1. Multiple-staged operation
2. Preoperative embolization of feeding arteries
3. Intra- or postoperative induced hypotension and barbiturate therapy
4. Intraoperative embolization combined with feeding artery ligation followed by surgical excision
5. Ligation of several feeding arteries followed by excision at a later date
6. Flow-regulated one-stage surgery with partial occlusion of internal carotid or middle cerebral artery, using intraoperative cortical blood-flow monitoring

Gradual stepwise reperfusion of the surrounding ischemic hemisphere after a staged reduction of shunt flow seems a reasonable approach to reestablish autoregulation. However, the hemodynamic change induced by preoperative embolization may cause a disastrous or fatal outcome. Some surgeons question the benefits of staged surgical excision of AVMs, a process which may induce acute intraoperative hypoperfusion superimposed on chronic preoperative hypoperfusion. The authors advocate a one-stage operation for large, high-flow AVMs, utilizing the modulation of blood flow.[16]

Flow-Regulated One-Stage Excision of Supratentorial Giant High-Flow Arteriovenous Malformations by Carotid Clamp

Case Example

The patient was admitted to our hospital because of transient gait disturbances, bruit in the right ear, and dizziness. There were no neurological deficits. Computerized tomography scan revealed a large enhanced mass in the right temporal and parasylvian area, and angio-

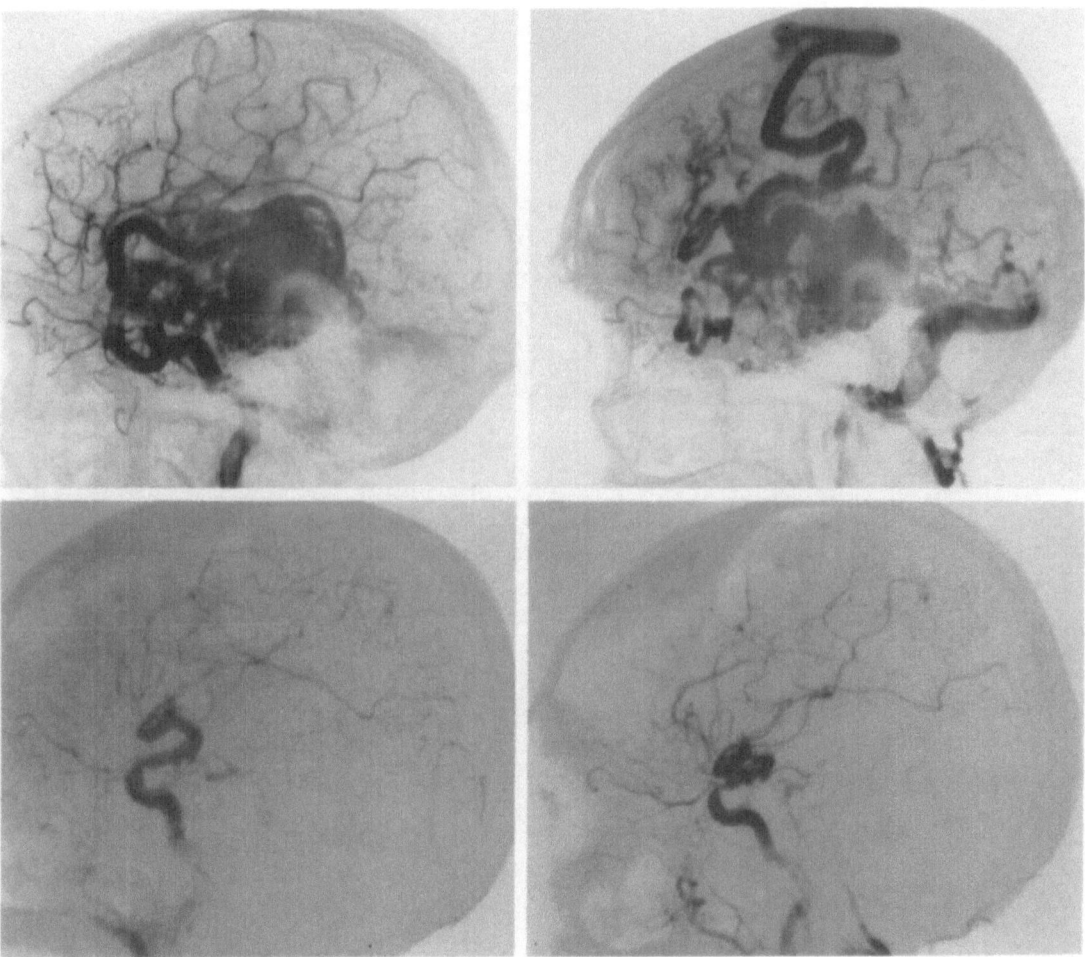

Figure 5.7. Right carotid angiograms of case 1 of the early (upper left) and late (upper right) arterial phase. Postoperative carotid angiography on the eighth postoperative day (lower left). Postoperative retrograde brachial angiography on day 35 after the operation (lower right). (From ref. 16)

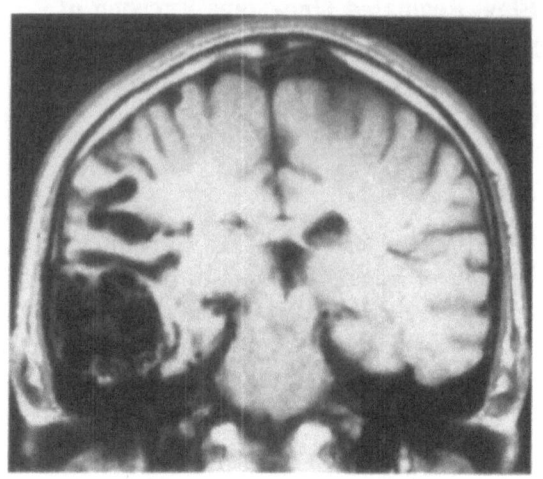

Figure 5.8. Magnetic resonance imaging of 1-weighted images of case 1.

graphy showed a large AVM fed through the middle cerebral, anterior choroidal, and posterior cerebral arteries (Fig. 5.7, upper right and upper left). The size of the nidus was 8 × 7 × 5 cm and drained into the superior sagittal sinus, internal cerebral vein, basal vein, vein of Labbé, and superficial sylvian vein. Magnetic resonance imaging (MRI) clearly demonstrated the anatomical relationship of the nidus, drainer of the AVMs, and surrounding cerebral structures (Fig. 5.8).

After exposure of the right common and internal carotid arteries, a Selverstone clamp was placed on the common carotid artery. A large h-shaped skin incision was made in the right frontoparietotemporal area, and the bone flap was made in the frontoparietotemporal

AVM   Dura   Vein

II

ica

M2-mca

Rt. temporal lobe

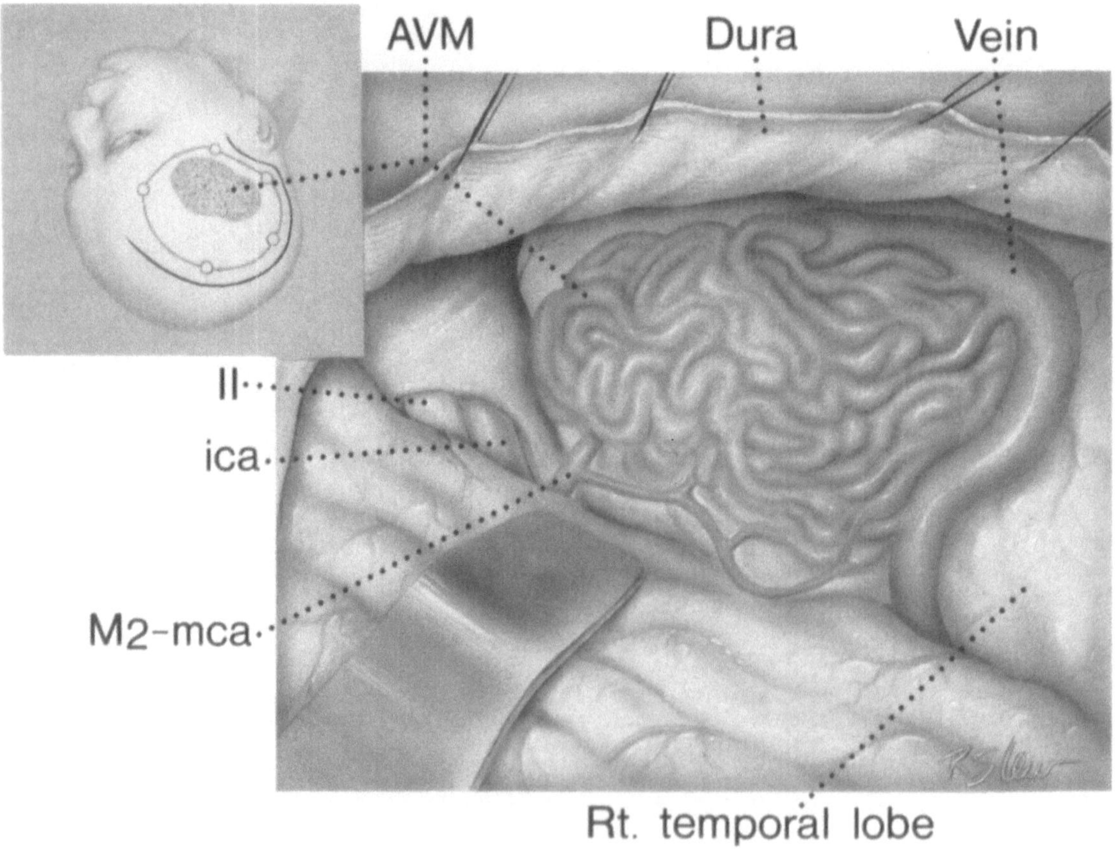

Figure 5.9. Dissection of right internal and middle cerebral arteries. The nidus was shown on the surface of the temporal lobes in case 1.

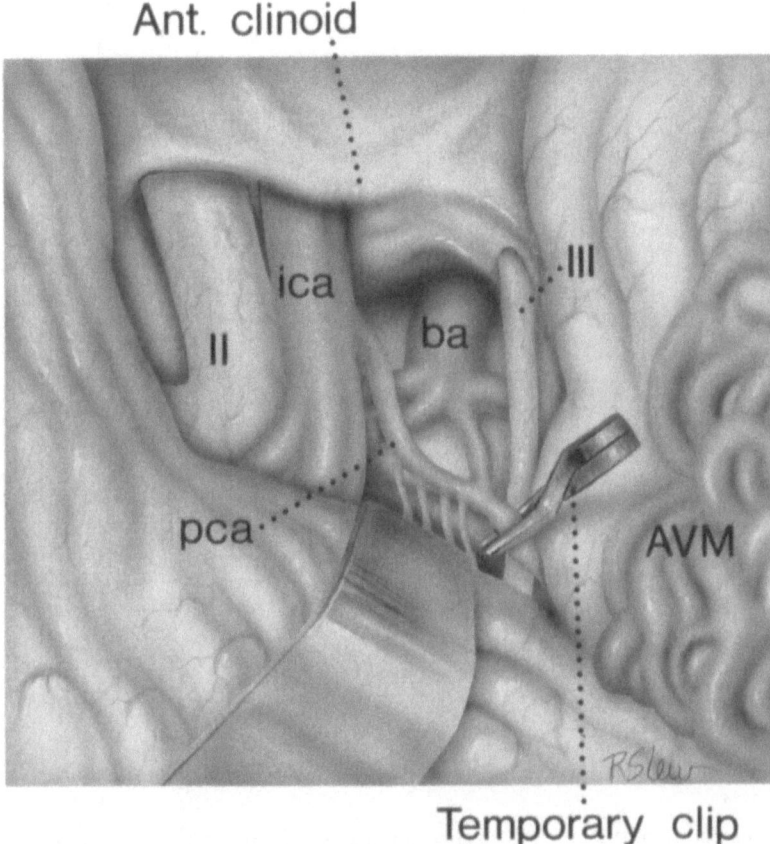

Figure 5.10. Identification and temporal clipping of P2 portion of the posterior cerebral artery.

area. The dura was opened after administration of 300 ml of mannitol solution, exposing the huge arteriovenous malformation and many enlarged, red-draining veins on the lateral surface of the right temporal lobe and the parasylvian surface of the frontoparietal lobe. The right frontal lobe was gently elevated, and the carotid cistern was exposed. Right carotid and middle cerebral arteries were identified (Fig. 5.9). A small aneurysm was found at the M1–M2 junction. Opening the sylvian fissure, two main feeding arteries were identified, dissected, and clipped. The posterior cerebral artery was exposed by retracting the internal carotid artery medially through a pterional transsylvian approach (Fig. 5.10). Temporary clipping of P2 was done with a Sugita temporary clip. Then the two main feeding arteries of the middle cerebral artery were coagulated around the nidus of the AVM. The anterior border of the nidus of the

AVM was dissected from the frontal lobe. Then, the nidus was dissected from surrounding yellowish gliotic brain tissue (Fig. 5.11). After clipping and cutting the largest drainer, the AVM was completely removed. An intraoperative cortical thermogradient blood flowmeter showed marked elevation of blood flow from 49 to 110 ml/100 g/min after excision. A Selverstone clamp was applied to the common carotid artery, so as to reduce the cortical blood flow to 69 ml/100 g/min. After complete hemostasis and removal of all temporary clips, the skin was closed.

The patient recovered completely, with only a minimal visual field defect. Right carotid angiography on the eighth postoperative day showed delayed circulation and so-called stagnated arteries, which suggested dysautoregulation (Fig. 5.7, lower left). The carotid clamps were removed on postoperative day 33. Angio-

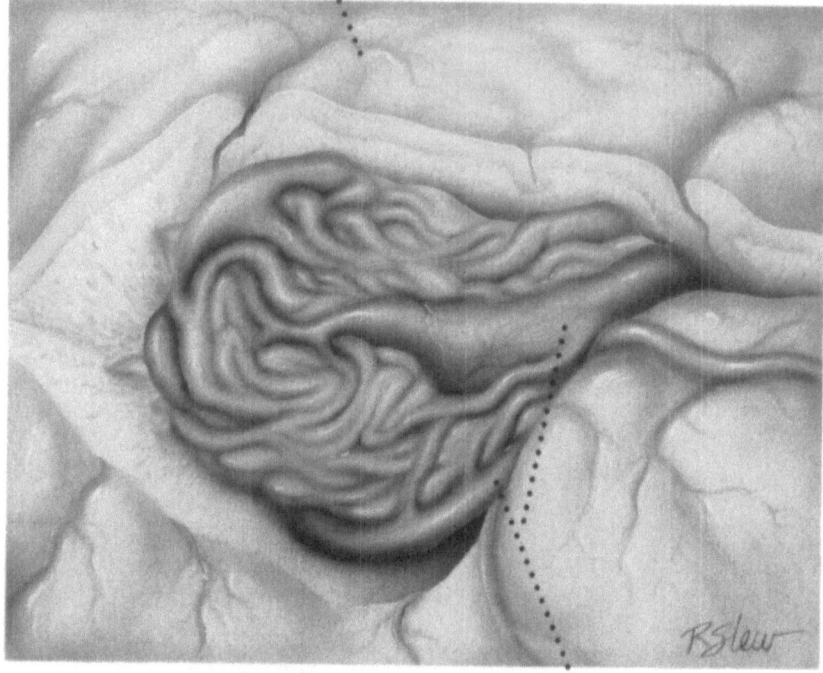

Figure 5.11. Dissection of the nidus from surrounding gliotic tissue. Largest drainer remains intact.

graphy on postoperative day 35 demonstrated a normal cerebral circulation pattern and complete removal of the AVM (Fig. 5.7, lower right). The patient was discharged without neurological deficit, except for a left homonymous quadrantanopia.

Flow-Regulated One-Stage Excision of Supratentorial Giant High-Flow Arteriovenous Malformations by Elective Temporary Stenosis of Middle Cerebral Artery

Case Example

This patient had a history of focal seizures. Computerized tomography abnormalities were discovered following the last seizure, which occurred 3 months before admission. There were no neurological deficits. Angiograms revealed an AVM, in the right parietal region, which was 3.5 × 2.5 × 2.5 cm in volume and was fed by the

right angular, posterior parietal, and parietooccipital arteries (Fig. 5.12, upper right and left). Venous drainage was through the superficial veins and into the superior sagittal sinus.

After the right temporoparietal craniotomy, the proximal portion of the middle cerebral artery was exposed. The brain surface around the AVM was also exposed. Before excision of the AVM, cortical blood flow was measured in several portions of the cortex about 2 cm away from the AVM, using a thermal blood-flow monitor (Biomedical Science, Inc., Tokyo, Japan). After the AVM was totally excised, blood flow was measured in the same areas. The maximal value of preexcision flow was 33 ml and postexcision flow was 93 ml/100 g/min. Since the postexcision flow increased to greater than twice the preexcision flow, an encircling clamp made from a silicone rubber tube with absorbable threads was placed around the M2 portion of the right middle cerebral artery (Fig. 5.12, lower left). The middle cerebral artery (MCA) was constricted by tying the threads attached to this

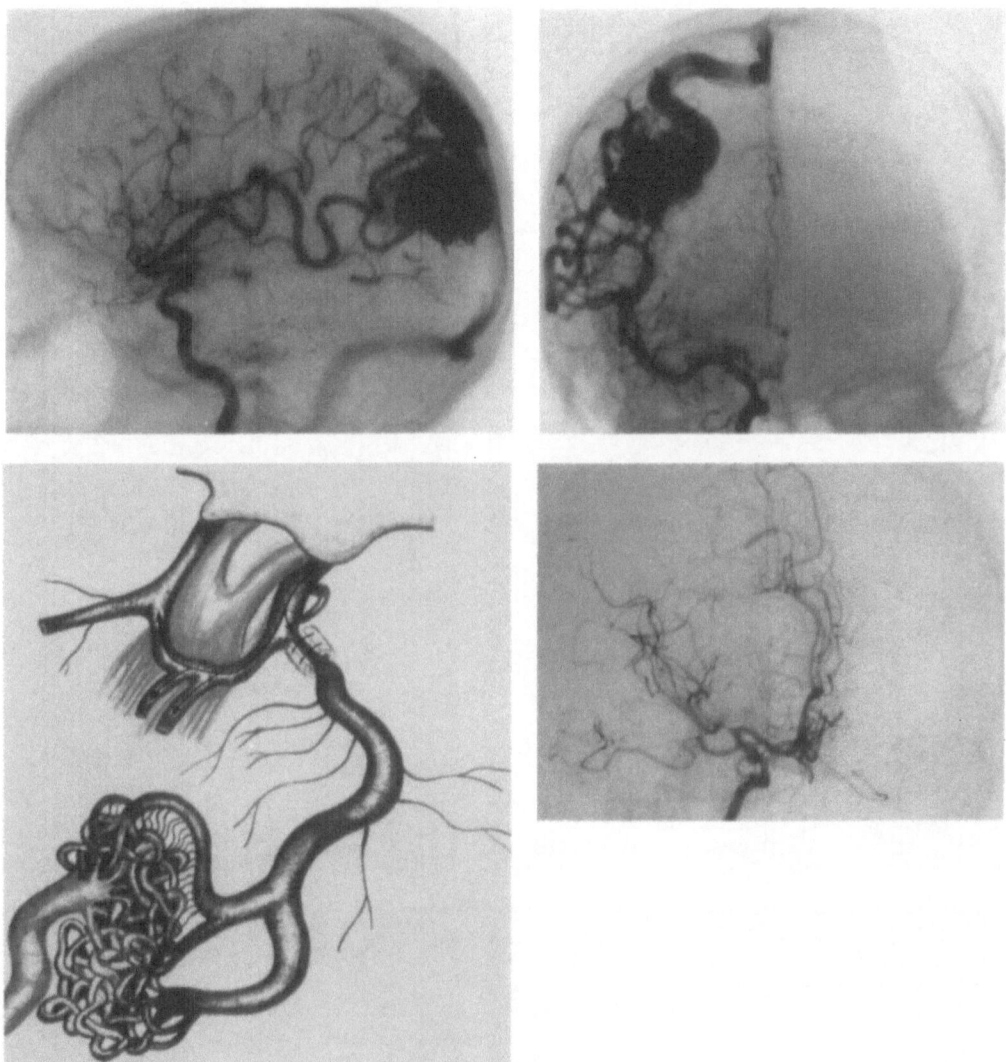

Figure 5.12. Right carotid angiograms of case 2 (upper right and left). After resection of AVMs, a specially designed silicone clamp was applied for reducing the flow of the middle cerebral artery (lower left).

Postoperative right carotid angiogram showed complete removal of the AVM and the partially occluded middle cerebral artery (lower right).

clamp until the cortical flow dropped to 150% of the preexcision level.

The patient's postoperative course was uneventful. The postoperative angiogram, done 20 days after the operation, demonstrated that the AVM was totally excised and the proximal segment of the M2 portion remained constricted (Fig. 5.12, lower right).

Multistaged Excision of a Corpus Callosum Arteriovenous Malformation

Case Example

The girl had a sudden attack of loss of consciousness and was subsequently admitted to the hospital. A computerized tomography scan

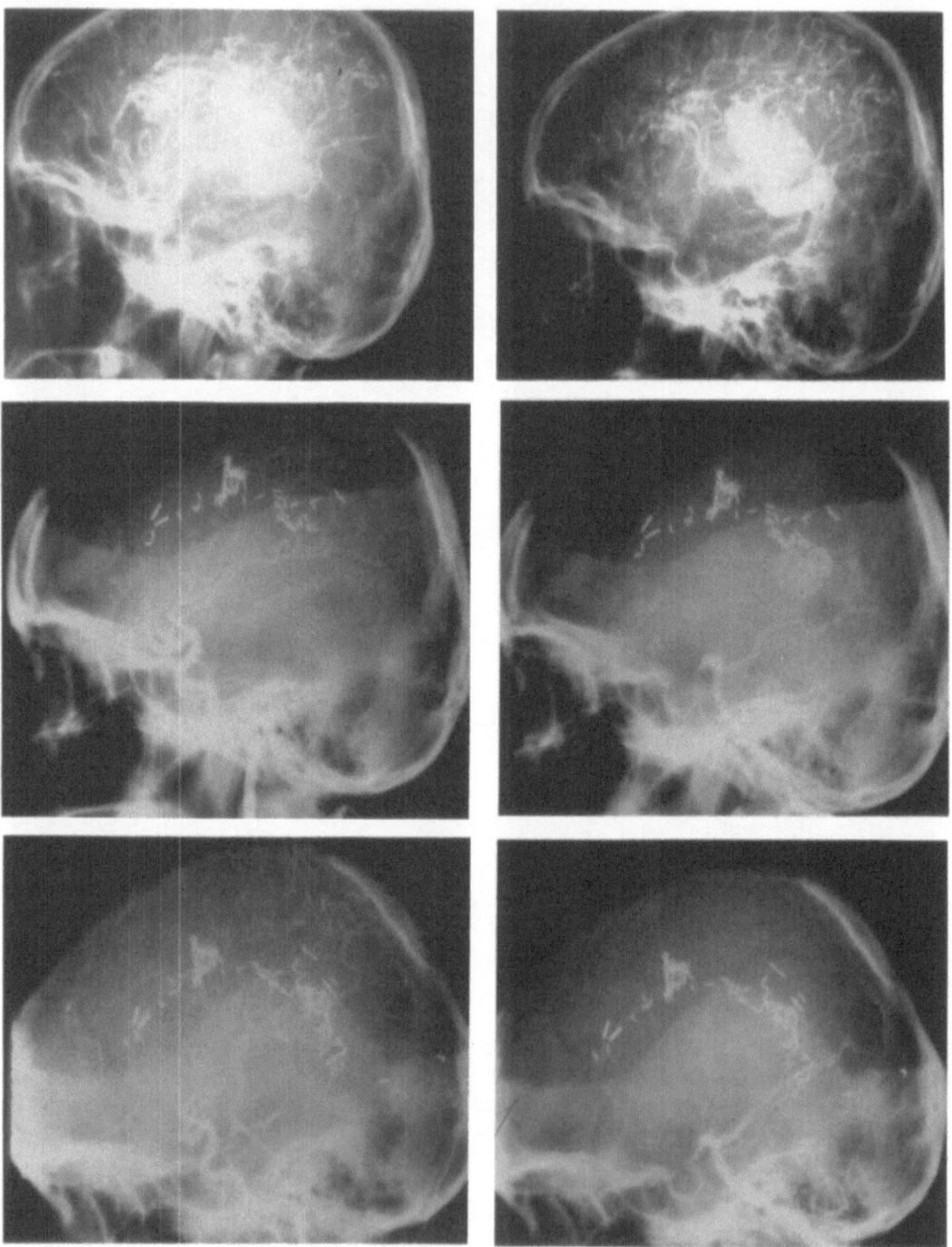

Figure 5.13. Preoperative left carotid angiogram (upper left) and left vertebral angiogram (upper right) of case 3. Postoperative left carotid and left vertebral angiogram after second operation (middle left and right). Postoperative angiograms after the third operation (lower left and right).

revealed intracerebral and intraventricular hemorrhages and emergency hemotoma removal and ventricular drainage were done on the same day. Angiography showed a large AVM occupying the entire corpus callosum, posterior part of the body of the left lateral ventricle, and superior part of the left thalamus (Fig. 5.13, upper right and left). Consciousness was recovered, but mild right hemiparesis, right homonymous hemianopia, and alexia persisted.

Second Operation

The left carotid artery was cannulated for intraoperative angiography, and then a horseshoe-shaped skin incision was made in the left frontoparietal area crossing the midline. After incision of the dura, the right pericallosal artery was identified through the interhemispheric fissure. Several feeders from this artery to the nidus of the corpus callosum were coagulated, clipped, and cut. After incision of the lower end of the falx, the right pericallosal artery was isolated. Then many small, tortuous feeding arteries from both pericallosal arteries were clipped and cut along the corpus callosum. Dissection of the AVM was begun from the anterior part of the nidus and the splenium of the corpus callosum, which was then completely split, and the AVM was followed into the body and trigone of the left lateral ventricle. After cutting feeding arteries from the posterior choroidal and the posterior cerebral arteries, the nidus seemed to have been completely removed. Intraoperative carotid angiography revealed disappearance of the AVM.

She recovered without additional neurological deficits. However, postoperative vertebral angiography showed residual AVM on the posterior inferior part of the corpus callosum, the quadrigeminal cistern, and the superior surface of the thalamus (Fig. 5.13, middle right and left). A third operation was scheduled 2 months later.

Third Operation

A skin incision was made in the parietooccipital area and the left occipital lobe was retracted laterally. The residual AVM was found at the posterior inferior part of the corpus callosum

and in the cistern of the vein of Galen. The nidus of this part of the AVM was then removed. Drainers into the vein of Galen were cut and both basal veins were identified. Both internal cerebral veins were followed forward, and at this time another residual AVM was found in the roof of the third ventricle along the tela choroidea and the AVM was at this time completely removed (Fig. 5.13, lower right and left). Postoperative angiography showed complete removal of the AVM. She recovered well, without additional neurological deficit, graduated from high school, and then went on to work in an office.

Excision of Posterior Fossa Arteriovenous Malformations

Case Example

This boy was admitted to an emergency hospital because of sudden onset of headache, nausea, and a loss of consciousness. A computerized tomography scan revealed a small intracerebellar hematoma. The patient recovered consciousness. One month later, neurological examination revealed only mild truncal ataxia. Angiography revealed an AVM in the inferior vermis, fed by the left posterior inferior and the right superior cerebellar arteries (Fig. 5.14, right and left). The size of the nidus was approximately 2 cm in diameter, and it drained into the superior vermian vein and the petrosal sinus.

After a suboccipital craniectomy, temporary clips were placed on the distal portion of the right superior cerebellar and left posterior inferior cerebellar arteries. Cerebellotomy was done at the lower vermis, and the hematoma was aspirated in the vermis. The nidus of the AVM

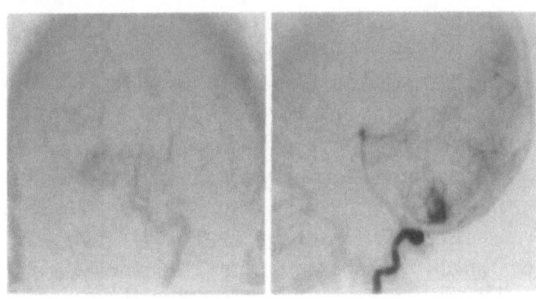

Figure 5.14. Left vertebral angiograms of case 4.

was dissected from the surrounding gliotic tissue and both feeding arteries were clipped. After cutting the drainers along the cerebellar surface, the AVM was completely removed. The patient recovered fully and returned to his home without any neurological deficit.

Nonsurgical Treatment

If AVMs are resected completely, the patients may be expected to be cured of this disease. However, if the risk of the operation is high, radiosurgery or interventional neuroradiology should be considered. Stereotactic radiosurgery or the proton beam have the limitation of lesion size.[17,18] For these reasons, small brainstem AVMs (less than 2 cm) respond well to this treatment. Interventional neuroradiology, utilizing a detachable balloon, glue, or pellet embolization, does not always succeed in occluding the AVM completely. This procedure is recommended for surgically inaccessible feeding arteries or inaccessible AVMs,[19] and also to reduce the surgical risk of a large, high-flow AVM.

References

1. McCormick WF: The pathology of angiomas. In: Fein JM, Flamm ES (eds.). Cerebrovascular Surgery, Vol. IV. Springer-Verlag, New York, 1985, pp. 1073–1095.
2. Yasargil MG: Classification of vascular malformation. In: Microneurosurgery, Vol. III-A. Georg Thieme Verlag, Stuttgart, 1987, pp. 57–62.
3. Fujita K, Ehara K, Kimura M, Matsumoto S, Arima M: Nationwide investigation of intracranial arteriovenous malformations in children. Nerv Syst Child [Shoni No Noshinkei (Japan)] 13:229–236, 1988.
4. Graf CJ, Perret GE, Torner JC: Bleeding from cerebral arteriovenous malformations as part of natural history. J Neurosurg 58:331–337, 1983.
5. Ondra SL, Troupp H, George ED, Schwab K: The natural history of symptomatic arteriovenous malformations of the brain: a 24-year follow-up assessment. J Neurosurg 73:387–391, 1990.
6. Tamaki N, Ehara K, Lin TK, Kuwamura K, Obora Y, Kanazawa Y, Yamashita H, Matsumo-

to S: Cerebral arteriovenous malformations: Factors influencing the surgical difficulty and outcome. Neurosurgery (in press).
7. Luessenhop AJ, Gennarelli TA: Anatomical grading of supratentorial arteriovenous malformations for determining operability. Neurosurgery 1:30–35, 1977.
8. Spetzler RF, Martin NA: A proposed grading system for arteriovenous malformations. J Neurosurg 65:476–483, 1986.
9. Spetzler RF, Wilson CB, Weinstein P, Mechdoron M, Townsend J, Telles D: Normal perfusion pressure breakthrough theory. Clin Neurosurg 25:651–672, 1978.
10. Barnett GH, Little JR, Ebrahim ZY, et al.: Cerebral circulation during arteriovenous malformation operation. Neurosurgery 20:836–842, 1987.
11. Nornes H, Grip A: Hemodynamic aspects of cerebral arteriovenous malformations. J Neurosurg 53:456–464, 1980.
12. Pertuiset B, Ancri D, Clergue F: Preoperative evaluation of hemodynamic factors in cerebral arteriovenous malformations for selection of radical surgery tactic with special reference to vascular autoregulation disorders. Neurol Res 4:209–233, 1982.
13. Sugita K, Kobayashi S: Arteriovenous malformation. In: Microneurosurgical Atlas. Springer-Verlag, Berlin, 1985, pp. 136–177.
14. Yamada S, Brauer FS, Knierim DS: Direct approach to arteriovenous malformations in functional areas of the cerebral hemisphere. J Neurosurg 72:418–425, 1990.
15. Marshall LF U HF: Treatment of massive intraoperative brain swelling. Neurosurgery 13:412–414, 1983.
16. Tamaki N, Lin T, Asada M, Fujita K, Tominaga S, Kimura M, Ehara K, Matsumoto S: Modulation of blood flow following excision of a high-flow cerebral arteriovenous malformation. J Neurosurg 72:509–512, 1990.
17. Steiner L: Radiosurgery in cerebral arteriovenous malformations. In: Cerebrovascular Surgery, Vol. IV: Springer-Verlag, New York, 1986, pp. 1161–1215.
18. Kemeny AA, Dias P, Forster DM: Results of stereotactic radiosurgery of arteriovenous malformations: an analysis of 52 cases. J Neurol Neurosurg Psychiatr 52:554–558, 1989.
19. Wilson CB, Hieshima GB: Preoperative balloon occlusion of arteriovenous malformations. Neurosurgery 22:301–308, 1988.

CHAPTER 6

Malformations and Aneurysmal Dilation of the Lesser and Greater Veins of Galen and the Medial Prosencephalic Vein

Anthony J. Raimondi and Claude Lapras

Introduction

During the past 10 years diagnostics have, once more, set the pace for and established the basis upon which treatment of what has heretofore been considered an ominous, if not incurable clinical entity, has been structured. The detailed angiographic (arteriographic) analyses of the vascular alterations (malformative, ectatic, fistulous) first reported by Raybaud and subsequently elaborated upon and put into clinical perspective by Lasjaunias, have brought us to a point where we may now understand and treat properly both the vascular alterations and their secondary complications.

As so very often occurs here, too, progress proceeding from diagnosis to treatment has been the direct result of ever-increasing specialization. Without the identification of neuroradiology as a distinct specialty, and the subsequent evolution of pediatric neuroradiology, the obliteration or exclusion of arteriovenous malformations and aneurysmal dilation of the Galenic system would have made no progress. Following Schechter's suggestion that the term "aneurysm of the vein of Galen" either be abolished or qualified,[1] since it is not an aneurysm, Raimondi classified his series of cases into *arteriovenous fistulae of the galenic (lesser and greater) system* and identified specifically the entity of *aneurysmal dilation of the vein of Galen* as a consequence of arteriovenous fistulization from anterior (pericallosal) and posterior (choroidal, retrosplenial, perforating, etc.)[1-3] circulation arteries. The aneurysmal dilation of the lesser,

greater, or both galenic systems was described by him to be the direct result of arteriovenous fistulization. In fact the primary fistulizing arterial system (pericallosal, retrosplenial, choroidal) served as the basis upon which the specific surgical approach (parietal, infratemporal, suboccipital) was based. Though this facilitated greatly identification of the tributary arteries to the aneurysmal dilation of the galenic system, it represented no qualitative basis upon which entirely new technical procedures could be structured. Indeed, it was not until the already mentioned works by the two French neuroradiologists, first Charles Raybaud and subsequently Pierre Lasjaunias, were reported that arteriovenous malformations and aneurysmal dilation involving the embryonic and fetal deep venous circulations could be effectively managed.

Presently, we have the theoretical and technical wherewithal to diagnose and treat, effectively in the majority of cases, arteriovenous malformations and aneurysmal dilation of the galenic system in children. We also have full clinical knowledge of the complicating problems: cardiac failure, hydrocephalus, mental retardation. It remains now for the clinicians diagnosing and managing these childhood anomalies to select which entities should be managed by endovascular interventional neuroradiology, which by classical neurosurgical techniques. It also remains for us to decide whether children with complicating hydrocephalus should be shunted and, if so, whether this should be performed before or after exclusion of the fistula and/or aneurysmal dilation.

Anatomical Basis for Classification, Diagnosis, and Treatment

The median prosencephalic vein (medial vein of the prosencephalon), a single midline structure, drains the choroid plexuses (of both the lateral and third ventricles) from the seventh through the twelfth weeks of intrauterine life. Subsequent to this, the medial vein of the prosencephalon disappears and the two internal cerebral veins may be identified. It is, in fact, the persistence of the medial vein of the prosencephalon, an embryonic structure, and the occasionally abnormal arterial pattern located over the cerebral hemispheres, which permit one to distinguish arteriovenous fistulae ("vein of Galen aneurysm") from the arteriovenous malformation of the cerebral hemispheres, the basal ganglia, and the brainstem[4] (see Chapter 7 by Lasjaunias et al. in this volume).

The medial vein of the prosencephalon, in fact, when it persists, has been considered by Raybaud[5] to be the aneurysmal sac of the arteriovenous malformation of the galenic system, identifying the time of occurrence as the third month of intrauterine life: some time between the disappearance of this (embryonic) prosencephalic vein and the appearance of the choroidal vessels.

This fundamental anatomical concept separates arteriovenous fistulae of the galenic system from the arteriovenous malformations, chronologically, in that the latter pathologic entity is characterized by the presence of normal arterial and venous structures.[6] Consequently, the arteriovenous malformation develops after the normal vasculature has formed; the arteriovenous fistula of the galenic system is a true pathological alteration of vascular development.[4] An additional morphologic characteristic of arteriovenous fistulae of the galenic system is the retention of the embryonic venous pattern, most commonly represented by a plexus or sinus of the falx. The straight sinus may or may not be patent.

Of extreme interest to the clinician is the fact that the dural sinus and the deep venous system, "draining" the aneurysmal dilation of the medial prosencephalic vein, are often subject to thrombophlebitis; consequently, the combination of extensive deep venous anomalies, persistence of such embryonic venous structures as the medial prosencephalic vein, single or plexiform sinuses in the falx, nonpatent straight sinus, very significant changes in blood flow and turbulence through the area of the arteriovenous fistula, all contribute to thrombophlebitis.[3,7] The result: thrombotic occlusion of the major tentorial sinuses (transverse) and draining veins.[2,3]

In fact, the progressive occlusion of the tentorial sinuses (straight, transverse, sigmoid) results from the high flow of arterial blood producing a mechanical thrombophlebitis first and thrombotic occlusions subsequently. When, as in some cases of arteriovenous malformations of the galenic system, the straight sinus is congenitally absent, the thrombophlebitis is all the more marked and deep venous drainage through tentorial sinuses impaired steadily, as collateral flow develops into and through the cavernous sinuses and ophthalmic vein. In these cases, with absence or occlusion of the sigmoid sinus and jugular bulb, the flow through the superior and inferior petrosal veins is obstructed, accentuating collateral flow through the orbital venous system. The result is quite obvious clinically: low-grade hemorrhagic conjunctivitis, varying degrees of venous distention of the palpebrae, serpiginous venous ectasia of the scalp over the frontal and temporal areas. One may palpate pulsatile flow through these venous systems, which emit an audible bruit. The impairment of visual acuity is not rare in children with this marked degree of collateral flow, and very often mental retardation also results.

One, consequently, immediately becomes aware of the need to distinguish between arteriovenous malformations (the classic AVMs which are so common in adults, so very rare in children under 15 years of age, and extremely rare in children under 10 years of age) on one hand, and the arteriovenous fistulae of the galenic system on the other. The next distinction to be made is between true malformations of the galenic system and "false" ones. Lasjaunias et al.[8] identified arteriovenous shunts draining into a venous structure ("venous pouch"), but without reflux into hemispheral veins (which Raimondi called "aneurysmal dilation of the great vein of Galen"; see Fig. 7.24 in ref. 3), from those characterized by drainage into the pouch and then retrograde flow into hemispheral and midline veins, which generally drain into the great vein of Galen. It was the latter group that they designated "cerebral AVM with vein of Galen ectasia" (and which Raimondi had already called "arteriovenous malformation of the galenic system"; see Figs. 7.20A and 7.23 in ref. 3). Another name they gave to this anomaly was "vein of Galen aneurysmal dilatation." The former group, arteriovenous shunting into a venous pouch without reflux, was called "vein of Galen aneurysmal malformation." Hence, the "vein of Galen aneurysmal dilation" consists of just that: dilation of the great vein of Galen to such an extent that the adjective aneurysmal could be applied. The second form is considered by them to be a true malformation: "vein of Galen aneurysmal malformation."

The above classification is not to be considered an escape into intellectual gymnastics, since it provides very precise and complete criteria upon which the clinician may base decisions regarding occlusion or exclusion of the pathology from the arteriovenous circulatory system. Consequently, what Raimondi called aneurysmal dilation of the great vein of Galen is currently best considered an arteriovenous shunt draining into a venous pouch, but not having reflux drainage into hemispheral veins. This venous pouch may easily be resected surgically, since the procedure consists of nothing more than isolating the pouch and then occluding the os at its point of entry into the pouch, a simple and safe surgical procedure. However, the very factors that make it a simple procedure from an operative point of view apply to endovascular occlusion. What Raimondi had referred to as arteriovenous malformation of the galenic system, on the other hand, is presently best termed "vein of Galen aneurysmal dilation," since the arteriovenous malformation is not necessarily limited to the galenic system but,

rather, *drains* into the galenic system. In fact, any arteriovenous malformation draining exclusively or predominantly into the galenic system causes dilation of the lesser, the greater, or both galenic systems; therefore, the term "vein of Galen aneurysmal dilation" is most appropriate, and most directly indicates the procedure to be performed. In these cases, the endovascular approach is preferable.

Probably one of the most significant contributions to the current status of knowledge on this subject, which is far from clear and certainly about which there is no unanimity, was made by Raybaud et al.[5] These authors made the point that the venous structure that becomes ectatic (aneurysmally dilated) is the medial vein of the prosencephalon, and that it, in fact, is the structure that involutes as the great vein of Galen is formed.

The vein of Galen aneurysmal dilation may occur in association with any arteriovenous malformation of the brain the draining structures of which are tributaries to the great vein of Galen. The vein of Galen aneurysmal malformation, on the other hand, *has no* vein of Galen. It is the medial vein of the prosencephalon that persists and becomes dilated secondary to the presence of the arteriovenous fistula feeding into it. Hence, the *true* malformation is the blind pouch of the medial prosencephalic vein, from which blood is not shunted into other arteries or veins: the medial prosencephalic vein is malformed. The *false* malformation is ectasia, dilation of the normally formed vein of Galen, which is enlarged because it serves as a conduit for the passage of blood from any cortical or centrencephalic vascular malformation into the other arteries or veins.

In a more recent work, Lasjaunias reviewed his total series of vein of Galen aneurysmal malformations and vein of Galen aneurysmal dilations.[4] Excluding the vein of Galen aneurysmal dilations from the study, he was able to document that the very first anatomical anomaly of the arterial and venous systems to occur embryologically is the vein of Galen aneurysmal malformation. He did this on the basis of the presence of alternate patterns of vessels draining the deep cerebral structures, corresponding to the 80-mm stage. In this work, he was able to confirm the hypothesis put forth by Raybaud, adding support to the theory that the vein of Galen aneurysmal malformation develops before the vein of Galen aneurysmal dilation. He also observed that other arteriovenous malformations of the brain occur after the cerebrovascular structure is completely formed. Furthermore, it was suggested that vein of Galen aneurysmal malformations, as already stated, consist of persistence and dilation of the medial vein of the prosencephalon and arteriovenous shunts involving either the choroidal arteries or mural shunts.[4]

With regard to children, one of the most common fistulae found is the arteriovenous fistula between branches of the posterior circle (and, occasionally, the pericallosal artery) and the galenic system, commonly referred to as "aneurysms of the vein of Galen," but which should for simplicity of expression be called vein of Galen aneurysmal dilation. Although, most certainly, aneurysmal dilation of one of the galenic veins invariably occurs when such a fistula develops, it is not truly an aneurysm. This distinction is important, since its surgical treatment is directed toward excluding the arterial flow into the galenic system, and not occlusion or resection of the "aneurysmal" dilation or malformation of the vein of Galen.

The galenic system of veins consists of the paired, paramedian, and internal cerebral veins located within the tela choroidea of the roof of the III ventricle (the lesser veins of Galen), and the single large anastomotic vein (the great vein of Galen), which receives the internal cerebral veins and the veins of Rosenthal. Fistulae between the choroidal arteries in the roof of the III ventricle (medial posterior choroidal branches of the posterior cerebral artery) and the internal cerebral veins (lesser veins of Galen) may occur as independent entities. Similarly, inferior retrosplenial, quadrigeminal, and superior cerebellar arteries may establish fistulous communications directly with the great vein of Galen. Unnamed branches of the internal occipital and superior cerebellar arteries may also penetrate the great vein of Galen directly. The terminal (splenial) branches of the pericallosal artery often enter the superior surface of the aneurysmal dilation or malformation (of

the vein of Galen) when such an arteriovenous fistula is present.

One may, then, observe an arteriovenous fistula with aneurysmal dilation of (1) only the internal cerebral veins (lesser galenic system), (2) only the great vein of Galen, or (3) the entire galenic system (lesser and greater veins of Galen).

Heart Failure, Arteriovenous Shunting, Thrombophlebitis, and Hydrocephalus

One may observe progressive, intractable, high-output failure without hydrocephalus in the newborn, and communicating or obstructive hydrocephalus with or without high-output failure in the infant and toddler. When the great vein of Galen is either simply dilated or an integral part of the malformation, hydrocephalus may occur as an associated condition secondary to compressive occlusion of the aqueduct of Sylvius by the dilated vein of Galen; as the result of a dramatic increase in venous flow and pressure; and/or as the consequence of progressive thrombosis secondary to thrombophlebitis of the major venous draining structures.

Despite the absence of signs of collicular plate compression in any of the heretofore reported cases of hydrocephalus in children with dilation or malformation of the galenic system, most authors, erroneously in our opinion, attributed the hydrocephalus to compressive occlusion of the aqueduct by the dilated vein of Galen. Nevertheless, it is, in the absence of definite evidence to the contrary, best to consider that this may be a pathogenetic factor. More common, and very much more probably as causes, are the coexistence of dramatic increases in cerebral intravascular flow and pressure along with such clear evidence of progressive venous thrombophlebitis of the dural sinuses and major draining veins. These latter pathological events are associated with (we think pathogenic of) the communicating hydrocephalus so very commonly complicating aneurysmal dilation or malformation of the galenic system.

Confronted with the child, with either a vein

of Galen arteriovenous malformation or a vein of Galen aneurysmal dilation, who has ventriculomegaly, one must determine whether the hydrocephalus is pathogenic or simply anatomic. In the event it is pathogenic, the next decision that must be made concerns shunting. Unless there is megacephaly and/or a bulging anterior fontanel, in an infant, we may not *a priori* diagnose pathogenic hydrocephalus. Of course, grade III ventriculomegaly,[1,9,10] the setting-sun sign, a shrill cry, paraparesis, delayed development of milestones, etc., are all clear-cut clinical indications of pathogenic hydrocephalus. On the other hand, distention of the subarachnoid spaces and the fissures, grade I or grade II ventriculomegaly, in the absence of clinical signs of cerebral embarrassment, are not indicative of pathogenic hydrocephalus.

Either the arteriovenous malformation or the arteriovenous dilation of the galenic system may give ventriculomegaly. Arteriovenous shunts, especially those involving the centrencephalic system, may cause ventriculomegaly (hydrocephalus) because of shunting of arterial blood, under arterial pressure, into the venous system, thereby increasing the venous outflow pressure. Aneurysmal dilation of the great vein of Galen, associated with these centrencephalic arteriovenous fistulae, deceptively indicates a compressive factor, suggesting to the clinician that the aqueduct of Sylvius is either compressed or occluded, thereby causing obstructive hydrocephalus. This is not the case. Aneurysmal dilation of the great vein of Galen may compress the superior portion of the cerebellum, shifting it downward, thus causing dislocation of the cerebellar tonsils across the line of the foramen magnum (Chiari I malformation), resulting in constrictive hydrocephalus.[1,2] It is doubtful that simple transforaminal herniation of the cerebellar tonsils in children with anomalies of the galenic system is the sole cause of hydrocephalus. *Rather, it is more likely that the centrencephalic arteriovenous shunting, increased venous outflow pressure, and resultant occlusion of tentorial sinuses represent the true pathogenesis of hydrocephalus in these children.*

In light of the fact that the hydrocephalic process in these children is most likely hemodynamic, there is little reason to suggest

that the most desirable approach to managing the hydrocephalus is a ventriculo-peritoneal shunt prior to correction of the vascular pathology. Rather, the most rational approach seems to be exclusion of the arteriovenous shunt first. If, thereafter, hydrocephalus persists and is symptomatic, one may safely proceed to a ventriculo-peritoneal shunting procedure.

The thrombophlebitic changes are the most insidious, potentially the most damaging, and those which make it mandatory for some of these arteriovenous fistulae to be treated rapidly and surgically: to eliminate the high-flow/high-pressure dynamics, the causes for both the potential cardiac failure *and* the even more damaging cerebral infarction secondary to thrombophlebitic occlusion of the major venous drainage pathways. Waiting 6 to 18 months may be acceptable, and even preferable, in children without evidence of hydrocephalus and some degree (need for digitalization) of cardiac failure. However, either of these pictures of clinical decompensation, and especially the presence of both simultaneously, indicates an urgent situation requiring relatively immediate exclusion of the arteriovenous shunt, whether into a dilated or malformed galenic system.

It is essential to determine whether the lesser or greater galenic system is involved in the fistula and to identify specifically the arterial flow into the fistula. Aneurysmal dilation of the internal cerebral vein, secondary to arteriovenous fistula, is characterized by hypertrophy and increased number of both the anterior choroidal and the middle posterior choroidal arteries. The latter vessels penetrate the tela choroidea of the roof of the III ventricle and shunt into the internal cerebral vein at that point. Branches of the anterior choroidal artery shunt into the choroid plexus along the choroidal fissure. The aneurysmal dilation of the entire internal cerebral vein and retrograde dilation of the terminal and subependymal veins may occur in the absence of involvement of the greater vein of Galen. The retrograde filling may also extend into the terminal and subependymal veins.

The choroid plexuses and subependymal veins are almost invariably distended and both the anterior and postero-lateral choroidal arteries are hypertrophied as a result of the increased flow into the centrencephalic venous system. It is generally difficult to identify the posteromedial choroidal arteries. The hypertrophy of the choroidal vessels and the choroid plexuses of the lateral ventricles along with the distention of the subependymal veins (which contain arterial blood) are additional factors that contraindicate insertion of a shunting system prior to exclusion of the vascular anomaly.

The fistulous communication may exist exclusively between arterial branches of the posterior circle and the great vein of Galen. In this instance, only the great vein of Galen dilates, without retrograde filling of the lesser vein, and the posterior communicating and posterior cerebral arteries may be remarkably dilated along with the posterior choroidal arteries. Similarly, the superior cerebellar arteries may shunt directly into the great vein of Galen. In these conditions, there is a complete aneurysmal malformation of the vein of Galen or of the galenic system.

There is no general rule concerning degree of shunt, aneurysmal dilation of the lesser galenic system, aneurysmal dilation of the greater galenic system, aneurysmal malformation of the entire galenic system, presence of hydrocephalus, and age. In fact, the newborn may have progressive, intractable, high-output failure or aneurysmal dilation of the great vein of Galen in association with arterial shunting into it. Therefore, in considering the congenital anomaly "arteriovenous malformation of the galenic system"/"aneurysmal dilation of the great vein of Galen," it is advantageous to distinguish between the onset of signs and symptoms in the newborn and those at a later age, since the cardiac changes, caliber of the carotico-vertebral systems, arterial tributaries to the galenic system, and size of the venous outflow structures are quite different.

In children diagnosed when newborn, heart failure is invariably present, and intractable high-output failure is the most common type, so that the arteriovenous fistulae of the galenic system are generally diagnosed by the cardiologist who is evaluating the child for the cause of the heart failure at birth. The carotico-vertebral systems are widely dilated, and the major

tributary arteries to both the lesser and greater galenic veins are generally perforating branches of the carotid and basilar arteries, although the pericallosal artery may occasionally shunt directly into the galenic system at the splenium. The middle cerebral system distal to its perforators does not shunt into the malformation. The lesser vein of Galen (internal cerebral vein) very often is widely dilated and opens directly into the great vein of Galen. The great unknowns: do the branches coming from the posteromedial and posterolateral perforating complexes pass through the midbrain and posterior floor of the III ventricle? around it? are they vessels "dedicated" to the fistula or hypertrophied perforators?

Open Surgery or Endovascular Interventional Neuroradiology?— Indications

Though there are as yet no hard and fast rules that permit one to determine whether an individual patient should be treated neurosurgically or with endovascular interventional neuroradiology, it appears at present that the large majority of children with arteriovenous anomalies involving the galenic system are being treated with endovascular techniques. Until approximately 1985, however, open surgical procedures or no operative treatment were the alternatives. Since that time, the truly dramatic progress in interventional neuroradiology has permitted some centers to accumulate truly remarkable experience![4,11] The only reports of extensive operative neurosurgery experience hold material treated prior to 1980, and group arteriovenous malformations and aneurysmal dilations of the galenic system together.[3,12]

Consequently, it is not presently possible to compare the two approaches, but it appears that the pediatric neurosurgical world has, with definite exceptions, chosen to recommend endovascular management. Those infants and children with either malformation or dilation involving the galenic system should initially be evaluated for endovascular treatment, though children with the pouch-like dilation of the medial prosencephalic vein may successfully and with extraordinarily low morbidity be treated with operative neurosurgery.

Surgical Indications and Technique

It is the opinion of the authors that the newborn with intractable high-output failure is not a candidate for either surgical or endovascular treatment because the cerebral parenchyma is, for all intents and purposes, the vascular anomaly. Consequently, even if one were able successfully to exclude the vascular anomaly, the brain has no potential for normal development.

In the event clinical indications or circumstances exclude endovascular management, neurosurgical treatment is directed toward resection of the blind pouch in vein of Galen arteriovenous malformation, which is best performed through a postero-medial occipital flap.

For surgical considerations, in infants and children, arteriovenous malformations of the galenic system may conveniently be subdivided anatomically into three categories, since such a classification permits the surgeon to plan approximately the operative approach. The categories are "superior," when the tributary arteries enter the superior surface of the galenic veins; "inferior," when they enter the ventral surface of the great vein of Galen; and "posterior," when they course around the aneurysmal dilation of the great vein of Galen to enter its postero-lateral (tentorial) surface. This classification permits the surgeon to plan a biparietal craniotomy approach along the falx cerebri for the superior group; a two-stage bilateral temporal craniotomy and supratentorial approach to the tributaries on either side, in the inferior category; and suboccipital craniotomy with fratentorial supracerebellar approach in the posterior category. It may safely be stated that in the very young child, an occipital flap with tentorial incision (Lapras procedure) may offer equally convenient access to all three categories.

In either event, the efferent (tributary) arteries are identified, clipped, and transected, as far from their entry into the aneurysmal dilation as possible. After all tributaries have been occluded and cut, the galenic system is left as is, without any attempt to diminish its size either by inserting imbricating sutures or opening and reconstructing it.

Superior Category—Figures 6.1 to 6.3

In the superior category, the pericallosal and posterior cerebral arteries enter the aneurysmally dilated lesser and/or greater vein(s) of Galen along median and paramedian planes. Careful study of the lateral and half-axial arteriographic projections permits identification of the point of entry of the tributaries into the aneurysm and, most importantly, the planning of the operative procedure. If all afferent vessels enter the aneurysm in the median (sagittal) plane, a unilateral parietal flap suffices for exposure and surgical access to tributaries from both the right and left pericallosal and posterior cerebral systems. If, however, the tributaries enter in a parasagittal or superior lateral plane, bilateral parietal flaps are necessary: it is not possible to work safely and effectively along the opposite

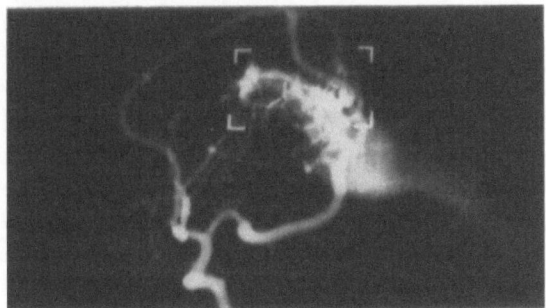

Figure 6.1.

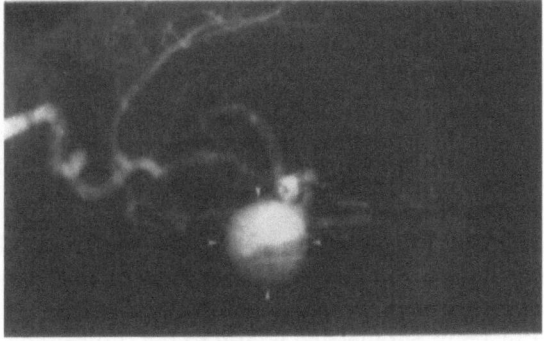

Figure 6.2.

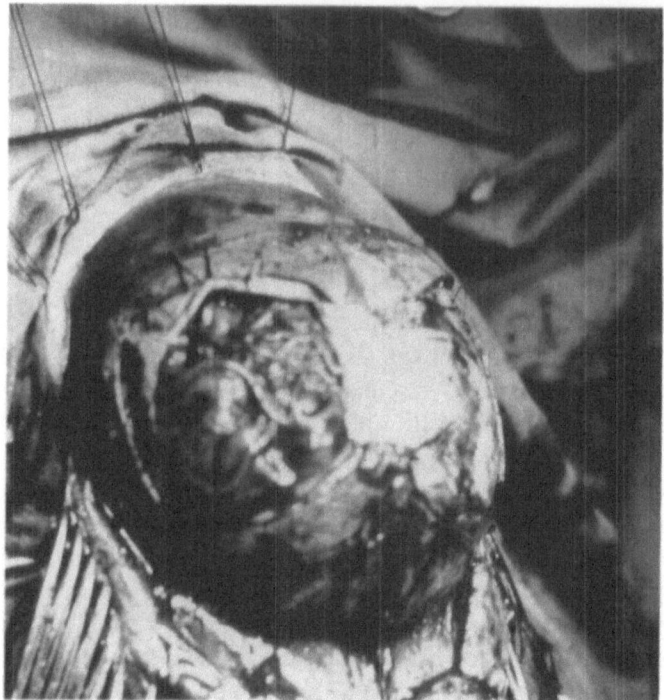

Figure 6.3.

superolateral surface of the aneurysm. Tributaries must be dissected over a distance of at least 6 mm. Consequently, those coming from the posterior cerebral system and the medial posterior choroidal artery course infero-superiorly, nestled within the wall of the aneurysmal dilation of the great vein of Galen. One cannot expose an adequate length by working over the dome of the aneurysm, so that one is obliged to be in position to expose the lateral surface without compressing or excessively retracting the dome.

If a biparietal flap is indicated, then it is best to do this in one stage, rather than to perform a two-stage operation. Access to the corpus callosum and galenic system is facilitated somewhat by the fact that children with arteriovenous fistulae involving the galenic system generally have a paucity of bridging cortical veins: most of the arterial blood is being shunted into the fistula.

In reflecting a biparietal flap in an infant, one should leave the superior sagittal suture (SSS) intact, cutting the parietal bone approximately 3 to 4 mm parallel and lateral to the suture. This affords protection to the SSS and permits the surgeon to prevent kinking (and, consequently, diminished flow) of the sinus during the operative procedure. If a toddler or juvenile is being operated on, the biparietal flap should be such as to leave a strip of bone over the superior sagittal sinus.

After reflection of the flaps and opening of the dura, one may observe a cerebrum that has the appearance of a ball of vessels containing oxygenated blood in the newborn who is in high-output failure, or a normal-appearing cerebrum with few cortical veins and arteries (the toddler and juvenile). The parasagittal surface of the parietal lobe is separated from the superior sagittal sinus and Telfa lain over it for protection as the falx is identified and then the parietal lobe retracted laterally. The pericallosal cistern is generally obliterated because of the posterior displacement and compression of the corpus callosum by the aneurysm. One notes immediately the remarkable size of the pericallosal artery(ies). These vessels are dissected from the corpus callosum and covered with fluffy cotton, which is kept moist, as the splenium and/or body of the corpus callosum is opened in the midsagittal plane. A Penfield No.

4 dissector is used to split the corpus callosum, since this instrument does so bloodlessly and also allows the surgeon to feel the underlying aneurysm. Once the corpus callosum has been sectioned, it is stripped from the aneurysm with the use of wet fluffy cotton, exposing the insertion of the pericallosal tributaries into the galenic aneurysm. Each tributary should be dissected over as long a distance as possible from its point of entry into the aneurysm, and then covered with Telfa. Once all pericallosal tributaries have been identified and dissected, one moves lateralward along the superior surface of the aneurysm to identify the tributaries coming from the medial posterior choroidal and posterior cerebral systems. This approach should be along the homolateral side, so that exposure of the tributaries, for example, coming from the right medial posterior choroidal artery, should be approached along the right side of the falx cerebri. This gives excellent visualization of the superior lateral surface of the aneurysm and provides the surgeon adequate access to these tributaries along a sufficient length of vessel to permit dissection, clipping, and transection. The entire superior lateral surface must be inspected for tributaries.

After all tributaries, on both sides (median and paramedian along the homolateral side, paramedian on the contralateral side), have been isolated, one proceeds to clip and transect. Depending upon the size of the tributaries, either small or medium hemoclips are applied. The recommended technique for application is to bring the jaws of the hemoclip over the surfaces of the afferent vessels, and then to close them very gradually, taking care to observe the jaws of the applicator as this is done to be sure that the clip closure does not skew. This could result in cutting rather than occluding the tributary. It is preferable to apply two clips, separated from one another by 1 mm, at the aneurysmal extremity of the vessels; and then, two more, separated from one another by a similar distance, approximately 3 mm away. The vessel is cut at the center of this 3-mm distance, allowing approximately a 1-mm stump on either end. This clipping technique provides maximum assurance of vascular occlusion.

Inferior Category—Figures 6.4 and 6.5

The "inferior" category is characterized by tributary branches from the posterior cerebral and posterior choroidal arteries entering the galenic system along its inferior lateral surface. Consequently, access to these tributaries is obtained through a temporal flap, elevating the temporal lobe, and entering the ambient cistern after exposing the rim of the tentorial foramen. This permits exposure of all afferent vessels to the galenic aneurysm within the ambient cistern, so that they may be occluded proximal to entry into the aneurysm. The temporal lobe must be elevated from the tentorium, so that the hippocampal gyrus and ambient cistern may be exposed.

Since the vein of Labbé is so very variable in anatomical location and size, no generalities concerning its management exist. However, if one follows the tentorium from the petrous apex to the ambient cistern, gradually elevating the temporal lobe while proceeding, correct orientation is maintained. At the rim of the tentorial

Figure 6.4.

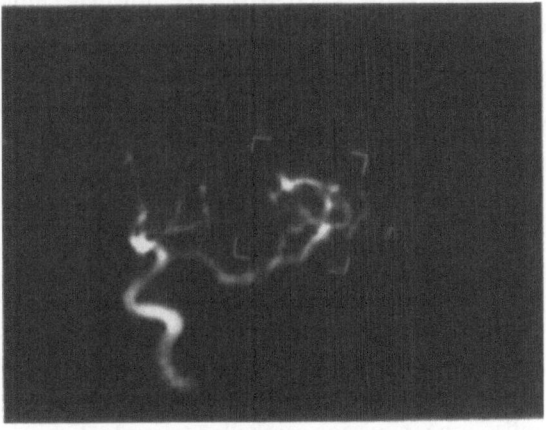

Figure 6.5.

foramen, the ambient cistern bulges prominently. Once opened, there is a gush of cerebrospinal fluid and the IV cranial nerve comes immediately into view, with the tributaries to the galenic aneurysm being located deep to this cranial nerve. These tributaries are branches of the posterior cerebral system.

Though the inferior supply to galenic aneurysms is almost invariably bilateral, the degree of dilation and number of tributary vessels vary from one side to the other, so that no rules apply. Consequently, one may find it necessary to operate bilaterally. When this is the case, surgery should be staged, with the most extensive system of tributaries being operated on first, and with a period of 3 to 5 months intervening.

After the temporal flap has been reflected and the dura opened, the temporal lobe is elevated until the ambient cistern is identified and opened. This gives egress to cerebrospinal fluid and brings the superior cerebral and medial posterior choroidal arteries into the center of the operative field. One may follow them posteriorly, superiorly, and medially in order to identify their tributaries to the galenic aneurysm. It is best to orient oneself by exposing these vessels along the lateral surface of the pontomesencephalic junction, and then to coagulate them along their course toward the aneurysm. The larger tributaries should be dissected along their entire course from the major nourishing vessel to the aneurysm. Generally, this system of tributaries has a more fragile vascular wall than those entering the superior surface of the galenic aneurysm. Some afferent vessels, however, have a rather rigid wall. The fragile vessels need only be coagulated and transected. Those vessels with a relatively rigid wall must be dissected over an extensive (5 to 7 mm) area, double clipped on either end, and transected.

Posterior Category—Figs. 6.6 and 6.7

When the tributary vessels to the arteriovenous fistulae of the galenic system enter the aneurysm along its postero-inferior surface, the surgical approach is through the posterior fossa, reflecting a superior cerebellar triangle flap and approaching the feeders along the infra-

tentorial, supra-cerebellar plane. This approach provides excellent exposure of the posterior and inferior lateral surfaces of the galenic aneurysm at the point of entry of the afferent vessels.

The significant anatomical characteristics are an almost complete absence of bridging tentorial veins, running from the superior surfaces of the cerebellar hemisphere and vermis to the transverse sinus and tentorium. The superior cerebellar cistern is often surrounded by thickened arachnoid, as is the quadrigeminal cistern. Both of these are densely adherent to the galenic aneurysm superiorly, the culmen monticuli of the cerebellar vermis postero-inferiorly, and the dorsal pontomesencephalic surface antero-inferiorly.

The great vein of Galen, converted into an enormous aneurysm, fills the entirety of the tentorial opening at its most posterior and superior surface, so that one sees only this structure after the superior cerebellar and quadrigeminal cisterns have been opened. In fact, the aneurysmal dilation of the great vein of Galen fills the tentorial opening posteriorly, at times compressing the collicular plate as it is displaced anteriorly. The ambient cistern borders the galenic aneurysm on either side, filling the interval between this latter structure and the tentorial edge. Within the ambient cistern are located the posterior cerebral artery and its tributaries to the galenic aneurysm, superior and lateral to the ambient cistern are the isthmus of the hippocampal gyrus and the hippocampal formation.

After a superior cerebellar triangle free bone flap has been reflected, the dura is exposed and a single trap-door dural opening is made. Neither the transverse sinus nor the torcular Herophili should be exposed. The superior bridging veins are identified, coagulated, and transected. This allows the superior surfaces of the cerebellar hemispheres and vermis to fall inferiorly, so that one may expose the superior cerebellar cistern, open it, and then expose the quadrigeminal cistern. Once this is exposed, the aneurysm of the great vein of Galen falls immediately into the operative field. The tentorial edges are then identified and, subsequent to this, the ambient cisterns are opened, exposing the major trunks of the posterior

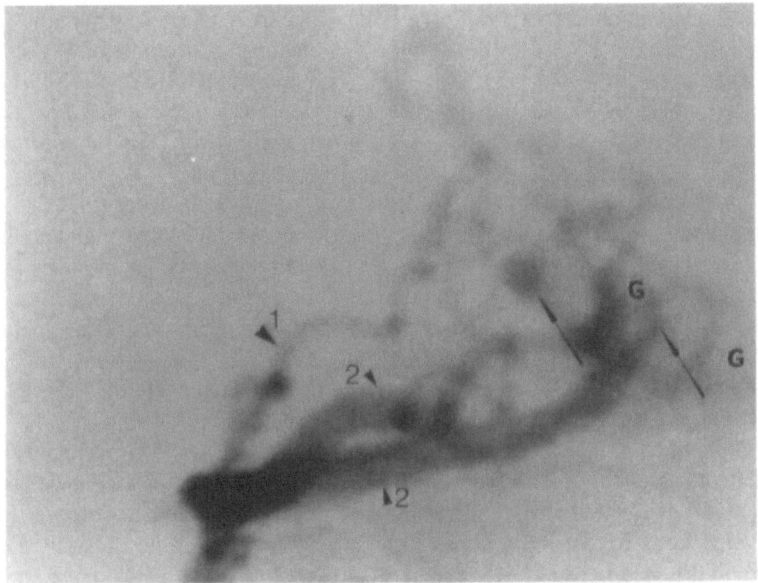

Figure 6.6.

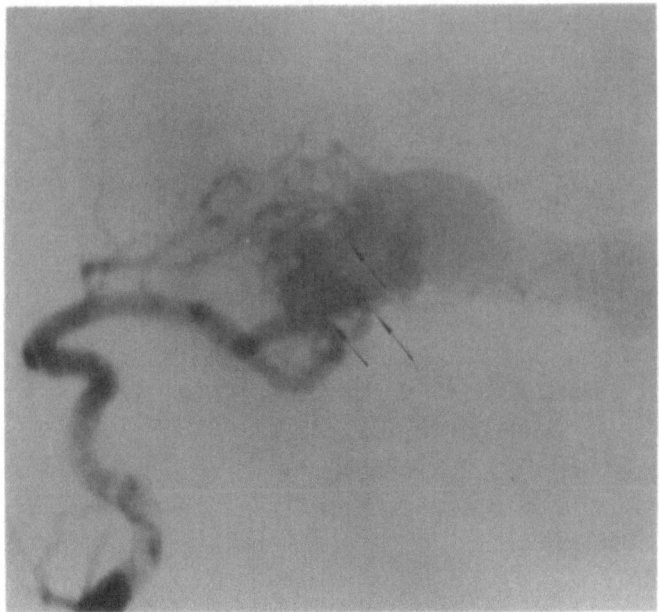

Figure 6.7.

cerebral arteries and their tributaries to the aneurysm. These tributaries nestle within the galenic aneurysm, so that it is necessary to dissect each from the aneurysm, using blunt dissection to separate one from the other, and taking great care to identify the point of entry into the aneurysm. Generally, there are afferent vessels coming from the internal occipital artery and the quadrigeminal branches of the posterior cerebral artery. These vary in number and size. After the tributaries have been identified, and dissected, bilaterally, they are double-clipped and transected, using the same techniques as for the superior and lateral categories. One will note gradual diminution in volume and distention of the galenic aneurysm as each set of tributaries is occluded. The aneurysm is not opened or imbricated.

References

1. Raimondi AJ: Pediatric Neuroradiology. W. B. Saunders, Philadelphia, 1972.
2. Raimondi AJ: Pediatric Neurosurgery—Theory and Art of Surgical Techniques. Springer-Verlag, New York, 1987.
3. Raimondi AJ, Cerullo LJ: Atlas of Cerebral Angiography in Infants and Children. Georg Thieme Verlag, Stuttgart, 1980.
4. Lasjaunias P, Garcia Monaco R, Zerah M, et al: Vein of Galen aneurysmal malformations—patient selection and endovascular management. In: Raimondi AJ, Choux M, Di Rocco C (eds.), Principles of Pediatric Neurosurgery III: Vascular Diseases, Ch. 7 Springer-Verlag, New York, 1992.
5. Raybaud, Ch, Hald JK, Strother CM, et al: Les aneurysmes de la veine de Galen. Etude angiographique et considerations morphogenetiques. Neurochirurgie 33:302–314, 1987.
6. Lasjaunias P, Terbrugge K, Lopes Ibor L, et al.: The role of dural anomalies in vein of Galen aneurysms: a report of 6 cases and review of the literature. AJNR 8:185–192, 1987.
7. Heinz ER, Schwartz JF, Sears RA: Thrombosis in the vein of Galen malformation. Br J Radiol 41:424, 1968.
8. Lasjaunias P, Rodesch G, Terbrugge K, et al.: Vein of Galen aneurysmal malformations. Report of 36 cases managed between 1982 and 1988. Acta Neurochir 99:26–37, 1989.
9. Raimondi AJ: A critical analysis of the clinical diagnosis, management and prognosis of the hydrocephalic child. Adv Pediatr 18:265–291, 1971.
10. Raimondi AJ: Hydrocephalus and the congenital anomalies associated with it: angiographic diagnosis. Semin Roentgenol 6:111–125, 1971.
11. Berenstein A, Lasjaunias P: Endovascular treatment of brain, spinal cord and spine lesions. In: Surgical Neuroangiography, Vol. 4. Springer-Verlag, New York (in press).
12. Litvak J, Yahr MD, Ransohoff J: aneurysms of the great vein of Galen and midline cerebral arteriovenous anomalies. J Neurosurg 17:945, 1960.

CHAPTER 7

Vein of Galen Aneurysmal Malformation: Patient Selection and Endovascular Management

Pierre Lasjaunias, Ricardo Garcia-Monaco, Michel Zerah, and Karel Terbrugge

Introduction

The literature has provided us with a large number of case reports and few series or reviews[1-6] of so-called arteriovenous malformations of the vein of Galen (AVMs of VG). All the cases regrouped presented with intracranial arteriovenous shunt (AVS) and an ectatic vein in the pineal region; however, the diseases involved were different and yet not differentiated. Clarisse[1] was among the first to suggest that true and false AVMs of VG could be distinguished, but still he included in the group of true malformations some cases that should have been excluded. In our earlier series[5] of patients, we separated the lesions draining into the venous pouch with no reflux into the cerebral veins from those where reflux from the pouch into the usual tributaries of the Vein of Galen was noted (Fig. 7.1). We proposed to call the latter cerebral AVMs with vein of Galen ectasia, or vein of Galen aneurysmal dilatation (VGAD). The remaining group corresponds to vein of Galen aneurysmal malformations (VGAMs). The only common point of all these cases was the concept of venous obstacle, either inborn or acquired[7] (Fig. 7.2).

Raybaud[8] sharpened further this anatomic classification when he stated, from pure arterial analysis, that the ectasia was the vein of Galen forerunner: the medial vein of the prosencephalon. Thereafter, of the 60 personal cases of intracranial AV shunt studied by us with a dilated venous channel in the pineal region we have distinguished two types: VGA dilatations (21 cases, 35%) and VGA malformations (39

cases, 65%). The former are not discussed in this chapter. They may occur in many cerebral AVMs, as long as these drain into a Galenic afferent and if the VG outlet is restricted (Figs. 7.1b and 7.2). The natural history of VGAD is that of any cerebral AVM with neurological manifestations (seizures, deficits, etc.) and hemorrhagic accidents. This type is seldom diagnosed in the newborn, and most of the time the onset of symptoms occurs in children or young adults (Table 7.1).

In VGAMs, the vein of Galen is absent. Its forerunner, the medial vein of the prosencephalon, persists and is dilated because of an arteriovenous shunt (AVS). Reviewing our cases with anatomic exclusion of the VGAM from the circulation, we were able to identify the alternate pattern draining the deep cerebral structures (Fig. 7.3). It corresponds to the 80-mm stage arrangement (third month), preceding the maturation of the internal cerebral veins and their confluence. This observation confirms Raybaud's hypothesis and gives further support to the concept of early (the earliest) development of the VGAM compared to any other brain AVM, including VGAD.

VGAM, which corresponds to a dilated medial vein of the prosencephalon, may be associated with either choroid fissure arteriovenous shunt(s) (choroidal type) (26 cases) or mural shunt(s) (mural type) (12 cases) (Fig. 7.4). In one newborn case definitive confirmation of its angioarchitectural type could not be made. He died in a few hours after birth. Both types are only encountered in the first years of life, and present clinically with systemic symptoms in

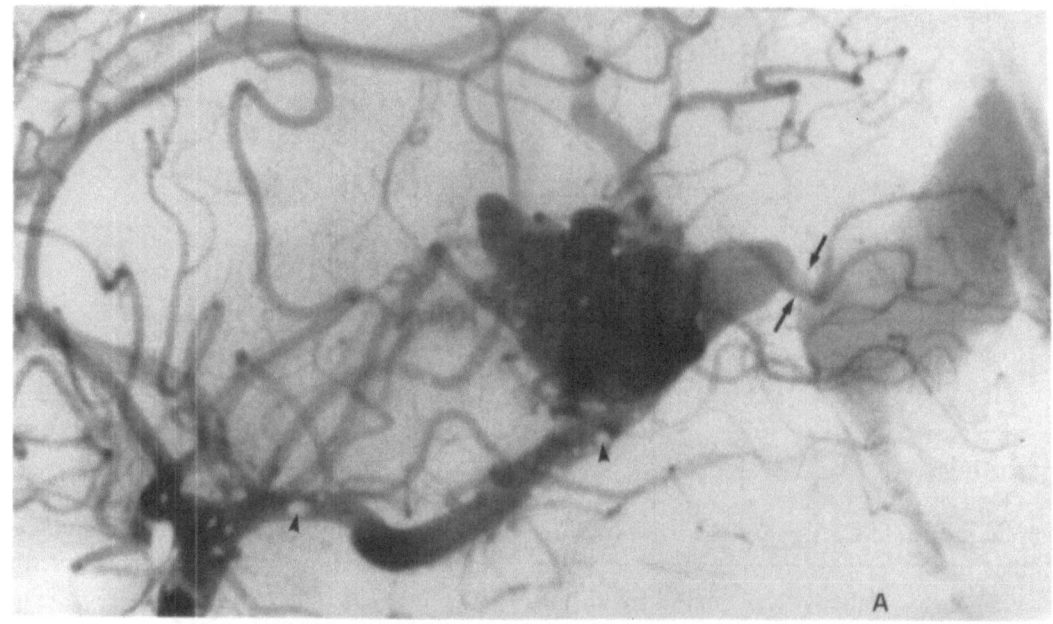

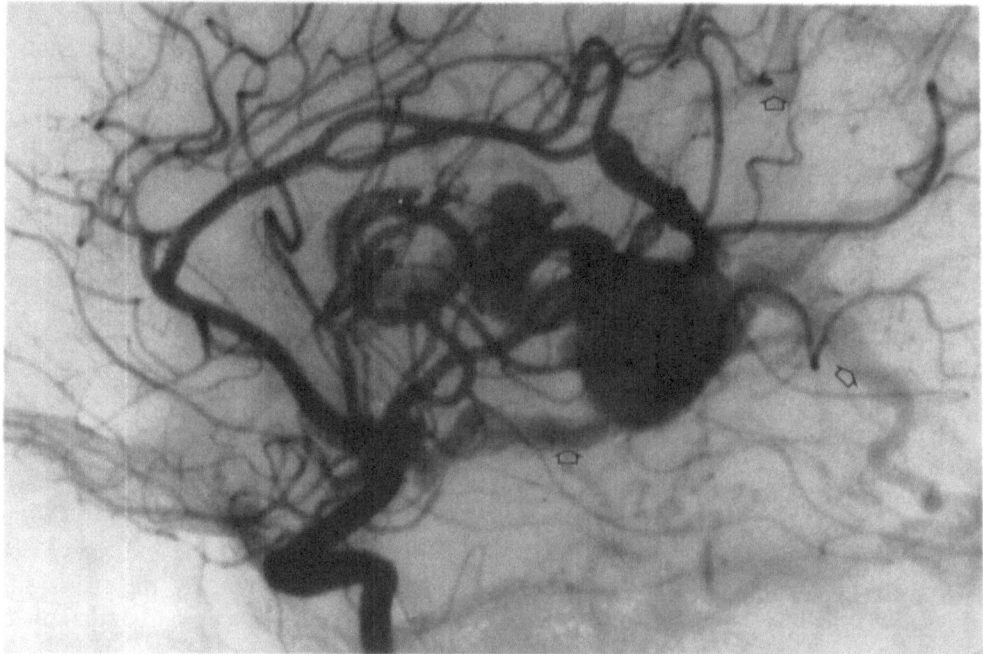

Figure 7.1. Internal carotid angiogram in lateral projection. (**A**) Typical aspect of VGAM with a narrow venodural junction (arrows). Note the Pantopaque droplets (arrowheads) from a previous diagnostic procedure. (**B**) Typical aspect of VGAD with retrograde opacification of vein of Galen afferents (open arrows). Reprinted in part from ref. 5 with permission.

neonates, cerebrospinal fluid (CSF) disorders in infants, and mental and neurological retardation in young children. They do not spontaneously produce hemorrhage because they do not communicate with the cerebral veins, unless distal thrombosis reroutes the AV shunt drainage from the superior sagittal sinus retrograde into the cerebral veins (Fig. 7.5). In

Table 7.1. Frequency of each type of arteriovenous malformation per age group.[a]

Aneurysmal malformation	Neo-nates	Infants	Children
VGAM (choroidal)			
VGAM (mural)			
VGAD			

Reprinted with permission from ref. 13.
[a] VGAM, Vein of Galen aneurysmal malformation; VGAD, vein of Galen aneurysmal dilatation.

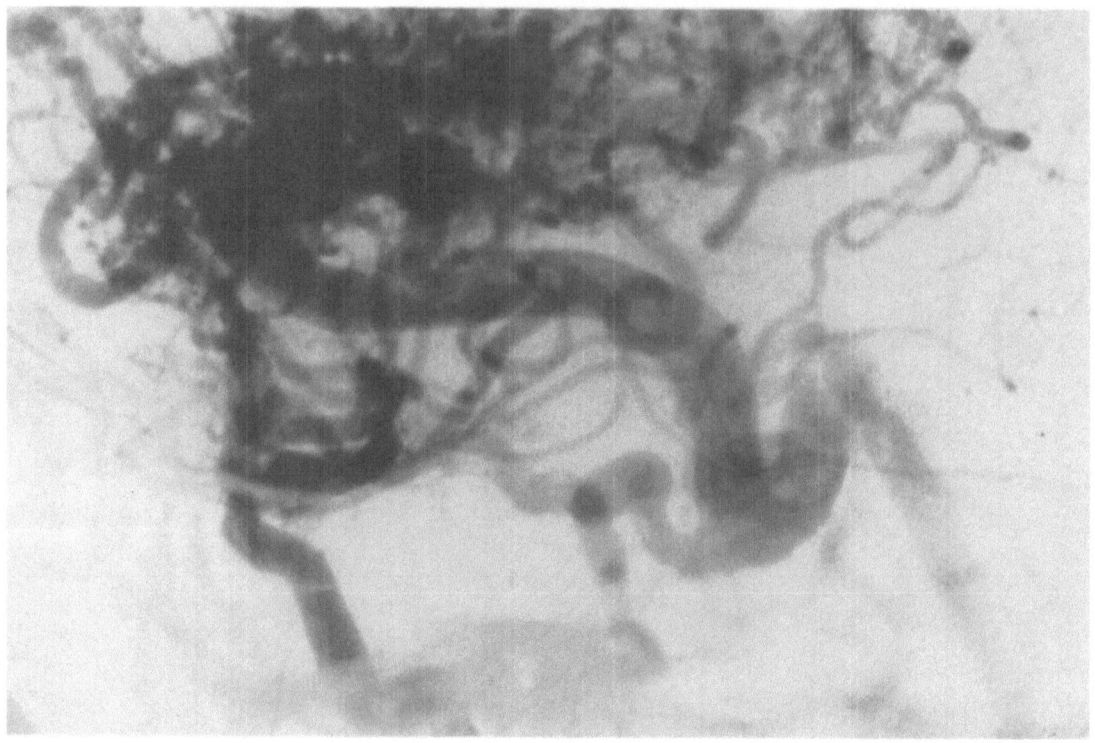

Figure 7.2. Internal carotid angiography in the lateral projection in a case of giant corpus callosum AVM. Note the enlarged internal cerebral vein, and the vein of Galen without dilatation. There is no hemodynamic constraint in the drainage of this malformation.

fact, the venous analysis of these lesions helps to understand the clinical manifestations but also to predict most of the natural history in a given case.[9] Usually, the confluens sinuum, which drains mainly the AVS, cannot drain properly the remaining brain (Fig. 7.6). The cortical and deep-seated veins will tend to join the deep and superficial sylvian collectors. However, at that stage, they do not yet open into the cavernous sinus, because the tentorial sinus (partial forerunner of these venous collectors) will only secondarily be supplanted by the cavernous sinus. This may occur either in utero or after birth. Clearly, the earlier this substitution the better for the brain: this opening represents a low-pressure venous outlet. Partial cavernous sinus occlusion recruits the vein of the foramen ovale. Complete occlusion permits collateral flow into the ophthalmic veins. The latter alternate flow is responsible for facial vein enlargement (Fig. 7.11), but also the exophthalmos and epistaxis mentioned in the literature. They are almost always encountered in infants (and not in the newborn), supporting the concept of postnatal maturation of the skull base venous channels.

Figure 7.3. (A) Schematic representation in superolateral view of a dissected brain. The deep venous system and its alternate pathways are indicated. 1, Internal cerebral vein; 2, thalamostriate vein; 3, transverse caudate vein; 4, septal vein; 5, lateral atrial vein; 6, superior striate vein; 7, inferior striate vein; 8, ventral diencephalic (posterior thalamic) vein; 9, hippocamposubtemporal vein; 10, infratemporal vein; 11, inferior ventricular vein; 12, sinus within the tentorium; 13, anterior pontomesencephalic vein; 14, medial parietal or occipital vein; 15, deep sylvian vein. **(B)** Late phase of an internal carotid angiography in a case of complete exclusion of the vein of Galen. Note the typical epsilon shape of the alternate pathways for the deep venous drainage: posterior thalamic vein (arrow); junction with the basal vein tributaries (double arrow). The collector opens into a tentorial sinus (double arrowhead).

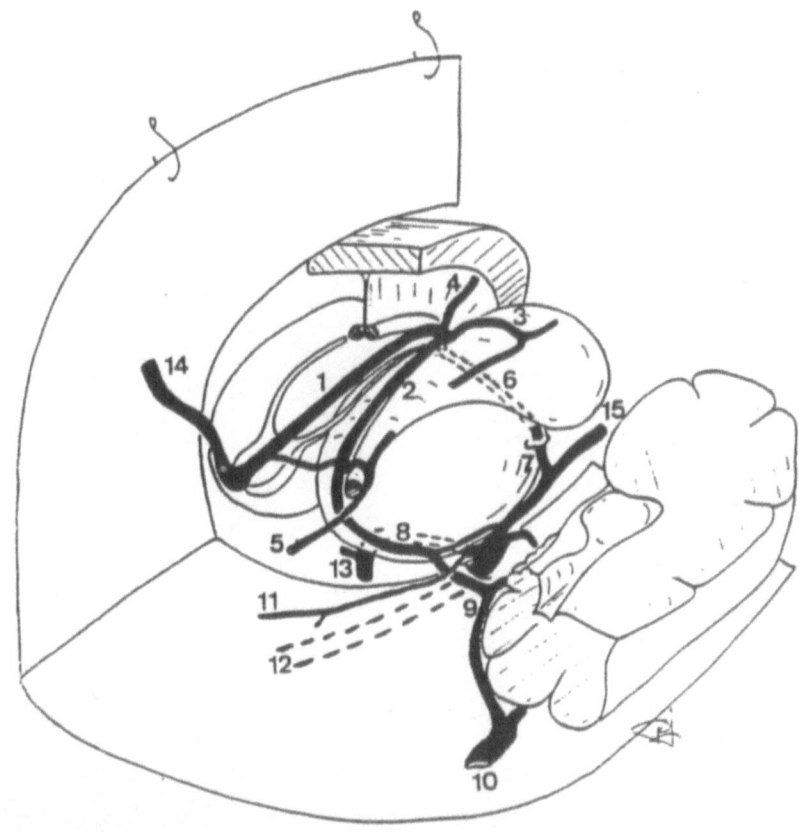

A

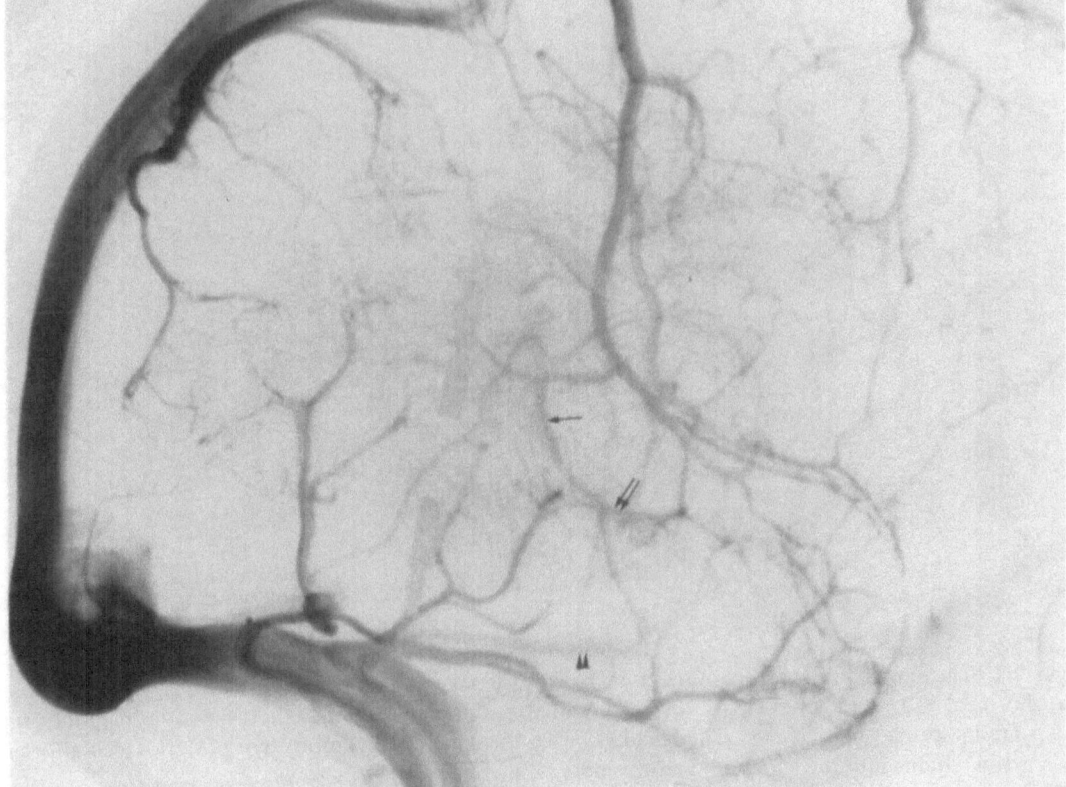

B

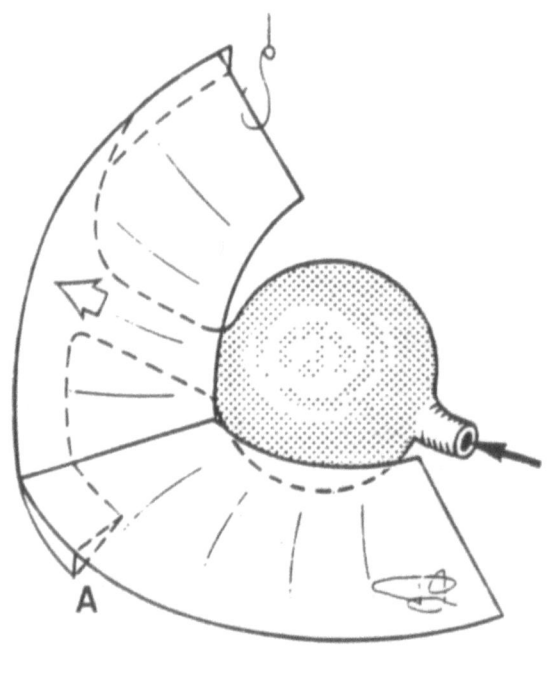

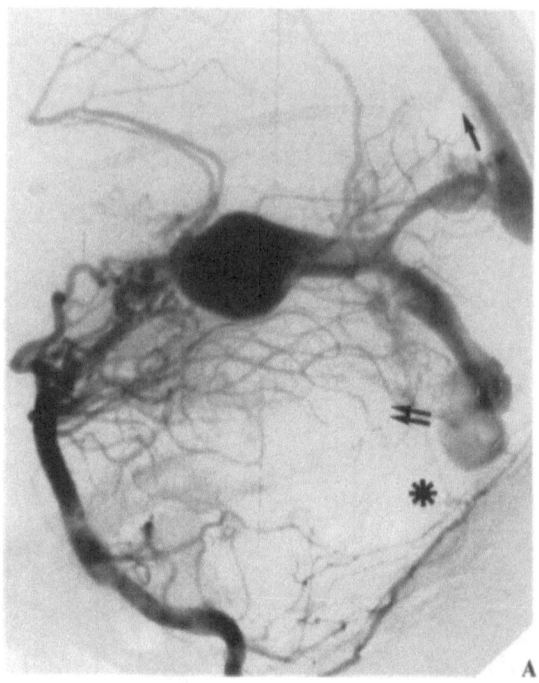

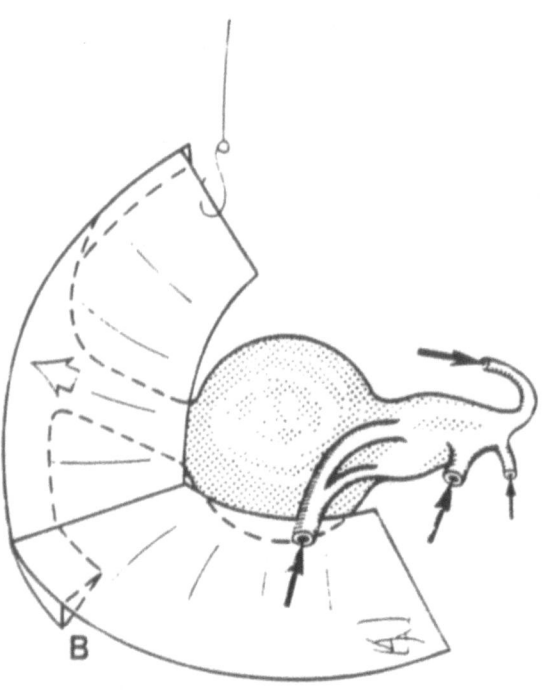

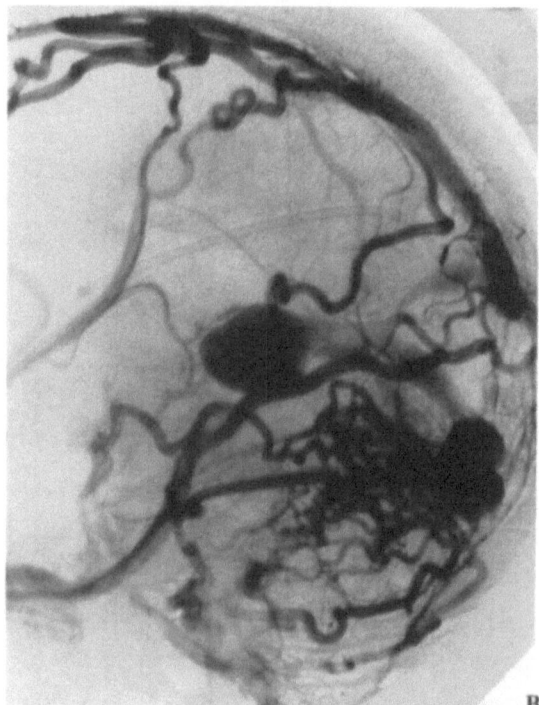

Figure 7.4. Schematic representation of the mural (**A**) and choroidal (**B**) types of VGAM. The arterial feeders are indicated (solid arrows). The falcine sinus (open arrow) drains into the superior sagittal sinus.

Figure 7.5. Vertebral angiography, early (**A**) and late (**B**) phases, in a case of VGAM with complete occlusion of the posterior sinuses (asterisk). The drainage of the malformation opacifies, in a retrograde fashion, the superior sagittal sinus afferents (arrow) and the posterior fossa-torcular afferents (double arrow).

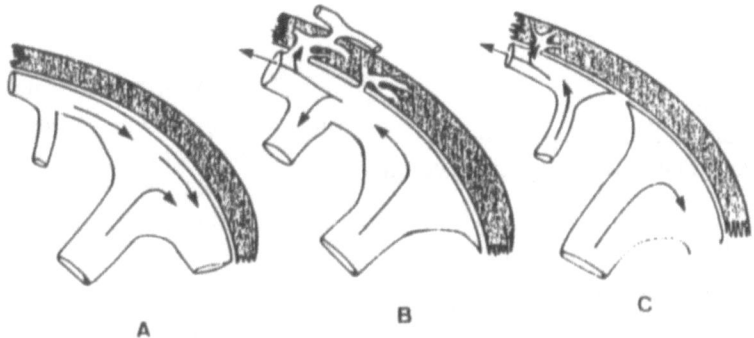

A   B   C

Figure 7.6. Schematic representation of the different types of dural connection of the malformation. (**A**) Common drainage between the brain and the arteriovenous lesion. (**B**) Reflux of the arteriovenous malformation drainage into the sagittal sinus and its afferents (see Fig. 7.5). (**C**) Separate drainage for the malformation and the remaining brain.

In addition to the "frozen venous pattern of the 3rd month stage,"[10] a primitive arterial disposition is also observed in VGAMs: the limbic arterial ring, bridging from the anterior cerebral artery to the posterior cerebral artery (Fig. 7.7).

Parallel to these anatomic advances, the technical breakthrough that permitted the development of miniaturized catheters for arterial approaches,[11] and the success obtained by venous approaches, created a tremendous hope.[12] However, the blind use of each method,

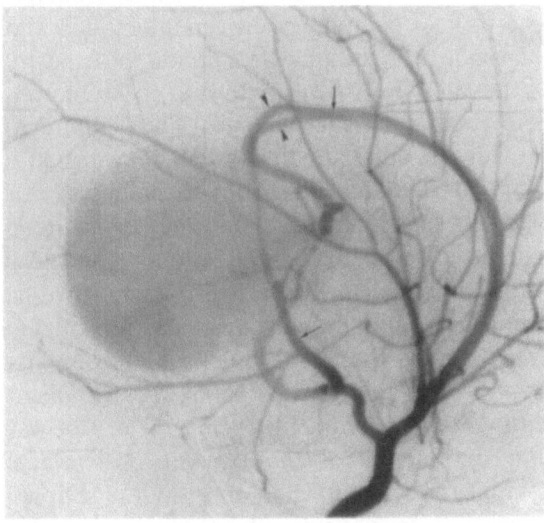

Figure 7.7. Internal carotid angiography in a lateral view in a case of VGAM. Note the limbic arterial ring (arrows) with the separate course for each right and left arterial branch (arrowheads).

or the systematic use of the venous approach because of the apparent ease of use, produced some predictable complications. In fact, from a careful anatomic observation of each case, the therapeutic choice may be conceptualized and performed with very low morbidity and mortality, and high chances of anatomic exclusion. The following sections represent a revisited review of the literature with this clarified anatomic approach.[13]

Clinical Manifestations

The classical four stages of the natural history of VG abnormalities result from the erroneous grouping of two different entities under the same name. From the experience acquired with the cerebral AVMs, and the dural AVMs, the outcome of each type may now be assessed. In a given patient, however, the search for prognostic factors is mandatory. As it has been demonstrated for all intracranial AV shunts, the venous pattern of the remaining brain provides the greatest amount of prognostic information. We herein present the clinical manifestations of VGAM.

From our experience, the anatomic disposition of the lesion indicates the specific technical details for its treatment, while changes in the remainder of the vascular tree are responsible for the clinical history.

Onset may be expressed either by age or by

type, since the clinical manifestations are grossly characteristic of an age group:

Cardiac failure in the newborn
Macrocephaly and CSF disorders in infants
Mental and neurological retardation in young children

Additional problems will occur later, or have been seen only following surgical ventricular shunting.

Cardiac Failure

When the diagnosis of VGAM is made in a newborn (Fig. 7.8), it is because of the presence of cardiac failure. From the multiorgan failure to mild cardiac overload diagnosed early and responding rapidly to medical treatment, all stages are possible.[14] We have never encountered major cardiac failure later than 2 weeks after birth, unless already present in the newborn. In infants, cardiac failure may require additional treatment because it produces a failure to thrive, or becomes medically resistant, but it does not appear nor worsen at that age. In none of the young children was cardiac failure prominent or even an indication for treatment. Later, mild cardiac overload previously overlooked may be noted from an increased

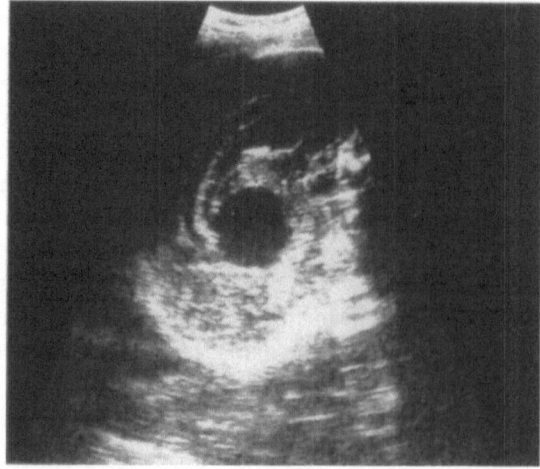

Figure 7.8. In utero ultrasonographic diagnosis of VGAM. Sagittal section of the fetal head at 34.5 weeks of gestation.

cardiothoracic index when exploring an infant or a young child for other symptoms of suggestive VGAM. Cardiac symptoms are, therefore, maximum within the first 2 weeks of age; their tolerance and response to medical treatment determine the type and timing for endovascular approach (Fig. 7.11).

Cerebrospinal Fluid Circulation and Resorption Disorders

Some neonates do present increased cranial circumference. However, it is most often in infancy that these symptoms come to the attention of a physician and the diagnosis is made. Mechanical compression (occlusion) of the mesencephalic aqueduct has been classically considered responsible for the ventricular enlargement. In our experience, this mechanism is not a significant cause. Each time MRI studies were obtained, the sagittal sections demonstrated patency of the aqueduct. Furthermore, the pericerebral spaces were clearly seen and often enlarged. Ventriculomegaly is probably more complex; very likely it involves the extracellular water compartment. Macrocephaly is, therefore, a multifactorial phenomenon related to an unfavorable anatomic venous disposition and an increased intrasinus (venous) pressure as the result of the AV shunt drainage. The lack of compliance of cerebral tissue and the venous congestion depend upon the capacity of the alternate venous pathways to accommodate venous pressure changes. Their failure to provide an outlet to the system may produce rapid internal and external hydrocephalus,[15] or even a slit ventricle syndrome in shunted patients. Ventricular shunting only "deflates" the CSF compartment. It does not improve the venous condition. In most instances, it probably even worsens the extracellular water compartment by creating a centripetal water gradient with cortico-subcortical ischemia. This observation accounts for all the frequent, postsurgical complications observed in our group of shunted patients. Surgical ventricular shunting may also enlarge the ectasia: a 30% increase in diameter has been seen in three of our cases, 1 to 2 months following surgery. The rapid reexpansion of the ventricles and correction of the macrocephaly

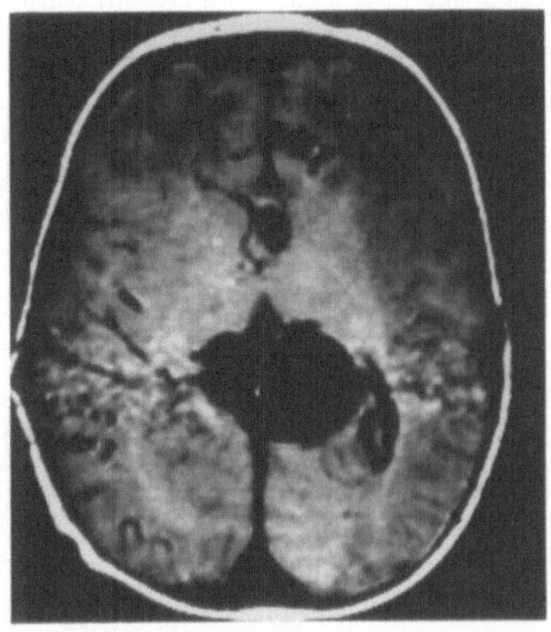
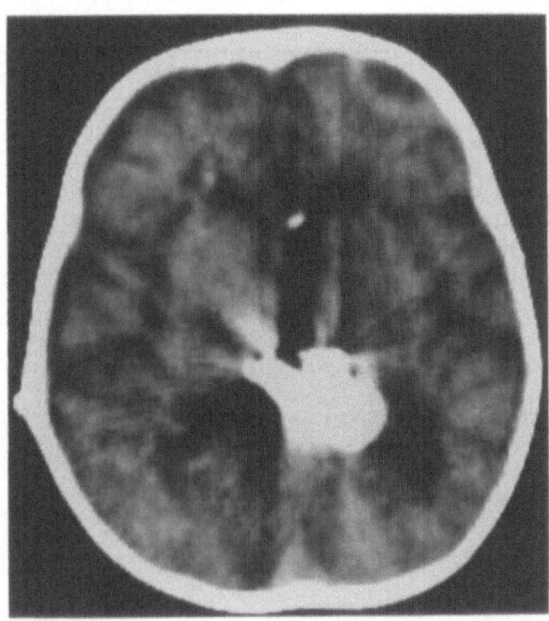

Figure 7.9. Magnetic resonance imaging (MRI) (**A**) and computerized tomography (CT) after embolization (**B**), in a case of a young infant presenting with rapid neurological deterioration. The child was shunted in another institution, and put under digitalo-diuretic medication for cardiac failure from VGAM. Note the slit ventricle and disappearance of the cisternal spaces around the brain. Following embolization (5 hr later), there is reexpansion of the ventricles and appearance of the cisternal space (**B**). Simultaneous dramatic clinical improvement was noted. The child is presently normal, and his digitalo-diuretic medication has been discontinued.

following embolization (without clinical manifestations) emphasize the need for urgent venous decongestion in case of liquid-related manifestations (Fig. 7.9). However, when surgical ventricular shunting has been done, endovascular treatment should not be done a few days later. Rather, it should be postponed, since complete exclusion of the AVS produces a rapid shrinkage of the ectasia, in addition to the diminution in size of the ventricles. Both of these rapid volume modifications in a few days' time may create a significant and acute decrease in the supratentorial pressure, leading to upward cerebellar herniation. These complex venous and water disorders[13,15] represent the most satisfactory explanation for white matter calcifications (watershed venous junction) which may develop in infancy (Fig. 7.11). In cases where therapeutic endeavors have been withheld for few months, careful search for these calcifications must be undertaken. Cerebral atrophy and delay in neurological maturation represent additional expressions of this complex disorganization of the choroido–venous–water equilibrium.[13,15,16]

Neurological Manifestations

VGAMs are chronologically represented by axial hypotony and delayed motor development, which are reversible if the malformation is treated early (Fig. 7.11). Correction of a 5-month delay at 13 months of age has been obtained in our series. The older the child, the lesser the chances to reverse or compensate the retardation even with complete anatomic exclusion of the lesion. Although we do not have the necessary long-term follow-up, the neurologic results obtained so far are very encouraging. The few cases in which neurological deficits or seizures were noted occurred in children who

Table 7.2. Differential characteristics between vein of Galen aneurysmal malformation (VGAM) and vein of Galen aneurysmal dilatation (VGAD).

Characteristics	VGAM		VGAD
	Choroidal	Mural	
Vein of Galen afferents	No	No	Yes
Dorsal vein of the prosencephalon	Yes	Yes	No
Falcine sinus	Frequent	Possible	Rare
Communication with cerebral veins	No	No	Yes
Most frequent age of onset	Newborn	Infant	Children
Congestive heart failure	Almost constant	Frequent	Rare
CSF disorders	Frequent	Frequent	Rare
Failure to thrive	Yes	Possible	Possible
Expected rate of cure per type with E°	High	Very high	Low
Natural history	Unknown	Unknown	Equal to deep-seated AVM with an already existing venous stenosis
Risk of future hemorrhage	If distal dural sinus thrombosis[a]	If distal dural sinus thrombosis[a]	Very high
Risk of future focal neurological symptoms	If ventricular shunting or calcification[b]	If ventricular shunting or calcification[b]	Very high

Reprinted with permission from ref. 13.

[a] Reflux of the AV shunt dural drainage into the cerebral vein.

[b] Mechanical and/or hemodynamic impairment of transcerebral venous drainage plus unfavorable anatomic disposition.

had had surgical ventricular shunting. In none of the cases that had only been embolized did these symptoms occur. One does not expect to see them unless calcification or postvenous ischemic gliosis creates epileptogenic foci.

Secondary spontaneous occlusion of the sinusal outlet of the VGAM by rerouting the flow of the shunt to the cerebral veins may rupture the fragile equilibrium of the remaining venous systems and produce cerebral or subarachnoid hemorrhages. However, this anatomic (asymptomatic) situation has only been encountered once in our series (Fig. 7.5) and we consider it unlikely that the ectatic vein would rupture spontaneously. Although hemorrhagic venous infarct may also occur, we have not seen a case where this diagnosis was plausible.

It is not (yet) possible for us to comment on the natural evolution of the VGAM, because we have never seen one in young adults, and because the cases reported in the literature refer in fact to VGADs. However, the symptoms projected from the present anatomic analysis so far seem reliable (Table 7.2).

Objectives of Treatment

Before undertaking treatment one should estimate, as objectively as possible, the chances of the child to grow normally in the expected family surroundings and in light of predictable care. The age of onset and dominant symptoms determine the objectives and the instrumentation.

Systemic Symptoms

Management of cardiac failure is controversial. However, we recommend the use of diuretics such as acetazolamide, which does not affect choroid plexus secretion. Digitalis is not

Table 7.3. Decision tree at the neonatal period.

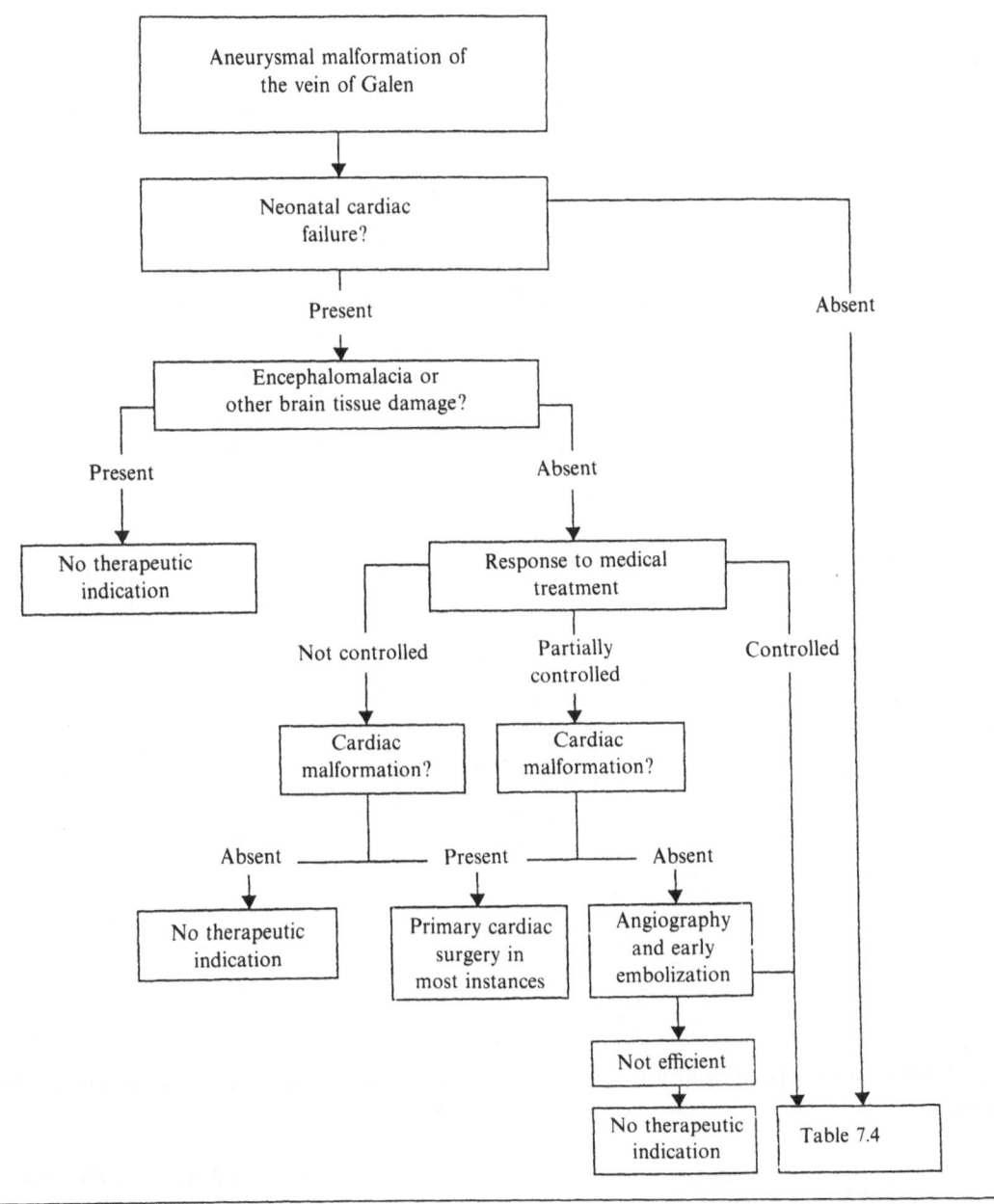

indicated because the heart is almost always normal (in our experience we found only two true, associated, cardiac malformations), and there may be an increase in blood volume. The results of partial embolization in these cases have been particularly rewarding. Table 7.3 illustrates our clinical contraindications for treatment in this age range.

Unstable response or absence of response will bring the child to the basic initial discussion of his neurological prognosis. It is clear from the literature than one can make these newborn survive almost regardless of the cerebral status. Therefore, newborn brain morphology must be assessed [ultrasound, computerized tomography (CT), and/or magnetic resonance imaging

Table 7.4. Decision tree for infants.

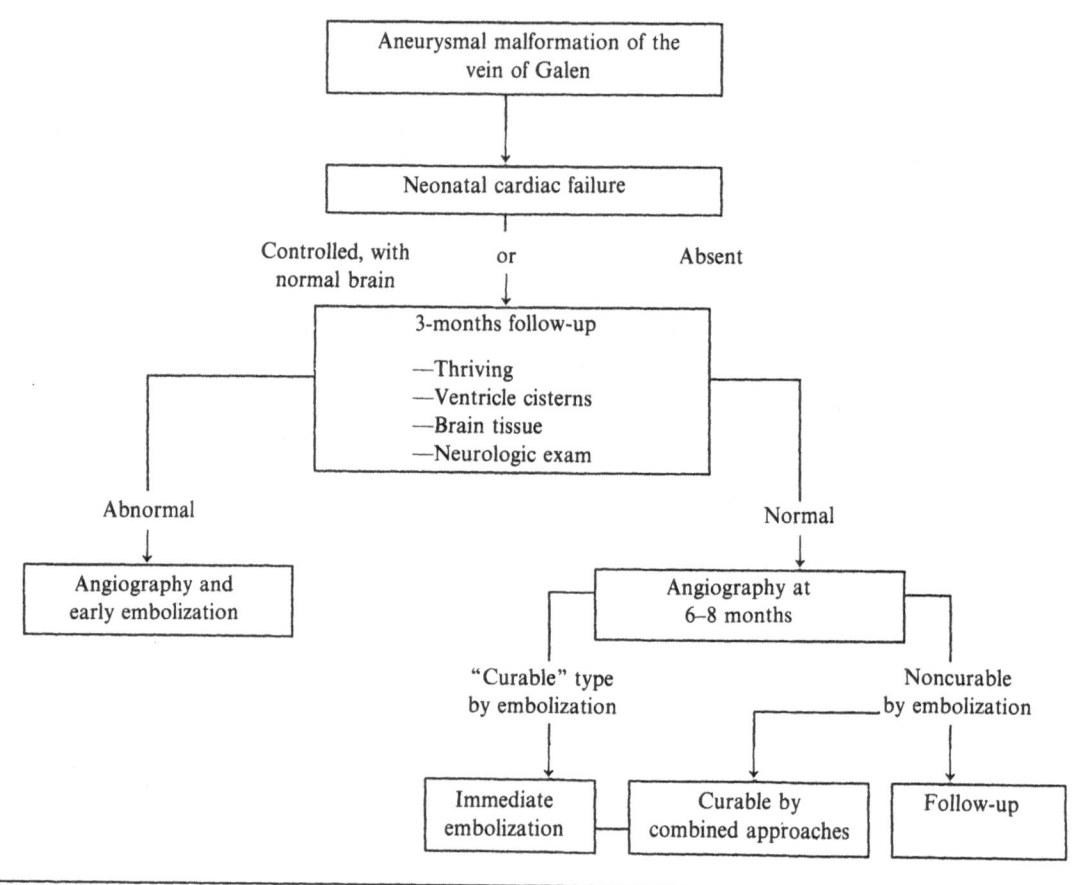

(MRI)] prior to undertaking any endovascular treatment.

Cerebrospinal Fluid Disorders

In case of CSF disorders, including macrocephaly, in infants one should not use ventricular shunting because it clearly creates cortico-subcortical ischemia, which may later produce seizures. Therefore, the objective of treatment of hydrocephalus and macrocephaly in VGAMs must be the urgent correction (even partial) of the venous disorder. Ventricular shunt should be done only when the endovascular management cannot be obtained

with the expected chances of success for the child.

Failure to Thrive and Mental Retardation

The objectives of treatment with failure to thrive and mental retardation are difficult, because they are not easily linked to a demonstrable dysfunction. Obviously, if the systemic symptoms are still prominent under medical treatment and compromise nutrition, correction of the arteriovenous shunt is required. If cerebral maturation delay is suspected to result from venous congestion, urgent occlusion of the arteriovenous malformation should be carried out (Table 7.4).

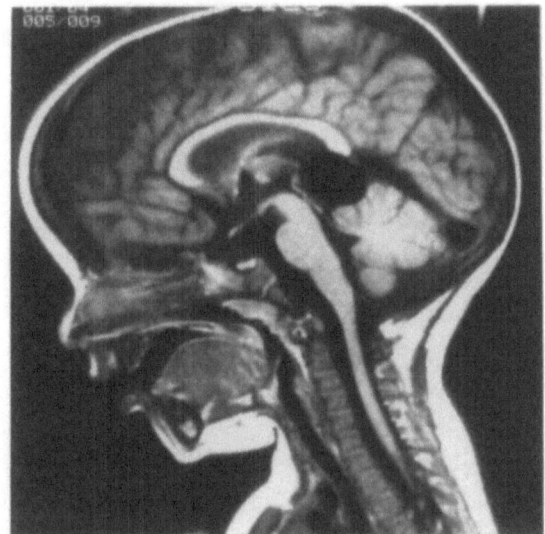

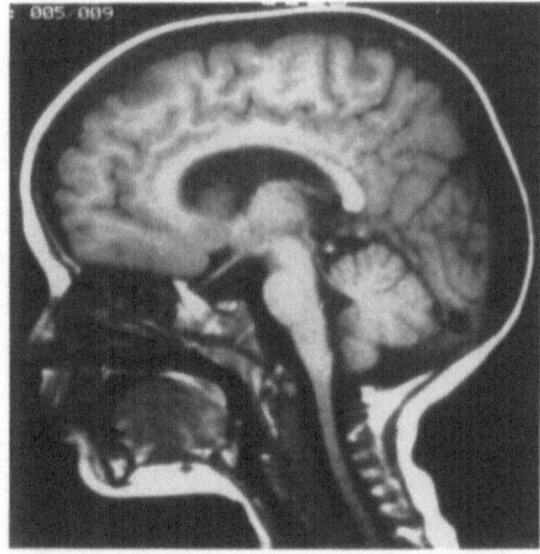

Figure 7.10. Sagittal section in MRI before (**A**) and after embolization (**B**) in a case of VGAM. Note the complete disappearance of the malformation 4 months following treatment. Reprinted from ref. 9 with permission.

Neurological Symptoms and Hemorrhages

Neurological symptoms and hemorrhages are not part of the natural history of VGAM, but belong rather to that of VGAD, with which they have been largely confused. Again, secondary thrombosis, or mechanical transdural manipulation in an incompletely controlled lesion, may

alter the architecture and produce seizures, hemorrhages, or deficits. But these observations are rare, and have not been registered in our series. At present, there is no rationale to treat an asymptomatic VGAM in an adult (if one encounters such a situation) on the assumption of a hemorrhagic risk, if the above-mentioned conditions are not encountered. Finally, one may question the value of shrinking the mass effect resulting from the venous ectasia, since compression of the neural tissue does not seem to be of any clinical significance. Nevertheless, we personally tend to obtain this morphological objective (Fig. 7.10). As a basic philosophy we attempt to limit our activity to attaining only what is necessary when we are forced to operate urgently. Otherwise, we prefer to choose the appropriate moment that would give us the best chances of treating entirely the VGAM. The moment will vary from one child to the other, but the technique used has in general been the same in our series (Fig. 7.11).

Methods of Treatment

Three types of approaches exist:

surgical
endovascular arterial
endovascular venous by femoral or transtorcu-
    lar approach

The surgical experiences are, in fact, a succession of case reports, or short series, in which the results have been anecdotally good, but in general very poor (Table 7.5). Since we did our first case of VAGM in 1984, we have had only one surgical exposure for torcular approach. All the others have been operated endovascularly.

The endovascular approach seems promising, but it requires further follow-up. We prefer the transarterial one, since in our hands it has given satisfactory results with lower risks (Tables 7.6 and 7.7). Comparative series with venous approaches were on different architectural analyses and objectives. However, as a technique we have used it in two instances, transtorcular and retrograde transfemoral. In the first case, the result was morphologically satisfactory, but the clinical evolution poor. The second case was

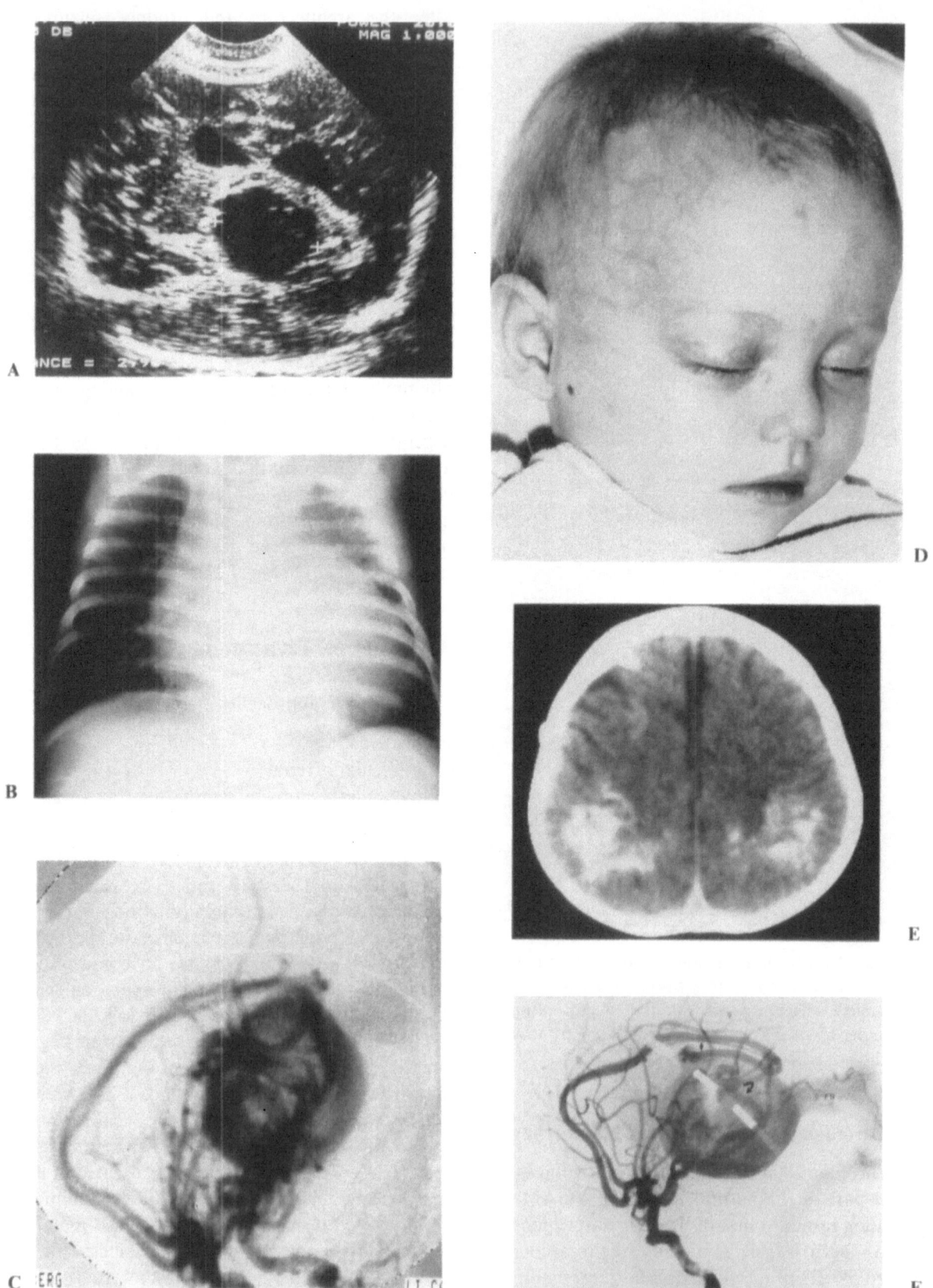

Figure 7.11.

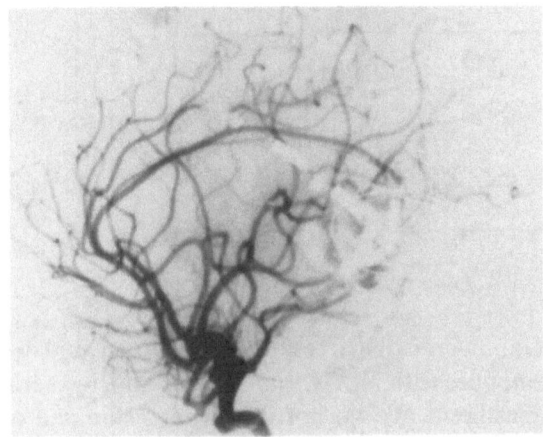

G

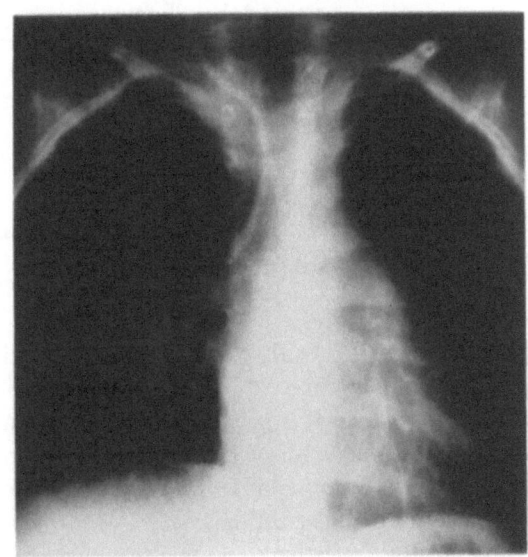

H

Figure 7.11. (**A**) Neonatal ultrasound in a case of a newborn presenting with cardiac failure. The frontal section demonstrates the VGAM. (**B**) Chest X-rays showing the cardiomegaly. (**C**) Angiography performed in another institution confirms the diagnosis. Due to the degree of cardiac insufficiency, the patient was referred to our institution and partial embolization done. Clinical improvement was immediately noted, and the patient was stabilized medically with small doses of digitalo-diuretics. Six months later, at the time of clinical follow-up (**D**), although the clinical evolution was felt to be satisfactory, bilateral calcifications in the parietal lobes were noted (**E**). The ventricles were moderately enlarged and without macrocephaly. The shunt was performed in the hospital of origin. Note (**D**) the venous collateral channels on the face. Carotid angiography, performed at the time (**F**), demonstrates the previous embolization and the remaining shunt (asterisk) fed by the choroidal branch of the anterior cerebral artery (arrow), and the posterior choroidal artery (bent arrow). The falcine sinus is well opacified (FS). Additional embolization was performed in three sessions, and complete occlusion finally obtained (**G**). Four years later, the chest rays (**H**) and the face of the child (**I**) look normal. Neurological examination and psychological tests are normal. Management of this newborn case illustrates the protocol of Tables 7.3 and 7.4.

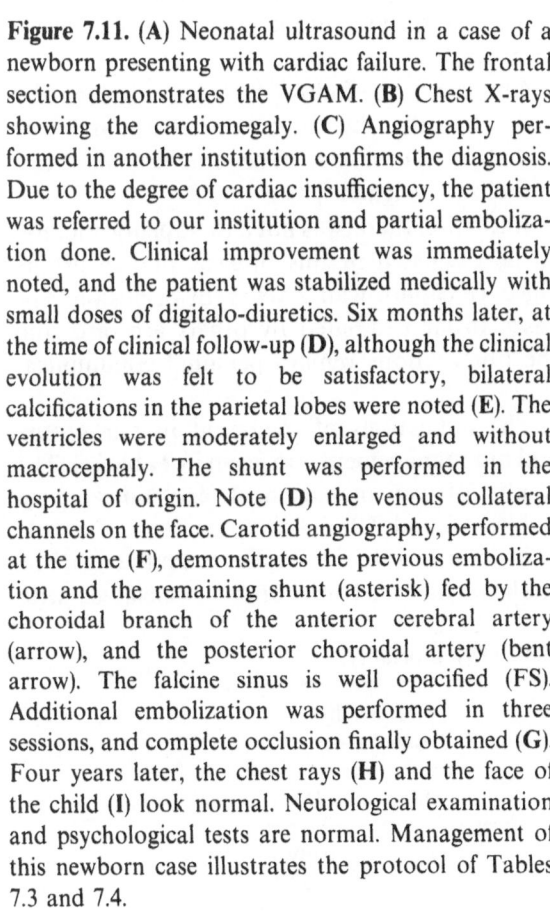

I

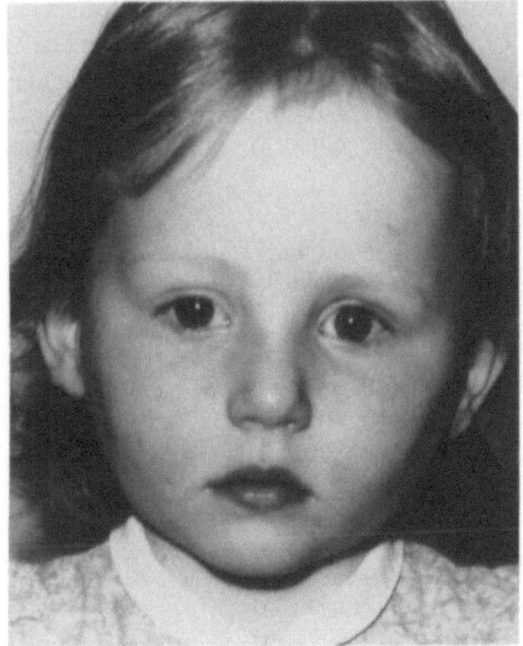

Table 7.5 Johnston's review of 167 cases: mortality in vein of Galen aneurysmal malformations.

Age	Number	Nontreated	Number	Treated
Newborns	12	100%	56	93%
Infants	11	72%	57	38%
Children below 5 years	6	66%	25	36%

[a] Data from ref. 3.

anatomically cured with addition transarterial approach and is clinically normal (Fig. 7.11). Both were managed since newborn. In both cases the venous approach had been chosen because of the impossibility to achieve a safe distal arterial catheterization.

Technically, we have used the femoral approach, with a 4F catheter, since we first started to accept children with this disease in 1984; we have never used any oversized sheath in newborns, infants, or children under the age of 3 years. We had three transient technical failures; we never had to perform a cut-down.

Table 7.6. Endovascular management: material (1984–1989).

VGAM	Cases embolization	Sessions	Arteries
VGF	19	48	65
VGM	9	12	14
Total:	28	60[a]	79

[a] Seventy-two percent of the sessions are performed in children below the age of 3 years.

Our microcatheter carries no balloon and we embolize with NBCA (liquid glue), under general anesthesia. We do not use hypotension and/or heparin, since we have no coaxial system. We have not had any perfusion breakthrough phenomena in our series, nor secondary cerebral venous thrombosis. In case of complete occlusion in one session, we keep the infant or newborn asleep for 24 hr before awakening him slowly. Blood pressure is kept at normal levels (Fig. 7.12).

Children are followed neuroradiologically and clinically by both ourselves and the pediatric neurologist. The smallest newborn embolized weighed 2.8 kg.

Radiation therapy is not a therapeutic method to be discussed in this disease, or age group, since we cannot wait 2 years for occlusion. The cases so far irradiated by others are rare, and the observations remain personal communications.

The indications of treatment in our group, and our management, are given in Table 7.4. The results of our management are indicated in Tables 7.8 and 7.9.

In conclusion, we believe that both the fatalism and heroics often associated with

Table 7.7. Patient management (1984–1989): mortality.

VGAM	Nontreated		Treated by embolization	
	Number	Dead	Number	Dead
VGF[a]	4	4 (100%)	19	0 (0%)
VGM	3	0 (0%)	9	2 (22%)
Total:	7	4 (57%)	28	2 (7%)

[a] Four are lost to follow-up.

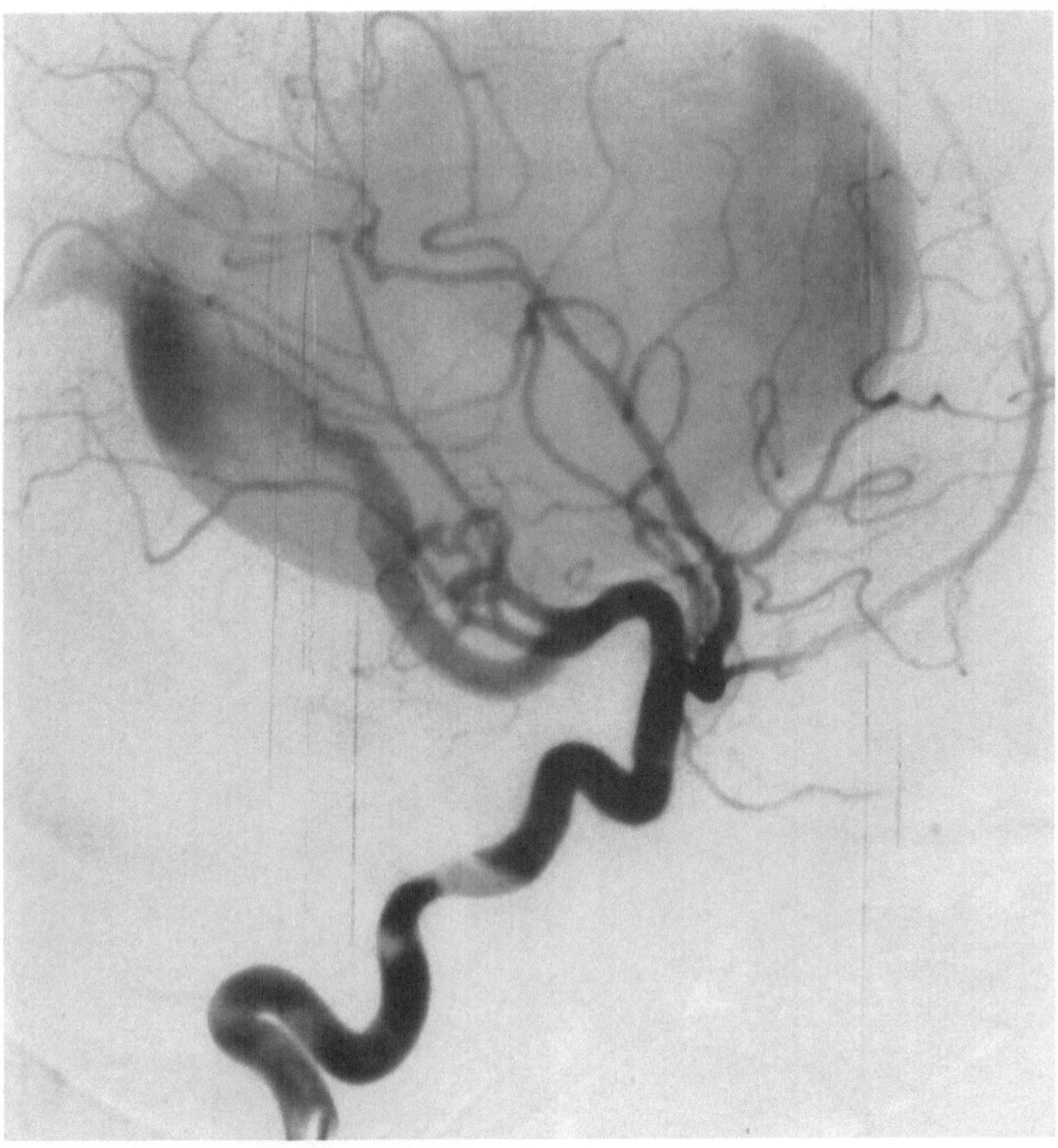

A

Figure 7.12. Giant VGAM with two separate fistulous sites. (**A**) Internal carotid in lateral projection. (**B**) Vertebral artery in frontal projection. Note the duplicated feeders (arrow and double arrow) converging into one of the fistulous locations. (**C**) Internal carotid angiography and (**D**) vertebral angiography 4 months after embolization; one session was performed. Although only one artery was used to deliver the glue (asterisk), regression of the other vessels was obtained. MRI in sagittal (**E**) and axial (**F**) sections demonstrates the immediate occlusion of the entire pouch. Clinical tolerance has been satisfactory and the postoperative course uneventful.

VGAM management should be left behind. It is of paramount importance to recognize the different groups of diseases within the classical AVM of VG entity, as outlined in this chapter.

In sum, the ectatic medial vein of the prosencephalon in VGAM "freezes" the remaining venous system at the 3-months stage. The arterial tree remains grossly normal. With strict patient selection, the results of embolization are excellent. We favor the arterial approach, so far it has given the best results. Our preference for embolization applies to the treatment of

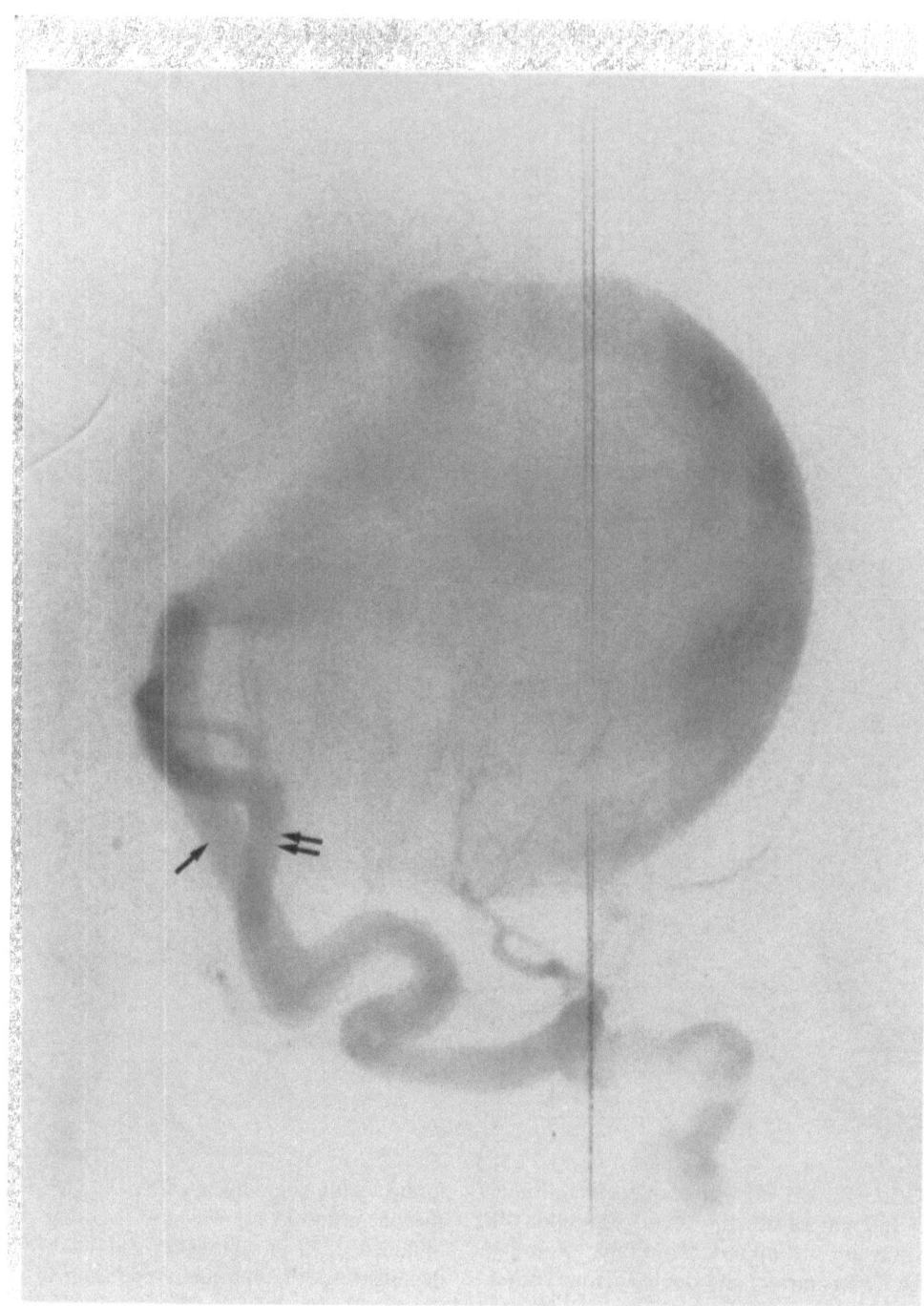

B

Figure 7.12. *Continued.*

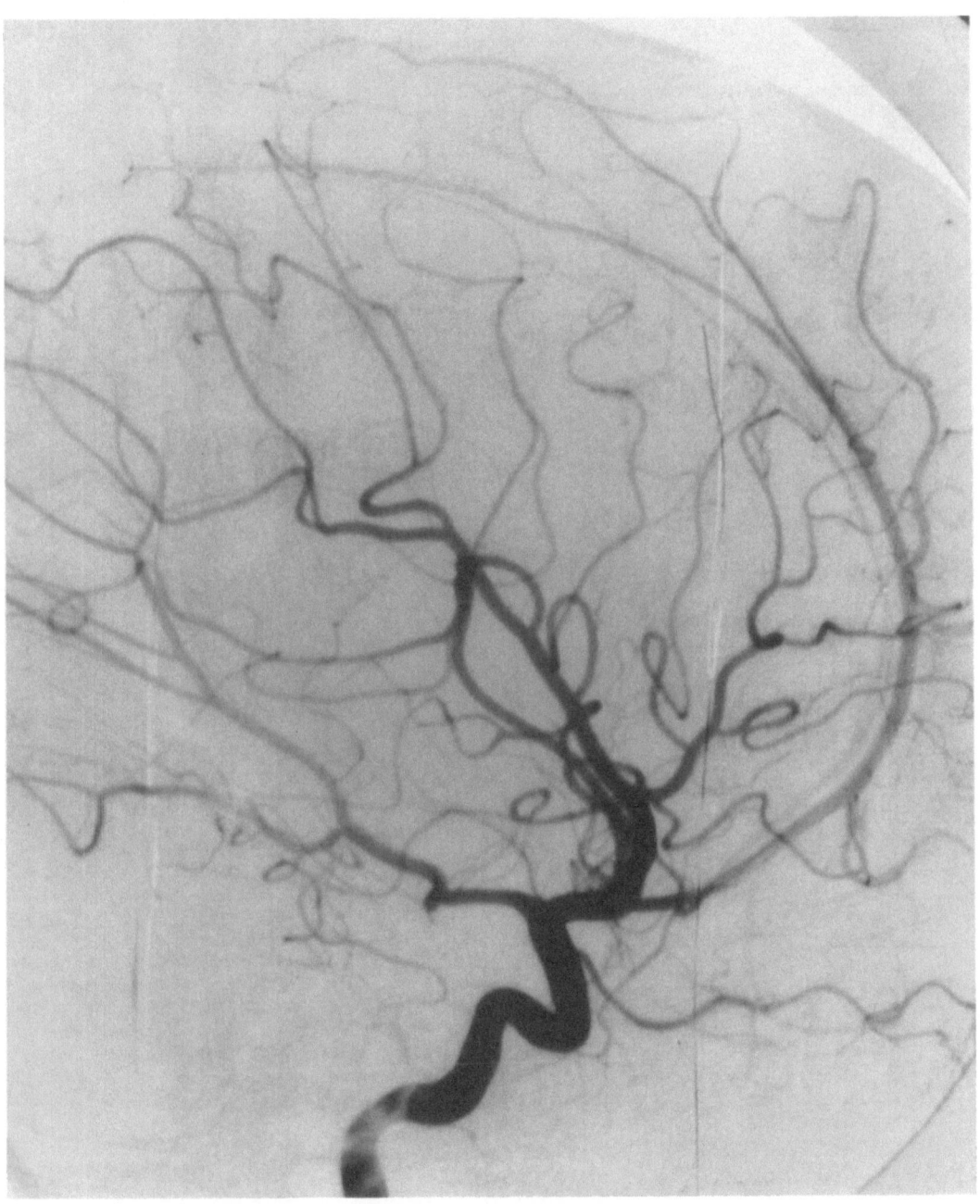

C

Figure 7.12. *Continued.*

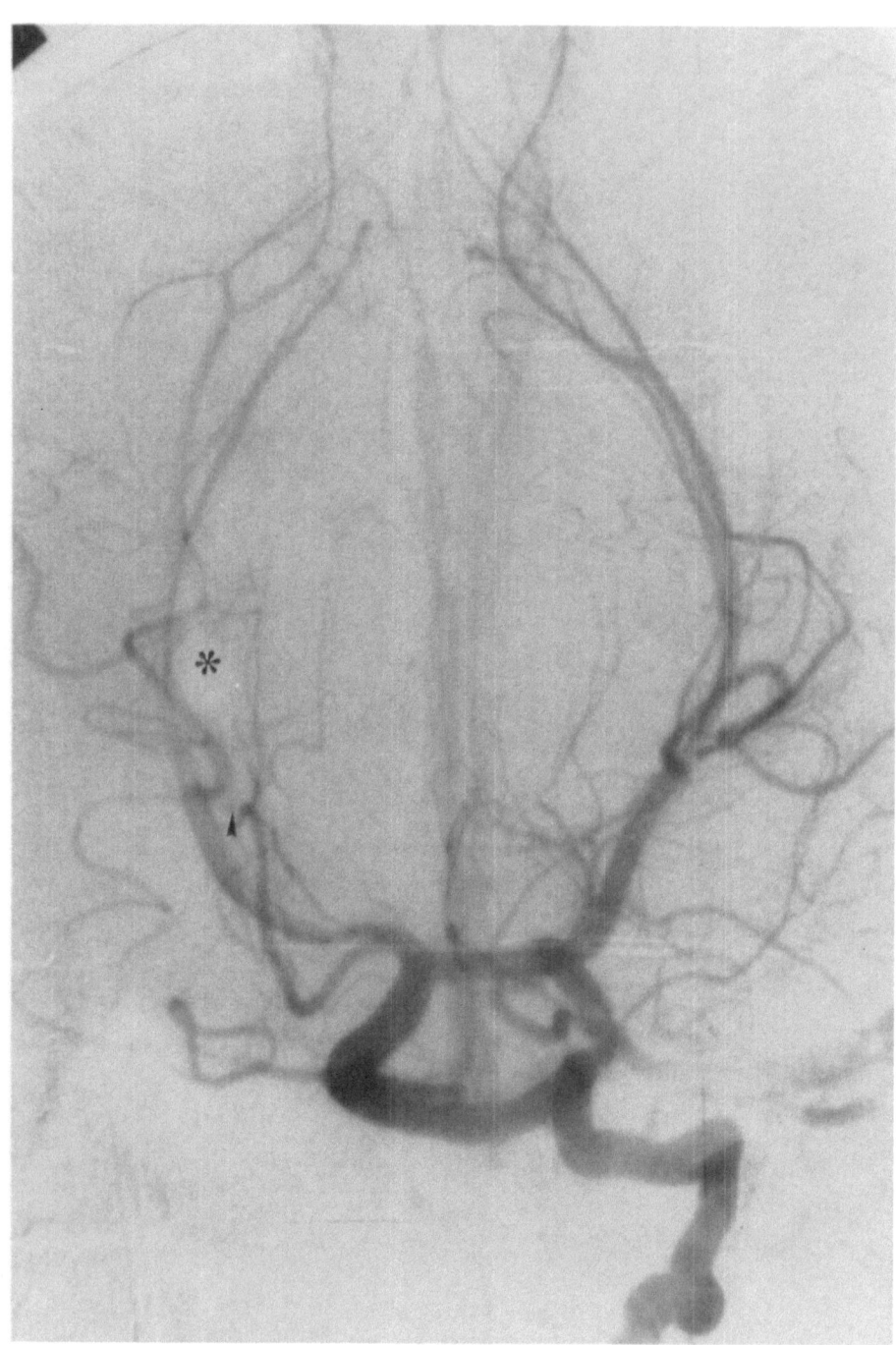

Figure 7.12. *Continued.*

D

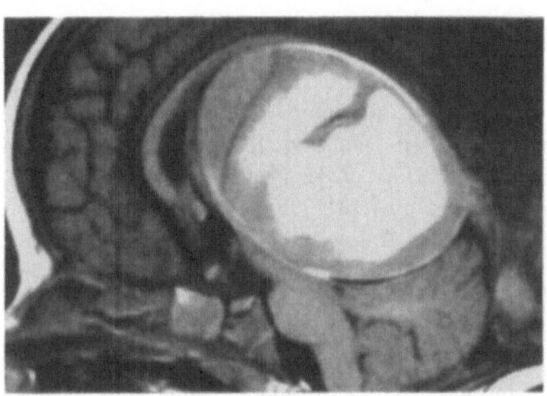 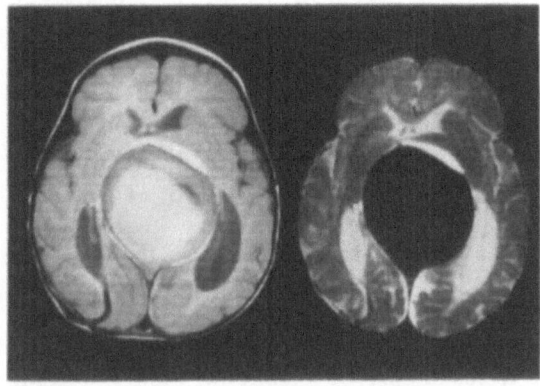

E F

Figure 7.12. *Continued.*

Table 7.8. Endovascular management (1984–1989): anatomic results and morbidity.

| VGAM | 100% by E° | Transient morbidity | | Permanent morbidity |
		Neurological	Nonneurological[a]	
VGF	5	0	2/48	0
VGM	7	0	3/12	0
Total:	12 (43%)	0	5/60 (8%)	0

[a] Transient headaches, urinary infection cases/sessions.

Table 7.9. Endovascular management (1984–1989) clinical results.

VGAM	Clinical cure	Improved	Stable	Total
VGF	6	12	1	19
VGM	4	1	2	7
Total:	10 (36%)	13 (46%)	3 (11%)	26 (93%)

associated CSF disorders (hydrocephalus) as well as the lesion (VGAM) itself.

References

1. Clarisse J, Dobbelaere P, Rey C, D'Hellemmes P, Hassan M: Aneurysms of the great vein of Galen. Radiological–anatomical study of 22 cases. J Neuroradiol 5:91–102, 1978.

2. Diebler C, Dulac O, Renier D, Ernest L, Lalande G: Aneurysms of the vein of Galen in infants aged 2 to 15 months. Diagnosis and natural evolution. Neuroradiology 21:185–197, 1981.

3. Johnston I, Whittle I, Besser M, Morgan M: Vein of Galen malformations: diagnosis and management. Neurosurgery 20(5):747–758, 1987.

4. Hoffman HJ, Chuang S, Hendrick B, Humphreys RP: Aneurysms of the vein of Galen. J Neurosurg 57:316–322, 1982.

5. Lasjaunias P, Rodesch G, Terbrugge K, Pruvost Ph, Devictor D, Comoy J, Landrieu P: Vein of Galen aneurysmal malformations. Report of 36 cases managed between 1982 and 1988. Acta Neurochir 99:26–37, 1989.

6. Maheut J, Santini JJ, Barthez MA, Billard C: Symptomatologie clinique de l'anévrysme de l'ampoule de Galien. Neurochirurgie 33:285–290, 1987.

7. Lasjaunias P, Terbrugge K, Lopez Ibor L, et al.: The role of dural anomalies in vein of Galen aneurysms: report of 6 cases and review of the literature. AJNR 8:185–192, 1987.

8. Raybaud Ch, Hald JK, Strother ChM, Choux M, Jiddane M: Les anévrysmes de la veine de Galien. Etude angiographique et considérations morphogénétiques. Neurochirurgie 33: 302–314, 1987.

9. Lasjaunias P, Rodesch G, Pruvost Ph, Grillot Laroche F, Landrieu P: Treatment of vein of Galen aneurysmal malformation. J Neurosurg 70:746–750, 1989.

10. Yokota A, Oota T, Matsukado Y, Okudera T: Structures and development of the venous system in congenital malformations of the brain. Neuroradiology 16:26–30, 1978.

11. Lasjaunias P, Terbrugge K, Chiu MC: Coaxial balloon-catheter device for treatment of neonate and infants. Radiology 159:269–271, 1986.

12. Mickle JP, Quisling RG: The transtorcular embolization of vein of Galen aneurysms. J Neurosurg 64:731–735, 1986.

13. Berenstein A, Lasjaunias P: Endovascular treatment of brain, spinal cord and spine lesions. In: Surgical Neuroangiography, Vol. 4. Springer-Verlag, New York, 1991.

14. Cumming GR: Circulation in neonates with intracranial arteriovenous fistula and cardiac failure. Am J Cardiol 45:1019–1024, 1980.

15. Stroobandt G, Harmant-Van Rijckevorsel K, Mathurin P, Dends C, De Ville De Goyet J: Hydrocéphalie externe et interne par malformation artério-veineuse chez un nourrisson. Neurochirurgie 32:81–85, 1986.

16. Quisling RG, Mickel JP: Venous pressure measurements in vein of Galen aneurysms. AJNR 10:411–417, 1989.

CHAPTER 8

Cavernous Malformations of the Central Nervous System

K. Stuart Lee and Harold L. Rekate

Introduction

A cavernous malformation or cavernous angioma is one of the four types of vascular malformations of the central nervous system. These lesions have been considered rare in the clinical setting, although they are not uncommon findings at autopsy.[1-3] The availability of magnetic resonance (MR) imaging has increased the number of cavernous malformations that have been diagnosed.[2]

In most series of cavernous malformations, adults greatly outnumber children. However, cavernous malformations do occur in children and have even been reported in neonates.

Epidemiology

Cavernous malformations have been estimated to account for 5 to 15% of all intracranial vascular malformations.[2,4] The incidence of cavernous malformations at autopsy has been quoted at 0.02 to 0.13% of cases, although in an autopsy series of 4069 brains, cavernous malformations were found in 16 brains (0.4%).[3-5]

Most patients with cavernous malformations are between 20 and 50 years old at the time of presentation, although patients at both extremes of life have been reported.[4,6] In a review of 138 cases of histologically verified cavernous malformations published since 1960, Simard et al. documented 28 cases (20%) in patients 19 years of age or younger.[4] Of 28 cases of intracranial cavernous malformations reported by Yamasaki et al. in 1986, 8 (29%) were in the first or second decades of life.[7] Herter et al. reported five cases of children with cavernous malformations and estimated that 25% of patients with cavernous malformations are younger than 18 years old.[8] The series by Rigamonti et al. is somewhat unusual, because 13 of 25 patients with pathologically documented cavernous malformations were in the first two decades of life.[9] In an extensive review of the literature, Gangemi et al. found that 20.6% of cavernous malformations were in patients 18 years of age or less, and only 3.24% of lesions occurred in children in the first year of life.[10]

Ferrante et al. analyzed 46 cases of children with cerebral cavernous malformations and noted two age peaks for presentation of these lesions. Children 1 to 2 years of age accounted for 28% of pediatric cases, and adolescents 14 to 16 years of age accounted for 33% of the cases.[11] Cavernous malformations do not appear to occur preferentially in males or females in either children or adults.[7-9,12]

Most intracranial cavernous malformations are located supratentorially, and it has been estimated that 75% of all cavernous malformations are supratentorial.[5,8] Supratentorial cavernous malformations are most frequently located in the subcortical white matter of the frontal and parietal lobes, the temporal lobes, and the periventricular regions.[5,8,13] Lesions have been reported within the ventricular system and in the pineal region.[8,14,15] Infratentorial cavernous malformations are most often located in the brainstem, and the pons is a common site.[5] Cavernous malformations do occur within the spinal cord, but these intramedullary lesions are rare.[16]

The familial occurrence of cavernous malformations has historically been considered uncommon.[2,4,17,18] However, recent reports indicate that the familial form of the disorder is more frequent than previously recognized and accounts for almost half of all cases of intracranial cavernous malformations.[2,19] The familial form of cavernous malformations is transmitted as an autosomal dominant trait with variable expression and is associated with a high incidence of multiple lesions.[2] The familial form of the disorder has been reported with increased frequency in Mexican–American families.[2,17,19]

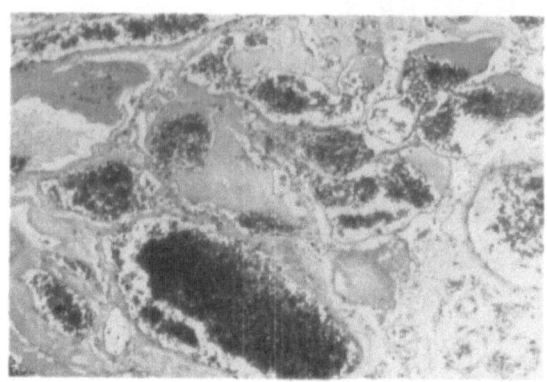

Figure 8.2. Microscopic section of a cavernous malformation demonstrates numerous vascular spaces of various sizes with absence of neural tissue between the vessels.

Pathology

Cavernous malformations have a characteristic gross and microscopic appearance.[1] The lesions vary greatly in size, but most cavernous malformations are 1 to 2 cm in diameter.[1,20] On gross examination, cavernous malformations are red or purple and lobulated and have therefore been likened to a mulberry or raspberry (Fig. 8.1).[1,20] Although cavernous malformations have no discrete capsule, the lesions are well circumscribed from the brain parenchyma by the presence of gliosis surrounding the malformation.[1,4,20] The surrounding brain parenchyma is usually stained yellow and orange from the deposition of hemosiderin from prior hemorrhage.[4,20] Almost all cavernous malformations demonstrate pathologic evidence of

prior hemorrhage (hemosiderin deposition) regardless of signs of overt clinical hemorrhage.[4]

On microscopic examination, a cavernous malformation is formed by numerous vascular spaces that vary in size and have contiguous walls (Fig. 8.2), which are formed by collagen and lined with a single layer of endothelial cells.[4,20,21] Brain parenchyma is not usually found between the vessels.[4,18,20,22] The absence of intervening neural tissue has been described as "a cardinal feature" that helps to differentiate cavernous malformations from capillary telangiectasias.[4] Thrombosis, organization, and calcification are often noted in cavernous malformations.[4,20,22] They do not, however, have abnormally enlarged arterial feeders and usually no enlarged veins.[20,22]

Cavernous malformations are dynamic lesions, and many patients have had documented enlargement of their cavernous malformations on serial imaging studies.[4,7,20,21,23] In the series of Yamasaki et al., for example, 9 of 27 patients were found to have enlarged lesions on serial computed tomography (CT).[7] The exact mechanism for growth of a cavernous malformation is unknown, but the most likely explanation is related to hemorrhage.[4,23] A small hemorrhage may be followed by organization and fibrosis, and even calcification can cause a malformation to enlarge.[4] In rats the polyoma virus can induce lesions similar to cavernous malformations, but they have characteristics of neoplasms.[4,23] Whether the cells of human cavernous mal-

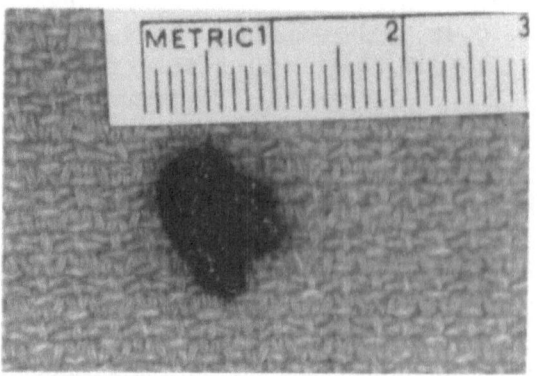

Figure 8.1. Gross specimen removed from the brainstem demonstrates the typical lobulated appearance of a cavernous malformation.

formations proliferate to account for growth of the malformations is not known.[24]

The coexistence of cavernous malformations and capillary telangiectasias in the same patient has been reported on numerous occasions and has led to the hypothesis that these two lesions may represent different stages in the evolution of the same pathological entity.[20,22,23,25,26] The presence of brain parenchyma between vessel walls, a characteristic of capillary telangiectasias, was noted in 61% of surgical specimens of cavernous malformations in one series.[25] The presence of transitional forms between the two lesions and the presence of multiple small lesions that resemble capillary telangiectasias in patients with clinically significant cavernous malformations have also been described.[25]

The association of a cavernous malformation and a venous malformation in the same patient has also been described, and this association is important from a clinical perspective.[27,28] Venous malformations represent anomalous venous drainage from an area of normal brain and have a low incidence of hemorrhage.[28] Therefore, hemorrhage from an adjacent cavernous malformation and venous malformation will most likely be related to the cavernous malformation.[28] Surgical treatment in this situation should be directed at removing the hemorrhage and the cavernous malformation, because removing the venous malformation could result in venous infarction.[28]

Clinical Presentation

The clinical manifestations of cavernous malformations are generally due to seizures, focal neurologic deficits, and hemorrhage.* Seizures are the presenting symptoms in 60 to 70% of patients with cavernous malformations; however, both Rigamonti et al. and Herter et al. noted that only about 50% of children with cavernous malformations have seizures as the initial manifestation.[8,9,22] Progressive or focal neurological deficits (with or without signs of intracranial pressure) are the presenting complaint in approximately 20% of patients with

cavernous malformations.[8,22] The exact number of patients with clinically symptomatic hemorrhage from cavernous malformations is not known but is less than 25%.[22]

Seizures are quite frequent with cavernous malformations, probably because the iron pigment in the hemosiderin deposited by hemorrhages from the malformation is epileptogenic.[31] Patients with seizures related to cavernous malformations often have a long history of a seizure disorder, although seizure frequency or difficulty in controlling the seizures may have increased more recently.[8,13,30] Pozzati et al. have noted that a long history of seizures, especially beginning in childhood and without focal neurological signs, would seem to exclude a surgical lesion as a cause of the seizures; however, a cavernous malformation should be excluded in such cases.[6]

Although pathological evidence of hemorrhage is present in almost all cavernous malformations, a clinically significant hemorrhage is relatively uncommon from cavernous malformations.[4,7,18,22,23,30] However, hemorrhage from these lesions can be fatal or neurologically devastating, depending on the location of the malformation. Recurrent clinical hemorrhages from cavernous malformations have been reported, although the incidence is unknown.[18] The incidence of hemorrhage from cavernous malformations in infants has been estimated to be higher than in older children or adults.[7,8,32]

Cavernous malformations have rarely been reported in very young children.[10] Many of these children presented with head enlargement from either hydrocephalus or cystic enlargement of the cavernous malformation.[10,14,15,33–35] As noted above, hemorrhage from the malformation appears more frequently in young children.[7,8]

The natural history of cavernous malformations remains unknown because they are relatively rare.[4,23] Numerous lesions found at autopsy were apparently asymptomatic during life.[3] An increasing number of incidental lesions have been diagnosed since the advent of MR imaging, particularly in family members of patients with the familial form of cavernous malformations.[2]

---

* See refs 4, 7–9, 12, 18, 21–23, 26, 29, 30.

Imaging Studies in the Evaluation of Cavernous Malformations

Skull X-rays may show calcification in cases of cavernous malformations, but this is obviously a nonspecific finding.[8,36] Cranial ultrasound may help detect hemorrhage from cavernous malformations in young children, but these lesions have no specific ultrasound characteristics.[8]

Arteriography may be normal in as many as 40% of cases of cavernous malformations.[37] Abnormalities that can be identified on arteriography include an avascular area, mass effect, mild capillary blush, or an occasional early draining vein.[36,37] None of these findings is specific for cavernous malformations and may occur with other vascular lesions or neoplasms. The lack of arterial supply, slowness of the circulation, and thrombosis of vascular channels in cavernous malformations can all contribute to the lack of angiographic visualization of these lesions.[18,37]

There are no pathognomonic features of cavernous malformations on CT scanning; however, CT scanning has greatly improved the ability to detect these malformations.[37] The most frequent CT finding is an area of increased density on a noncontrast scan without significant mass effect.[30,36,37] There is usually minimal enhancement of the lesion after the administration of intravenous contrast.

MR imaging has become the imaging modality of choice to evaluate a patient with a cavernous malformation (Fig. 8.3).[2,16,23,36] MR imaging is more sensitive than CT scanning for detecting lesions, which have a specific appearance on MR imaging.[36] On T1-weighted imaging, larger cavernous malformations appear as reticulated areas of mixed signal intensity; on T2-weighted imaging, these lesions have a prominent rim of surrounding decreased signal intensity that represents hemosiderin deposition around the lesion.[22,36] Smaller lesions appear in areas of decreased signal intensity on both T1- and T2-weighted imaging.[36] T2-weighted imaging is more sensitive for detecting lesions than T1-weighted imaging.[36]

MR imaging is particularly useful in the evaluation of patients with cavernous malformations of the brainstem and spinal cord and in the screening of relatives of patients with suspected familial cavernous malformations (Fig. 8.4).[2,16,19]

Treatment of Cavernous Malformations

The treatment of cavernous malformations must be related to the circumstances of each case, since the natural history of these malformations is poorly understood.[4,22,23] Several authors have recommended surgical excision for all surgically accessible cavernous malformations to prevent subsequent hemorrhage.[10,18,21] However, the increased number of incidental lesions that have been discovered with the availability of MR imaging warrants a more conservative approach, because many of these malformations can be treated conservatively provided there is clinical and radiographic follow-up.[7,22,23]

At our institution, the indications for surgery for a cavernous malformation are seizures that are poorly controlled medically, a single hemorrhage from a lesion in an accessible location, progressive neurological dysfunction related to a lesion, enlargement of the cavernous malformation on serial imaging studies, or multiple hemorrhages from a malformation even in a deep but surgically approachable location.

Surgery for cavernous malformations is greatly facilitated because the lesions are surrounded by a plane of gliotic tissue and are therefore well circumscribed.[5,8,9,12,16,18,21,30] The lack of arterial feeders and slow circulation within the malformation usually makes it possible to control intraoperative hemorrhage from a cavernous malformation.[5]

The role of radiation therapy in the treatment of cavernous malformations is unclear.[7,23] Although radiation therapy has been used, it was ineffective in at least some cases.[18] Stereotactic radiosurgery might prove beneficial in highly selected cases of small, deep cavernous malformations.

To a great extent, the prognosis after surgical removal of a cavernous malformation depends on the location of the malformation. Excellent

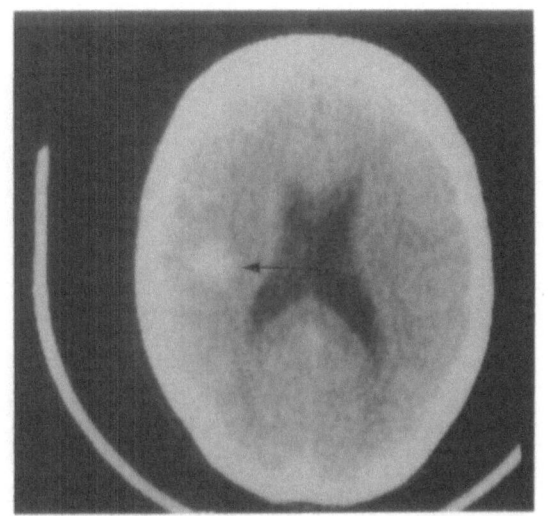

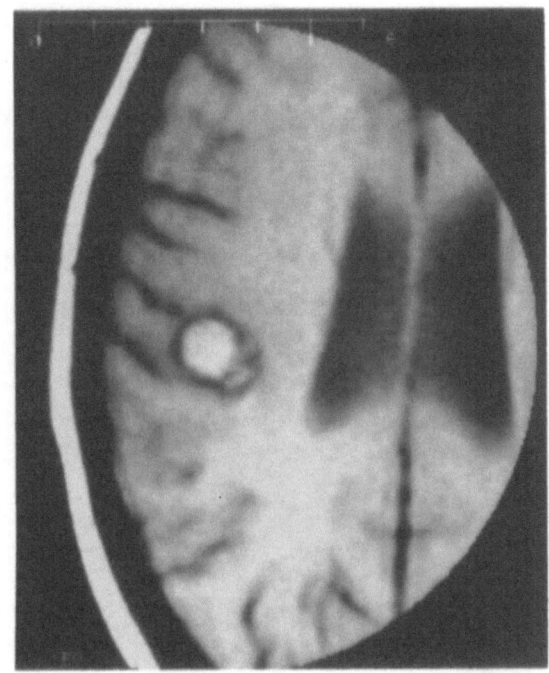

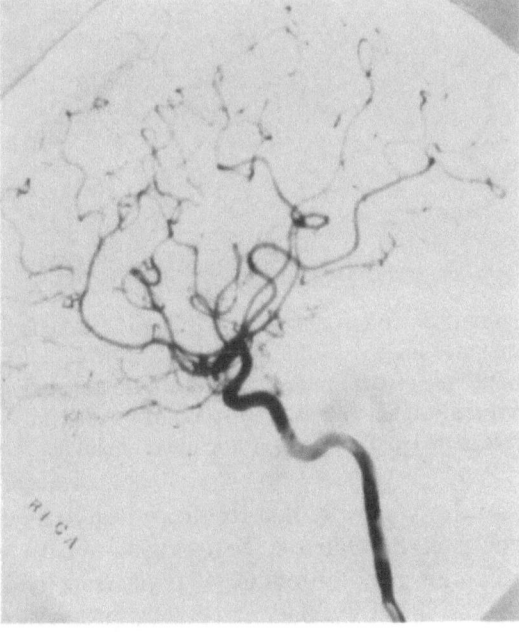

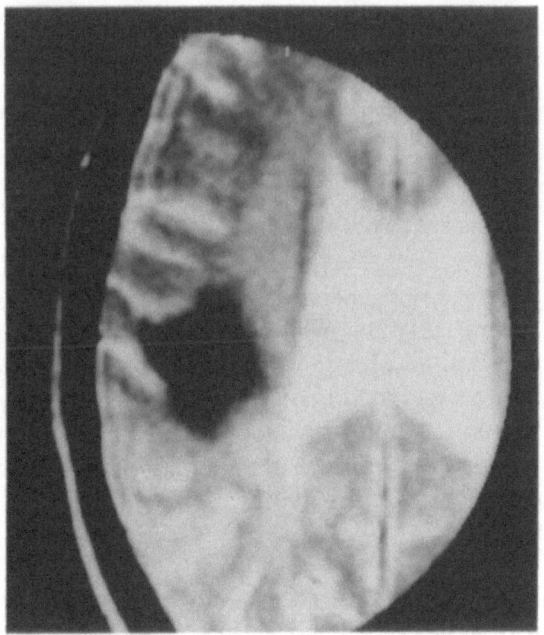

Figure 8.3. Multiple imaging studies of a patient with a right parietal cavernous malformation. (**A**) Non-contrast computerized tomography scan demonstrates a hyperdense mass. (**B**) Cerebral arteriography is normal. (**C**) T1 weighted magnetic resonance (MR) image (TR 750 msec, TE 20 msec) demonstrates an area of mixed signal intensity, and (**D**) a T2-weighted MR image (TR 1800 msec, TE 80 msec) demonstrates a prominent area of decreased signal intensity due to hemosiderin deposition.

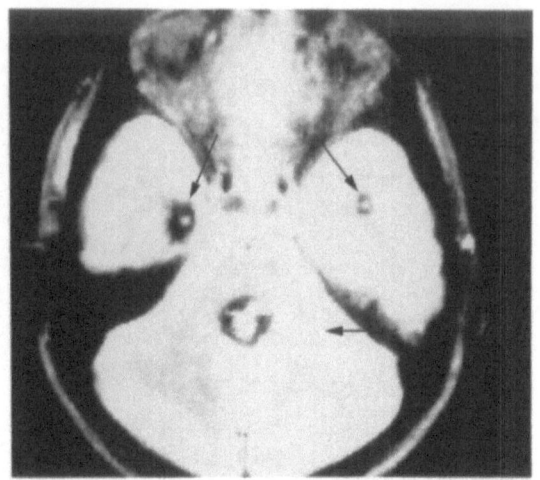

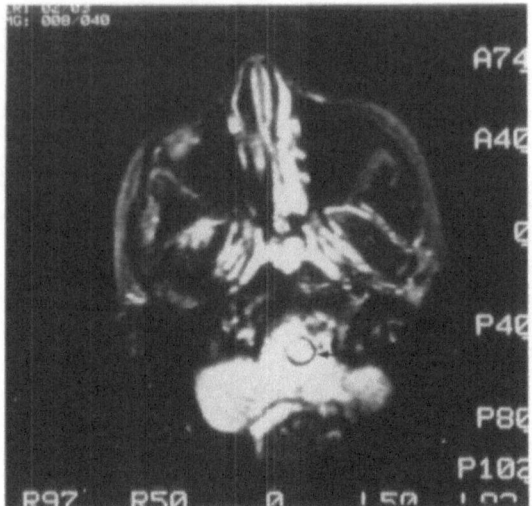

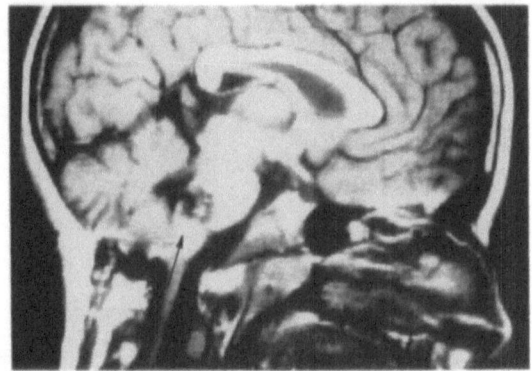

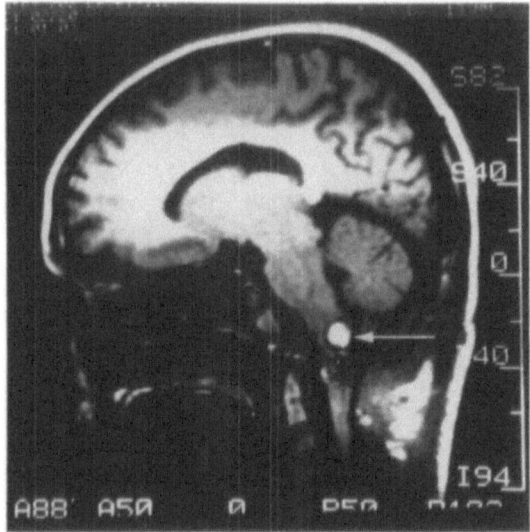

Figure 8.4. (A) Axial and (B) sagittal magnetic resonance images of a 14-year-old patient who had suffered multiple brainstem hemorrhages demonstrate a large cavernous malformation in the medulla and smaller lesions in both temporal lobes.

results are generally obtained with more superficial lesions, while outcome is poorer with deeply situated lesions.[30] Control of seizures in patients operated upon for epilepsy is typically excellent; up to 90% of patients have been reported to be seizure free after removal of their cavernous malformation.[23]

Experience with Cavernous Malformations in Children at the Barrow Neurological Institute

Between 1969 and June 1989, 19 (11 females and 8 males) patients in the first and second decades of life underwent surgical removal of 21

Figure 8.5. (A) Axial and (B) sagittal magnetic resonance images at the time of the patient's initial symptoms of hemiparesis demonstrate an area of increased signal intensity surrounded by a rim of decreased signal intensity in the lower medulla.

cavernous malformations of the central nervous system at the Barrow Neurological Institute. Presenting symptoms of the 19 patients included seizures in seven patients (37%), progressive focal neurological symptoms in six (32%), hemorrhage in four (21%), and symptoms of increased intracranial pressure in one (5%). One patient (5%) was asymptomatic and had a positive family history of massive hemorrhages related to cavernous malformations. A screening

after apparent total resection of the lesion and required another operation (Figs. 8.5 and 8.6).

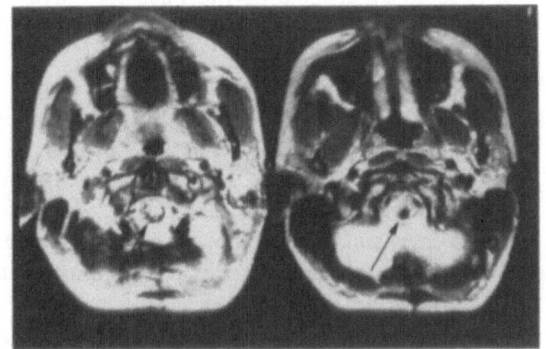

A

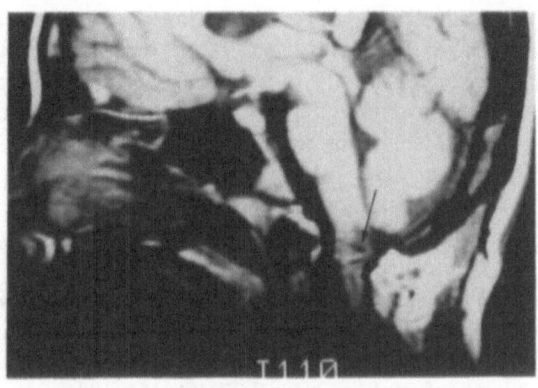

B

Figure 8.6. (A) Axial and (B) sagittal magnetic resonance images obtained when the patient's symptoms recurred 2 years postoperatively demonstrate an area of mixed signal intensity in the lower medulla. Enlargement of this area was noted on serial studies, and a recurrent cavernous malformation was removed.

MR image demonstrated a large frontal cavernous malformation with evidence of old hemorrhage.

Of the 21 surgically excised lesions, 8 were located in the frontal lobe, 4 in the parietal lobe, 2 in the temporal lobe, 1 in the pineal region, 3 in the cerebellum, 2 in the brainstem, and 1 in the spinal cord.

All patients did well following surgery. Only one patient had an increased neurologic deficit postoperatively. This deficit, transient diplopia, occurred in one of the patients with a cavernous malformation of the brainstem. All patients who were operated upon for seizures that had been difficult to control were markedly improved postoperatively. One patient with a cavernous malformation of the lower medulla had recurrence of her cavernous malformation 2 years

References

1. McCormick WF: Pathology of vascular malformations of the brain. In: Wilson CB, Stein BM (eds.), Intracranial Arteriovenous Malformations. Williams & Wilkins, Baltimore, 1984, pp. 44–63.
2. Rigamonti D, Hadley MN, Drayer BP, Johnson PC, Hoenig-Rigamonti K, Knight JT, Spetzler RF: Cerebral cavernous malformations. Incidence and familial occurrence. N Engl J Med 319:343–347, 1988.
3. Sarwar M, McCormick WF: Intracerebral venous angioma. Case report and review. Arch Neurol 35:323–325, 1978.
4. Simard JM, Garcia-Bengochea F, Ballinger WE Jr, Mickle JP, Quisling RG: Cavernous angioma: a review of 126 collected and 12 new clinical cases. Neurosurgery 18:162–167, 1986.
5. Martin NA, Wilson CB, Stein BM: Venous and cavernous malformations. In: Wilson CB, Stein BM (eds.), Intracranial Arteriovenous Malformations. Williams & Wilkins, Baltimore, 1984, pp. 234–245.
6. Pozzati E, Padovani R, Morrone B, Finizio F, Gaist G: Cerebral cavernous angiomas in children. J Neurosurg 53:826–832, 1980.
7. Yamasaki T, Handa H, Yamashita J, Paine JT, Tashiro Y, Uno A, Ishikawa M, Asato R: Intracranial and orbital cavernous angiomas: a review of 30 cases. J Neurosurg 64:197–208, 1986.
8. Herter T, Brandt M, Szüwart U: Cavernous hemangiomas in children. Child's Nerv Syst 4:123–127, 1988.
9. Rigamonti D, Rekate H, Pittman H, Spetzler RF: Cavernous malformations (angiomas) in children. J Pediatr Neurosci 4:55–59, 1988.
10. Gangemi M, Longatti P, Maiuri F, Cinalli G, Carteri A: Cerebral cavernous angiomas in the first year of life. Neurosurgery 25:465–469, 1989.
11. Ferrante L, Mastronardi L, D'Adetta R, Acqui M, Fortuna A: Cerebral cavernous angioma in children (abstract). Child's Nerv Syst 4:167, 1988.
12. Tagle P, Huete I, Méndez J, Del Villar S: Intracranial cavernous angioma: presentation and management. J Neurosurg 64:720–723, 1986.
13. Pozzati E, Galassi E, Giulianai G: Cerebral cavernous angiomas in children. Study of 13 treated cases (abstract). Child's Nerv Syst 4:167, 1988.

14. Iwasa H, Indei I, Sato F: Intraventricular cavernous hemangioma. Case report. J Neurosurg 59:153–157, 1983.

15. Sonntag VKH, Waggener JD, Kaplan AM: Surgical removal of a hemangioma of the pineal region in a 4-week-old infant. Neurosurgery 8:586–588, 1981.

16. McCormick PC, Michelsen WJ, Post KD, Carmel PW, Stein BM: Cavernous malformations of the spinal cord. Neurosurgery 23:459–463, 1988.

17. Bicknell JM, Carlow TJ, Kornfeld M, Stovring J, Turner P: Familial cavernous angiomas. Arch Neurol 35:746–749, 1978.

18. Giombini S, Morello G: Cavernous angiomas of the brain. Account of fourteen personal cases and review of the literature. Acta Neurochir 40:61–82, 1978.

19. Bicknell JM: Familial cavernous angioma of the brain stem dominantly inherited in Hispanics. Neurosurgery 24:102–105, 1989.

20. Russell DS, Rubinstein LJ: Pathology of tumours of the nervous system. Williams & Wilkins, Baltimore, 1989, pp. 730–736.

21. Voigt K, Yasargil MG: Cerebral cavernous haemangiomas or cavernomas. Incidence, pathology, localization, diagnosis, clinical features and treatment. Review of the literature and report of an unusual case. Neurochirurgia 19:59–68, 1976.

22. Rigamonti D, Spetzler RF, Johnson PC, Drayer BP, Carter LP, Uede T: Cerebral vascular malformation. Barrow Neurol Inst Q 3(3):18–28, 1987.

23. Farmer J-P, Cosgrove GR, Villemure J-G, Meagher-Villemure K, Tampieri D, Melanson D: Intracerebral cavernous angiomas. Neurology 38:1699–1704, 1988.

24. Fischer EG, Sotrel A, Welch K: Cerebral hemangioma with glial neoplasia (angioglioma?). Report of two cases. J Neurosurg 56:430–434, 1982.

25. Rigamonti D, Johnson PC, Drayer BP, Spetzler RF: Cavernous malformation and capillary telangiectases: two facets of the same pathological entity (abstract). J Neuropathol Exp Neurol 46:401, 1987.

26. Vaquero J, Leunda G, Martinez R, Bravo G: Cavernomas of the brain. Neurosurgery 12:208–210, 1983.

27. Goldberg HI, Grossman RI, Levine RS, Zimmerman RA: Association of venous and cavernous angiomas (abstract). AJNR 6:465, 1985.

28. Rigamonti D, Spetzler RF: The association of venous and cavernous malformations. Report of four cases and discussion of the pathophysiological, diagnostic, and therapeutic implications. Acta Neurochir 92:100–105, 1988.

29. Schneider RC, Liss L: Cavernous hemangiomas of the cerebral hemispheres. J Neurosurg 15:392–399, 1958.

30. Vaquero J, Salazar J, Martínez R, Martínez P, Bravo G: Cavernomas of the central nervous system: clinical syndromes, CT scan diagnosis, and prognosis after surgical treatment in 25 cases. Acta Neurochir 85:29–33, 1987.

31. Steiger HJ, Markwalder TM, Reulen HJ: Clinicopathological relations of cerebral cavernous angiomas: observations in eleven cases. Neurosurgery 21:879–884, 1987.

32. Yamasaki T, Handa H, Yamashita J, Moritake K, Nagasawa S: Intracranial cavernous angioma angiographically mimicking venous angioma in an infant. Surg Neurol 22:461–466, 1984.

33. Jain KK: Intraventricular cavernous hemangioma of the lateral ventricle. Case report. J Neurosurg 24:762–764, 1966.

34. Khosla VK, Banerjee AK, Mathuriya SN, Mehta S: Giant cystic cavernoma in a child. Case report. J Neurosurg 60:1297–1299, 1984.

35. Moritake K, Handa H, Nozaki K, Tomiwa K: Tentorial cavernous angioma with calcification in a neonate. Neurosurgery 16:207–211, 1985.

36. Rigamonti D, Drayer BP, Johnson PC, Hadley MN, Zabramski J, Spetzler RF: The MRI appearance of cavernous malformations (angioma). J Neurosurg 67:518–524, 1987.

37. Savoiardo M, Strada L, Passerini A: Intracranial cavernous hemangiomas: neuroradiologic review of 36 operated cases. AJNR 4:945–950, 1983.

CHAPTER 9

Carotid-Cavernous Fistulas

Gabriel Lena, Lorenzo Genitori, and Philippe Farnarier

Introduction

Carotid-cavernous fistula (CCF) is usually a rare complication of severe head injury. The incidence is less than 1%,[1] even in large series, and 72 to 75% are of posttraumatic origin.[1,2] Few series of CCFs were published and the great majority of cases concern adult patients.[3-7] Multiple sporadic cases were published, explaining probably the multiplicity of techniques used to treat these lesions. The details of four cases occurring in young children have been reported. The youngest was 7 weeks old with a spontaneous external CCF,[8] the other three were, respectively, 2.5[9] and 7 years of age.[10,11] Uncommonly, they were bilateral and in 1980 West[2] found, in analyzing the case of an 8-year-old boy with a bilateral CCF due to severe head injury, only 29 cases; among these two were children, 14 and 15 years old, respectively. Personally, we observed six cases in children during the last 12 years; four cases were of posttraumatic origin and two cases were spontaneous. The clinical data of these cases are described in Table 9.1.

Anatomy

Since Winslow first named the cavernous sinus in 1732, several and sometimes conflicting descriptions of this sinus have been proposed.[6,12-15] As had been suggested by Taptas,[14] Parkinson[6] came to the conclusion that the cavernous sinus is a venous plexus incompletely surrounding the internal carotid artery with various sizes of veins dividing and anastomosing with each other. For Harris and Rhoton[12] the cavernous sinus is an unbroken trabeculated venous channel with no plexus of veins. More recently, Rhoton et al.[13] described three major venous spaces located posterosuperior, medial, and anteroinferior to the intracavernous portion of the carotid artery. The intracavernous carotid artery divides into five branches: the meningohypophyseal artery, the inferior sinus artery, the McCornell's capsular arteries, the ophthalmic artery, and the dorsal meningeal artery, respectively, present in 100, 84, 28, 8, and 6% of cadavers.

Pathophysiology

There are two types of carotid-cavernous fistulas: The most usual are of posttraumatic origin. Generally, a wound of the carotid wall by a bullet or a basilar fracture[6] of the sphenoid bone or the petrous apex produce the lesion. A direct puncture through the orbit has also been described (Nélaton, quoted by Hamby[4]). Traumatic fistulas can be due likewise to tearing of the carotid artery and/or one or more of its intracavernous branches.[13] Usually, the wall of the carotid artery is partially disrupted, but a case of complete transection of the intracavernous carotid artery has also been published.[16] According to Parkinson[6] there are two types of posttraumatic fistulas: In type 1, there is a hole in the carotid artery itself, and in type 2, one of the cavernous sinus branches is torn, resulting in two arterial openings.

CCFs may also be spontaneous, of which two types are described.[17] The first is secondary to rupture of a weakened internal carotid artery

Table 9.1. Clinical data of our series.[a]

Case number	Age (years), sex	Etiology	Clinical manifestation	Angiogram	Treatment	Result
1	11, M	Posttrauma	Exophthalmos, oculomotor palsies, unilateral blindness	EC and IC fistula	Balloon occlusion	Recurrence
2	4, M	Spontaneous	Exophthalmos	EC fistula	Particle embolization	Good
3	16, M	Spontaneous	Exophthalmos	EC fistula	Particle embolization + surgery	Excellent
4	4, M	Posttrauma (bullet)	Moderate exophthalmos, unilateral blindness	IC fistula	No treatment	Good
5	13, M	Posttrauma	Drowsiness, hemiparesis	IC fistula + EDH	Trapping	Excellent
6	13, M	Posttrauma	Bilateral exophthalmos, oculomotor palsies	IC fistula	Balloon occlusion	Excellent

[a] EC, Exrernal carotid artery; IC, internal carotid artery; EDH, epidural hematoma.

wall in the area of the cavernous sinus; this weakness can be congenital or acquired. Intracavernous aneurysm,[18] syphilis,[19] fibromuscular dysplasia,[20] Ehlers–Danlos syndrome,[21] atherosclerosis,[22] and persistent primitive trigeminal artery[23–26] have been reported as causes of spontaneous CCFs, but these pathological associations are usually observed in adult patients. Bilateral spontaneous CCFs are very rare and only 10 cases have been reported,[4,17–19,21,22,27–29] but the youngest is 18 years old. The second, which is the more frequent type, is also encountered in children. This is characterized by a dural arteriovenous fistula involving the cavernous sinus. Several pediatric cases have been described.[7,8,30]

Signs and Symptoms

Usually, the diagnosis is late, the clinical manifestations coming on gradually in weeks or months; but, in one series[31] slightly less than half of the cases were recognized as early as 24 hr after injury. In one of our cases, the diagnosis was made from an emergency angiogram performed for an epidural hematoma. Unilateral headaches are rare but may be the first symptom. Exophthalmos is the most usual sign, frequently associated with an intracranial retroorbital or frontotemporal bruit, this latter found in most pediatric patients[30] presumably because children are disposed to high-flow lesions. Although the objective bruit is important, it may not be perceived by the child as an abnormality if it has been present since birth.[30] Clinical examination reveals a venous dilatation on the eyelid generally associated with chemosis. A thrill may be palpable, and orbital auscultation reveals a permanent bruit with a systolic reinforcement that decreases or disappears with carotid compression. Oculomotor nerves in the cavernous sinus may be involved, so diplopia is common. Less frequently vagus nerve damage produces facial pain or corneal hypoesthesia. Some authors[7,32] have proposed that venous occlusive factors are responsible for the cranial nerve manifestations in cases of spontaneous carotid sinus dural arteriovenous malformations (AVMs). Other authors[30] suggest that cranial nerve involvement in this location may be due to dural arterial "steal" mechanism or both mechanisms. A mechanical phenomenon may also be responsible for the pseudoextraocular motor palsies in cases of cavernous dural AVMs draining into the orbital venous system. In such cases, proptosis and muscle tension could be the causes of diplopia and poor movements of the eyeball. The optic nerve can be stretched by a major exophthalmia or compressed by huge ophthalmic veins, leading to loss of visual acuity. Visual failure may be due to retinal ischemia,[33] or to the development of cataracts, vitreous opacities, or glaucoma.[34] Lasjaunias,[30] analyz-

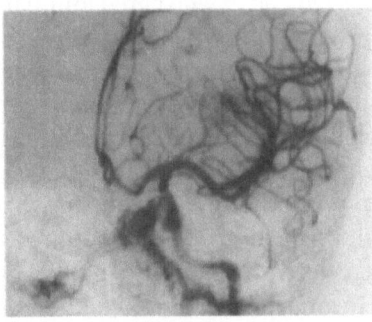

A

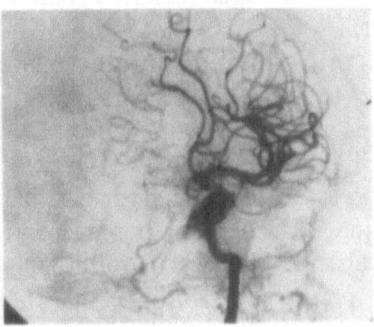

B

Figure 9.1. Case 5: (A) Internal carotid angiogram showing the direct CCFs and displacement of anterior cerebral artery. (B) Oblique view showing the frontal epidural hematoma (arrowhead).

ing 36 cases of cavernous sinus dural AVMs from the literature precised the respective incidence of the major symptoms: proptosis (83%), bruit (42%), visual deficits (28%), peripheral nervous system deficits (44%), and focal nervous system symptoms (3%). The clinical symptoms of our cases are unremarkable (exophthalmos, oculomotor palsies), except in one case: a 13-year-old boy admitted per emergency with hemiparesis, which developed several hours after suffering a traumatic head injury. A carotid angiogram was performed and showed a frontal epidural hematoma and a CCF (Fig. 9.1). The epidural hematoma was evacuated and the fistula was treated with Hamby's procedure. The follow-up was uneventful.

The natural history of CCFs is variable: a spontaneous cure by thrombosis of the fistula is a rare eventuality. This was observed in 5 to 10% of the cases.[19,35,36] Indeed, a cerebral ischemia due to a steal phenomenon may occur.[37]

The patient may die of an uncontrollable hemorrhage. Hamby,[4] analyzing 322 cases, reported that 9 patients died as a result of hemorrhage, 6 from fatal epistaxis, and 3 from intracerebral hemorrhage. Other authors have mentioned this hemorrhagic complication just as subarachnoid hemorrhage.[35,38-43] The pathophysiology of the hemorrhage consists of a high pressure in the dilated veins, particularly the pontomesencephalic and the peduncular veins, which are situated between the cavernous sinus and the vein of Galen.[44]

Finally, the patient may continue with the lesion and its consequences if the fistula is not treated or treated unsuccessfully.

Diagnosis

Usually, the diagnosis of CCF is easy to establish, particularly when the fistula is of posttraumatic origin. Sometimes, at the initial phase the diagnosis may be difficult when frontoorbital edema obstructs the local examination. Orbital and temporal auscultation with and without carotid compression is an important and mandatory diagnostic maneuver. The diagnosis of spontaneous fistulas may be more difficult, particularly when the clinical symptoms are mild. Nevertheless, a precise and complete diagnosis requires selective, and sometimes supraselective, angiography. It is necessary to study the exact anatomy of the fistula, and the anatomical variations, particularly of the circle of Willis. An external carotid angiogram can reveal smaller dural arteries feeding the shunt from branches of the maxillary artery, ascending pharyngeal artery, and middle meningeal artery. All these elements are essential to plan the best treatment.

Treatment

There is a great variety of therapeutic methods to treat CCFs. The goal of treatment is to preserve the patency of the carotid artery and to exclude the fistula. Even if 10% of low shunt flow fistulas close spontaneously after angiography,[4,20,35,36,45] or after intermittent compression of the carotid artery,[22] the great majority of CCF fistulas require some form of intervention.

Historically, the first therapeutic attempt was the ligature of the carotid artery, but the mortality was about 10%; the morbidity included extensive thrombosis, "steal" syndromes or transient ischemic attack. Most important, cures were obtained in only 25 to 30% of the cases.[46,47]

Trapping procedures were introduced by Hamby and Gardner in 1932. This technique consists of ligation of both the proximal and distal portions of the carotid artery, performed on the more symptomatic side. Hamby[4] mentions 94% success, Echols and Jackson[35] only 50%. Trapping associated with embolization allows the cure of the fistulas in 98% of the cases (Jaeger, cited by Hosobuchi[5]). Also, Eguchi et al.[27] used the Hamby procedure associated with a bilateral extraintracranial bypass. But all these methods involve the sacrifice of the carotid blood flow, with the risk of mortality and morbidity.

Surgical repair with the aim to preserve the carotid artery was initiated by Parkinson,[6] but this method requires profound hypothermia, circulatory bypass, and cardiac arrest.

More recently, some authors have simplified the surgical approach to the cavernous sinus, using microtechniques. Direct repair with a combination of three approaches (pterional, subtemporal, and the exposure of the intrapetrous carotid artery) is the method of

choice for Dolenc,[48] who cured four patients. He uses this method in low-risk groups and young patients. Another direct approach, packing the cavernous sinus with particles such as muscle or fibrin sealant[49] and oxidized cellulose[50] is also used. Thrombosis of the cavernous sinus may also be produced by introducing hemostatic material through a venous pathway[40] or by inducing electrothrombosis[5] of the cavernous sinus. Hosobuchi cured five children among 80 CCFs; all of these children did well after treatment.

Until the publication of Serbinenko's balloon catheter technique,[51] which reports successful results in over 95% of the cases, the treatment of CCFs was essentially surgical. Recent advances in catheter and detachable balloon techniques[3,7,52] make it possible to obliterate the fistulas; nevertheless, carotid patency is not always preserved: Debrun et al.[3] indicate 53 successful occlusions of the fistula in 54 cases, but the carotid artery was occluded in 21 cases (41%); Vinuela et al.[7] observed 2 complications, but 1 transitory and 2 failures among 20 cases.

In our series, two children underwent detachable balloon techniques, but a recurrence was observed in 1 case with an external carotid and internal carotid cavernous sinus fistula. The other one (Fig. 9.2) is neurologically intact and the carotid artery blood flow preserved. Two children with spontaneous external carotid

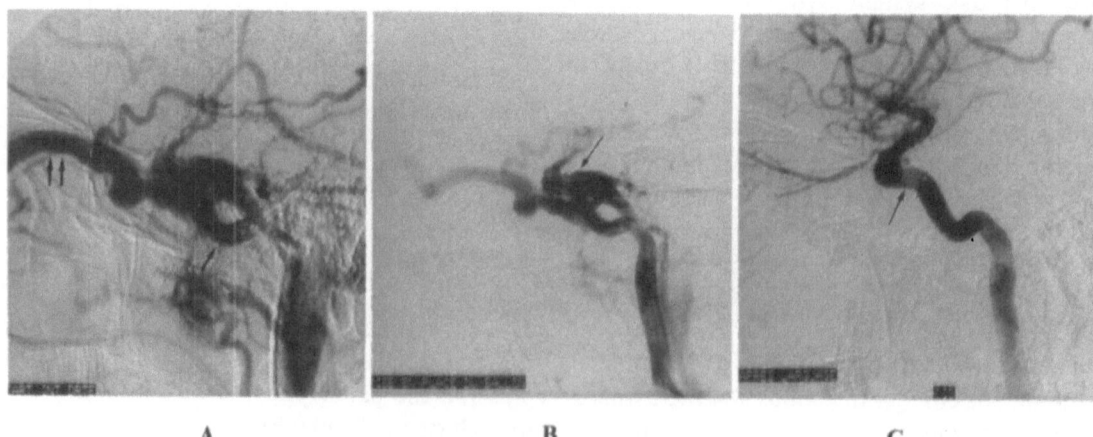

A   B   C

Figure 9.2. Case 6: (A) Internal carotid angiogram showing high-flow fistula. Simple arrow: internal carotid artery; double arrow: superior ophthalmic vein; large arrow: superior petrosal sinus. (B) During the embolization the balloon (arrow) is taking place. (C) At the end of embolization, the balloon (arrow) is inflated and the patency of carotid artery preserved.

cavernous sinus fistulas were treated by embolization with particles, and one also by surgical resection of the dural AVMs. The results were excellent. One case was treated by an entrapment procedure that was successful, and one young child with a moderate exophthalmos was not treated.

References

1. Vigouroux RP, Baurand C, Guillermain P, Reynier Y, Gomez A, Lena G, Vincentelli F, Gondim-Oliveira J: Traumatismes cranio-encephaliques. Encycl Méd Chir Paris Neurol 17785:A10,A15,A20, 1982.
2. West CGH: Bilateral carotid-cavernous fistulae: a review. Surg Neurol 13:85–90, 1980.
3. Debrun G, Lacour P, Vinuela F, Fox A, Drake CG, Caron IP: Treatment of 54 traumatic carotid-cavernous fistulas. J Neurosurg 55:678–692, 1981.
4. Hamby WB: Carotid-cavernous fistula. Charles C Thomas, Springfield, IL, 1966.
5. Hosobuchi Y: Electrothrombosis of carotid-cavernous fistula. J Neurosurg 42:76–85, 1976.
6. Parkinson D: A surgical approach to the cavernous portion of the carotid artery. Anatomical studies and case report. J Neurosurg 23:474–483, 1965.
7. Vinuela F, Fox AJ, Debrun G, et al: Spontaneous carotid-cavernous fistulas: clinical, radiological and therapeutic considerations. J Neurosurg 60:976–984, 1984.
8. Pang D, Kerber C, Biglan AW, et al: External carotid-cavernous fistula in infancy: case report and review of the literature. Neurosurgery 8:212–218, 1981.
9. Broughton WL, Gee W, Doppman J, et al: Nonpulsatile exophthalmos in carotid-cavernous sinus fistula. J Pediatr Ophthalmol 14:221–224, 1977.
10. Agnetti V, Pav A, Pinna L: Cerebral pseudo-angiomatous pattern in a case of carotid-cavernous fistula. J Neurosurg Sci 18:75–79, 1974.
11. Arseni C, Horvath L, Ciurea V, Simionescu N: Carotid-cavernous fistula in a child. Rev Roum Med Neurol Psych 16:29–32, 1978.
12. Harris FS, Rhoton AL Jr: Anatomy of the cavernous sinus. A microsurgical study. J Neurosurg 45:169–180, 1976.
13. Rhoton AL Jr, Harris FS, Renn WH: Microsurgical anatomy of the sellar region and the cavernous sinus. Clin Neurosurg 24:54–85, 1977.
14. Taptas JN: La loge du sinus caverneux: sa constitution et les rapports des élements vasculaires et nerveux qui la traversent. Sem Hop Paris 25:1719–1722, 1949.
15. Umansky F, Nathan H: The lateral wall of the cavernous sinus. With special reference to the nerves related to it. J Neurosurg 56:228–234, 1982.
16. Sbeih I and O'Laoire SA: Traumatic carotid-cavernous fistula due to transection of the intracavernous carotid artery. J Neurosurg 60:1080–1084, 1984.
17. Yamamoto I, Wanabe T, Shinoda M, Hasegawa Y, Sato O: Bilateral spontaneous carotid-cavernous fistulas treated by the detachable balloon technique: case report. Neurosurgery 17:469–473, 1985.
18. Poppen JL: Specific treatment of intracranial aneurysms: experiences with 143 treated patients. J Neurosurg 8:75–102, 1951.
19. Dandy WE: Carotid-cavernous aneurysms (pulsating exophthalmos). Zentralbl Neurochir 2:77–114, 1937.
20. Hieshima GB, Cahan LD, Mehringer CM, Bentson JR: Spontaneous arteriovenous fistulas of cerebral vessels in association with fibromuscular dysplasia. Neurosurgery 18:454–458, 1986.
21. Schoolman A, Kepes JJ: Bilateral spontaneous carotid-cavernous fistulae in Ehlers–Danlos syndrome. J Neurosurg 26:82–86, 1967.
22. Stolpmann E: Doppelseitige nicht-traumatische Carotis-Sinus-cavernosus-Fistel. Albrecht von Graefes Arch Klin Exp Ophthalmol 185:83–94, 1972.
23. Berger MS, Hosobuchi Y: Cavernous sinus fistula caused by rupture of a persistent primitive trigeminal artery. Case report. J Neurosurg 61:391–395, 1984.
24. Eadie MJ, Jamieson KG, Lennon EA: Persisting carotid-basilar anastomosis. J Neurol Sci 1:501–511, 1964.
25. Enomoto T, Sato A, Maki Y: Carotid-cavernous sinus fistula caused by rupture of a primitive trigeminal artery aneurysm. Case report. J Neurosurg 46:373–376, 1977.
26. Kerber CW and Manke W: Trigeminal artery to cavernous sinus fistula treted by balloon occlusion. J Neurosurg 58:611–613, 1963.
27. Eguchi T, Mayanagi Y, Hanamura T, Tanaka H, Ohmori K, Takakura K: Treatment of bilateral spontaneous carotid-cavernous fistula by Hamby's method combined with an extracranial-intracranial bypass procedure. Neurosurgery 11:706–711, 1981.

28. Rainer A, Haselbach H: Bedsetige spontane carotia-Sinus-cavernosus-Fistel. Laryngol Rhinol 54:163–168, 1975.

29. Voigt K, Sauer M, Dichgans J: Spontaneous occlusion of a bilateral carotidocavernous fistula studied by serial angiography. Neuroradiology 2:207–211, 1971.

30. Lasjaunias P, Chiu M, Terbrugge K, Tolia A, Hurth M, Bernstein M: Neurological manifestations of intracranial dural arteriovenous malformations. J Neurosurg 64:724–730, 1986.

31. Henderson JW, Schneider RC: The ocular findings in carotid-cavernous fistula in a series of 17 cases. Trans Am Ophthalmol Soc 56:123–141, 1958.

32. Brismar J, Lasjaunias P: Arterial supply of carotid-cavernous fistulas. Acta Radio (Diagn) 19:897–904, 1978.

33. Sanders MD, Hoyt WF: Hypoxic ocular sequelae of carotid-cavernous fistulae. Study of the causes of visual failure before and after neurosurgical treatment in a series of 25 cases. Br J Ophthalmol 53:82–97, 1969.

34. Biglan AW, Hiles DA: The visual results following infantile glaucoma surgery. J Pediatr Ophthalmol Strabismus 16:377–381, 1979.

35. Echols DH, Jackson JD: Carotid-cavernous fistula: a perplexing problem. J Neurosurg 16:619–627, 1959.

36. Speakman TJ: Internal occlusion of carotid-cavernous fistula. J Neurosurg 21:303–305, 1964.

37. Day AL, Rhoton AL Jr: Aneurysms and arteriovenous fistulae of the intracavernous carotid artery and its branches. In: Youmans JR (ed.), Neurological Surgery. W. B. Saunders, Philadelphia, 1982, pp. 1764–1785.

38. Ambler MW, Moon AC, Sturner WQ: Bilateral carotid-cavernous fistulae of mixed types with unusual radiological and neuropathological findings: Case report. J Neurosurg 48:117–124, 1978.

39. Dohrmann PJ, Batjer HH, Samson D, Suss RA: Recurrent subarachnoid hemorrhage complicating a traumatic carotid-cavernous fistula. Neurosurgery 17:480–483, 1985.

40. Mullan S: Treatment of carotid-cavernous fistula by cavernous sinus occlusion. J Neurosurg 50:131–144, 1979.

41. O'Reilly GV, Shillito J, Haykal HA, Kleefield J, Wang A-M, Rumbaugh C: Balloon occlusion of a recurrent carotid-cavernous fistula previousy treated by carotid ligations. Neurosurgery 19:643–648, 1986.

42. Sedzimir CB, Occleshaw JV: Treatment of carotid-cavernous fistula by muscle embolisation and Jaeger's maneuver. J Neurosurg 27:309–314, 1967.

43. Turner DM, Van Gilder JC, Mojahedi S, Pierson EW: Spontaneous intracerebral hematoma in carotid-cavernous fistula: report of three cases. J Neurosurg 59:680–686, 1983.

44. Matsushima T, Rhoton AL Jr, de Oliveira E, Peace D: Microsurgical anatomy of the veins of the posterior fossa. J Neurosurg 59:63–105, 1983.

45. El Gindi S, Andrew J: Successful closure of carotid-cavernous fistula by the use of acrylic. Case report. J Neurosurg 27:153–156, 1967.

46. Arutiunov AL, Serbinenko FA, Sklykov AA: Surgical treatment of carotid-cavernous fistulas. Prog Brain Res 30:441–444, 1968.

47. Rey A, Cophignon J, Thurel C, Djindjian R, Houdart R: Traitement des fistules carotido-caverneuses. Neurochirurgie 19:111–122, 1973.

48. Dolenc V: Direct microsurgical repair of intracavernous vascular lesions. J Neurosurg 58:824–831, 1983.

49. Isamat F, Ferrer E, Twose J: Direct intracavernous obliteration of high-flow carotid-cavernous fistulas. J Neurosurg 65:770–775, 1986.

50. Albert P, Polaina M, Trujillo F, Romero J: Direct carotid sinus approach to treatment of bilateral carotid-cavernous fistulas. Case report. J Neurosurg 69:942–944, 1988.

51. Serbinenko SA: Balloon catheterization and occlusion of major cerebral vessels. J Neurosurg 41:125–145, 1974.

52. Halbach VV, Higashida RT, Hieshima GB, Hardin CW, Pribam H: Transvenous embolization of dural fistulas involving the cavernous sinus. AJNR 10:377–383, 1989.

CHAPTER 10

Intracranial Aneurysms in Children

Maurice Choux, Gabriel Lena, and Lorenzo Genitori

The discovery of an intracranial aneurysm in children is a rare occurrence. The incidence of aneurysms in the pediatric population varies from 0.5% for Patel and Richardson[1] to 3.1% for Ostergaard and Voldby[2] (Table 10.1)[1-6] Matson,[7] in 1964, presented the first series of 15 cases of pediatric aneurysms. Following this only a few series were published. They are summarized in Table 10.2.[1,2,4-28] Recently, we have collected 448 cases from the literature, including 21 cases observed in the Department of Pediatric Neurosurgery in Marseilles. In this material, 316 cases are presumably of multifactorial origin, 32 are traumatic, and 48 are of mycotic origin. We studied (separately) 52 giant aneurysms, which raise different surgical problems.

Cerebral Berry Aneurysms

Among 316 cases of childhood cerebral berry aneurysms in the literature, it has been possible for us to review in detail 177 cases, including 13 personal cases.

Age

The majority (54.5%) are seen after 10 years of age and only 17.4% occurred in infants. Rare cases of neonatal aneurysms have been published.[29-31] Most of them were giant aneurysms. A 42-mm embryo with a basilar artery aneurysm was reported by Bremer[32] in 1943. Lipper et al.,[29] in 1978, collected 19 cases of so-called congenital saccular aneurysms in the first year of life. Since this publication, we have found nine other cases in the literature. In our personal series we have seen a neonate who presented with an intracerebral and intraventricular hemorrhage with a secondary hydrocephalus. A shunt was performed at the age of 1 month. A computerized tomography (CT) scan done 1 year later showed a huge aneurysm of the right internal carotid artery. It was clear that the initial hemorrhage originated from the ignored congenital aneurysm (Fig. 10.1a and b).

Sex

In all the series, boys present more frequently (60.5%). The male preponderance in most of the

Table 10.1. Incidence of aneurysms in children and adolescents.

Authors	Ref.	Number of aneurysms	Number of pediatric aneurysms
Locksley (1966)	3	6368	41 < 19 years (0.6%)
Patel and Richardson (1971)	1	3000	16 < 15 years (0.5%)
Ostergaard and Voldby (1983)	2	1368	43 < 19 years (3.1%)
Pasqualin et al. (1986)	4	1461	38 < 20 years (2.6%) < 15 years (1.2%)
Meyer et al. (1989)	5	1387	23 < 18 years (1.6%) < 12 years (1%)
Heiskanen (1989)	6	1346	16 < 20 years (1.2%)

Table 10.2. Series of aneurysms in childhood and adolescents.

Authors	Ref.	Number	Age (years)
McDonald and Korb (1939)	8	34	<15
Krayenbuhl and Yazargil (1959)	9	6	<15
Laitinen (1964)	10	9	<15
Taveras and Wood (1964)	11	4	<15
Lapras et al. (1964)	12	4	<15
Matson (1969)	7	15	<17
Patel and Richardson (1971)	1	58	<20
Suwanwela et al. (1972)	13	4	<15
Sedzimir and Robinson (1973)	14	50	<16
Thompson and Pribam (1973)	15	22	<16
Kunk (1974)	16	7	<15
Almeida et al. (1977)	17	11	<15
Sano et al. (1978)	18	3	<15
Becker et al. (1978)	19	14	<2
Amacher and Drake (1979)	20	32	<18
Arseni et al. (1980)	21	11	<15
Gerosa et al. (1980)	22	15	<15
Visudiphian et al. (1980)	23	5	<15
Granieri et al. (1980)	24	3	<15
Storrs et al. (1982)	25	29	<15
Schauseil-Zipf et al. (1983)	26	15	<18
Ostergaard and Voldby (1983)	2	43	<19
Hourihan et al. (1984)	27	87	<20
Mazza (1984)		15	<15
Pasqualin et al. (1986)	4	38	<20
Gutierez et al. (1987)	28	14	<16
Heiskanen (1989)	6	16	<20
Meyer et al. (1989)	5	23	<18
Choux and Lena (1990)		21	<15

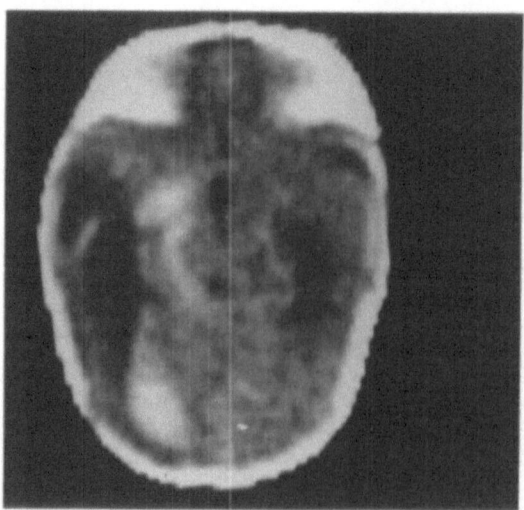
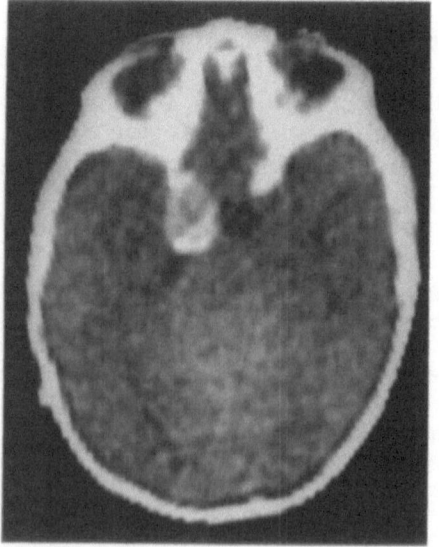

Figure 10.1. (A) CT scan of a neonate presenting with an intracerebral and intraventricular hemorrhage. **(B)** CT scan control at the age of 1 year in this shunted child, showing a huge right internal carotid aneurysm.

pediatric series is notable: see Matson[7] (12:1), Thompson and Pribam[15] (2.5:1), Amacher and Drake[20] (2:1), and Roche et al.[33] (3:1).

Clinical Presentation

Clinical presentation is unremarkable and mostly similar to adult series. A subarachnoid hemorrhage occurs in 80% of the cases. It is isolated in 40% or associated with coma (24.5%), mass effect (22.5%), or seizures (3%).

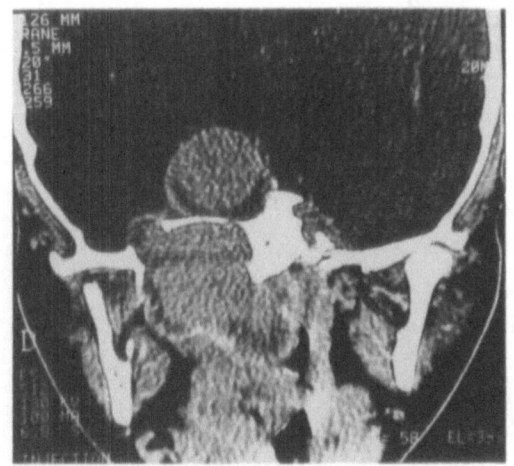

A

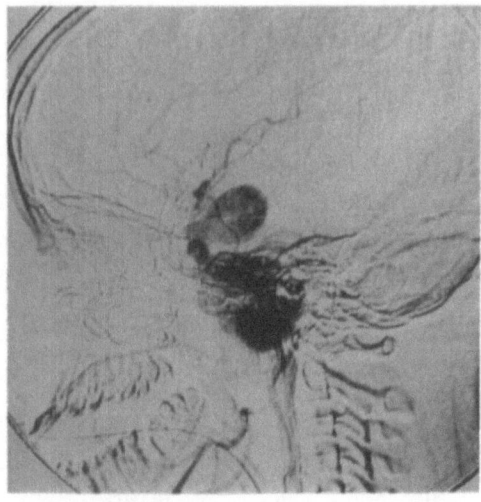

B

Figure 10.2. (**A**) Cerebral CT scan in a 14-year-old girl, previously treated for multiple aneurysms in the arms and legs. (**B**) The angiography shows the topography and extension of a polyglobular aneurysm of the internal carotid artery.

Only in three cases were seizures the initial symptom. Hydrocephalus was present five times, and three times it was the presenting symptom. Unusual initial symptoms, such as diabetes insipidus[34] or an exophthalmos,[35] may be present.

Associated with congenital malformations such as coarctation of the aorta (7.5%), polycystic disease of the kidneys (three cases), hyperplasia of the renal arteries, and even agenesis of the corpus callosum have been reported in the literature.[1,7,36–38] Childhood aneurysms may also be associated with such other diseases as collagen vascular disease, fibromuscular dysplasia, Ehlers–Danlos syndrome, Marfan syndrome, moyamoya disease, syphilis, or tuberous sclerosis.[39–43]

In one of our cases, a 14-year-old girl was operated on twice for multiple aneurysms localized in the arms and the legs. A routine angiographic study of the intracerebral circulation demonstrated a giant polyglobular aneurysm of the right internal carotid artery. The girl is now totally asymptomatic (Fig. 10.2a and b).

Topographical Distribution (Table 10.3)

One hundred and fifty-five (86.5%) were on the anterior circulation and 24 (13.5%) on the posterior circulation. In adult series only 5% are on the posterior system.[44] The large number of posterior circulation aneurysms in children is evident in all the series: see Amacher and Drake[20] (59%), Storrs et al.[25] (35%), Meyer et al.[5] (46%) and Roche et al.[33] (26%).

Some authors emphasize the preferential location to be at the internal carotid artery (ICA) bifurcation in children: see Pasqualin et al.[4] (37%), Patel and Richardson[1] (34%), Storr et al.[25] (31%), and Almeida et al.[17] (54%). On the contrary, our study finds a preferential location on the ICA, MCA, ACoA, and ICA bifurcation, in this order.

In this study, 175 aneurysms were single and 5 were multiple. Kojima,[45] in a series of 59 patients with multiple cerebral aneurysms (17%, among 356 patients with intracranial aneurysms) found 10 cases (2.8%) with more than one aneurysm on the same artery. Only one was a child. Multiple aneurysms are mostly associated

Table 10.3. Anatomical distribution of aneurysms in children.[a]

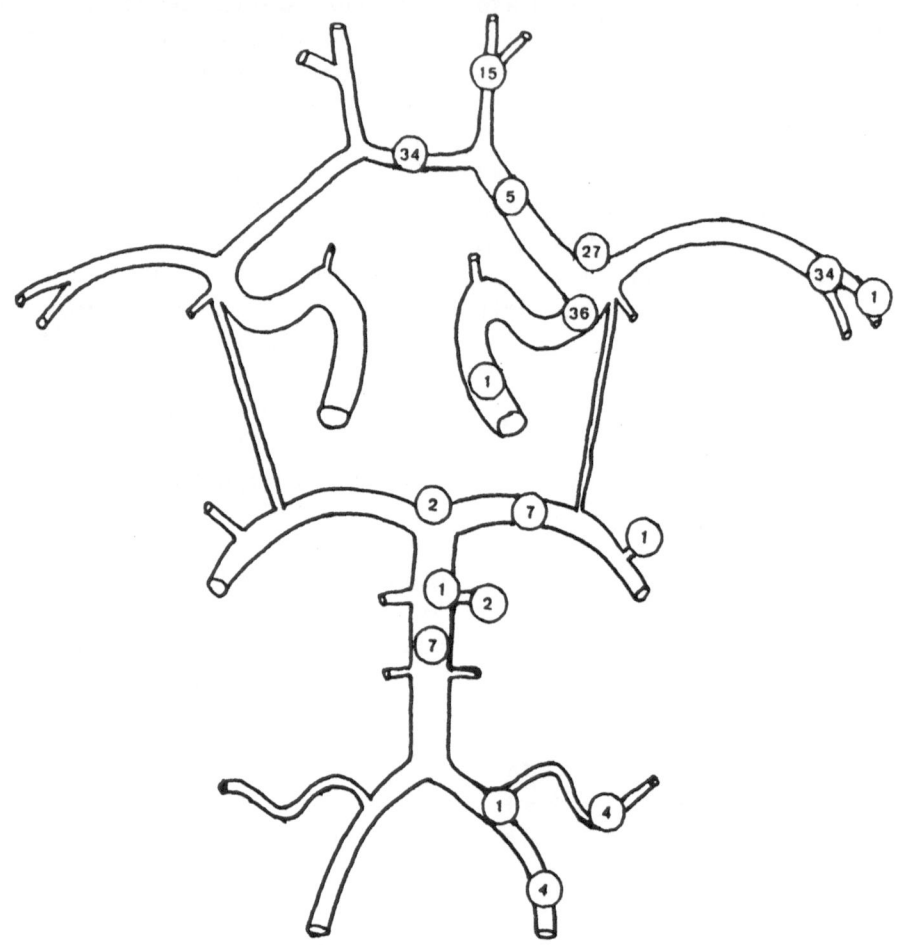

[a] In 182 cases of the literature.

Table 10.4. Results in 10 pediatric series.

Series[a]	Ref.	Normal	Minor sequeline	Severe handicap	Death
Matson (14)	7	7 (53.8%)	1	3	3 (23%)
Amacher and Drake (32)	20	21 (67%)	3	1	7 (22.5%)
Almeida et al. (11)	17	7 (70%)	1	1	2
Storr et al. (21)	25	9 (42.8%)	4	3	5 (23.8%)
Roche et al. (43)	33	27 (63.5%)	9	2	5 (12.2%)
Humphreys et al. (35)	48	15 (49%)	0	6	14 (40%)
Pasqualin et al. (38)	4	28 (73%)	1	1	8 (21%)
Gutierrez et al. (12)	28	6 (50%)		3	3 (25%)
Meyer et al. (24)	5	21 (87%)	1	1	1 (4%)
Choux and Lena (21)		12 (57%)	3	2	4 (19%)

[a] Number of parentheses indicate number of cases in series.

with systemic diseases. Cedzich et al.[46] have recently published the rare case of an 11-month-old boy with multiple middle cerebral artery aneurysms without systemic disease. An arteriovenous malformation was associated with an aneurysm in six cases.[21,24,26,30,39,47]

Management

Surgery was performed 130 times. In the good-risk group (107 cases) the surgical mortality was confined to 6.5%. In the bad-risk group (23 cases), 8 children had a good result, 6 are disabled, and 11 died. In the nonsurgical group (38 cases), 32 children in grade 4 or 5 died, 3 are alive, and 2 are disabled. The results of surgery in children are better than in adults, except for children in grade 4 or 5, where the mortality rate remains high. The results in 10 pediatric series are described in Table 10.4.[4,5,7,17,20,25,28,33,48]

Vasospasm in children appears earlier and, especially, has a better prognosis than in adults. Ostergaard and Voldby[2] find vasospasm in 53% of children who have had angiography in the first 3 days.

Giant Cerebral Aneurysms

In series covering all age groups, giant aneurysms represent around 5% of the cases. Some authors find a high proportion: 7.4%[49] or 13%.[50] In the pediatric age group the usual rate is higher, around 20%. Hacker, reviewing 500 cases of patients under the age of 20, found giant aneurysms in 20% of the cases.[51]

In our literature review study of nearly 300 cases in children under the age of 15, the proportion of giant aneurysms is 18%. Humphreys et al.[48] observed a higher proportion: 28.5%. Ten of the 18 aneurysms in the Gutierrez et al.[28] series were giant aneurysms.

In a recent study[52] we reviewed the literature, collecting 47 cases of giant aneurysms in children younger than 16 years. It is notable that 19.5% were discovered in patients under 1 year of age. In the adult population 60% of giant aneurysms are found in females.[44] On the contrary, in children, boys represent 62%. Signs

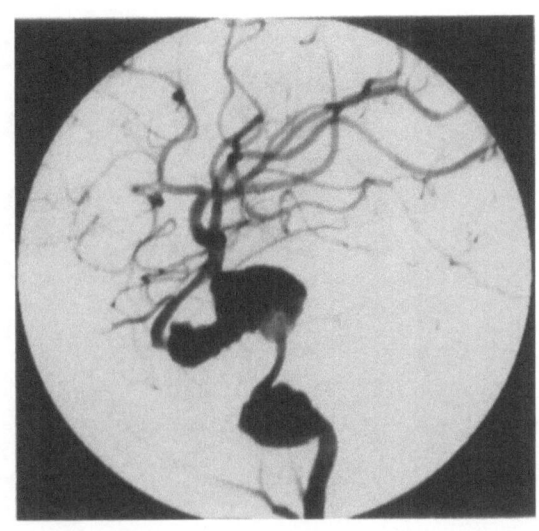

Figure 10.3. Angiogram in a 14-year-old boy presenting with a unilateral complete oculomotor deficit. A giant aneurysm of the internal carotid artery fills the cavernous sinus.

of subarachnoid hemorrhage are observed in 80% of the cases. Mass effect (brainstem compression, motor deficit, oculomotor palsy) is present in 44% of the cases. In one of our cases, a 14-year-old boy, with a giant aneurysm of the internal carotid artery, was discovered after a unilateral complete oculomotor deficit (Fig. 10.3).

In this series of 47 cases, hydrocephalus was found in 6 cases and 5 were infants. In four cases the aneurysm was totally asymptomatic and discovered incidentally on CT scan. It is interesting to mention that in one of our cases a rupture of a huge aneurysm of a middle cerebral artery was diagnosed after a severe head trauma. This 8-year-old girl presented with severe mental retardation since birth (Fig. 10.4).

Studying the localization, there is a clear difference between adult series of giant aneurysms, where the anterior system is much more affected, and the pediatric series, where, as Hacker[51] said, "there is approximately an equal distribution between the anterior and the posterior system." In this series of 51 cases, giant aneurysms in the anterior system represent 56% of the cases. Especially in young infants, giant

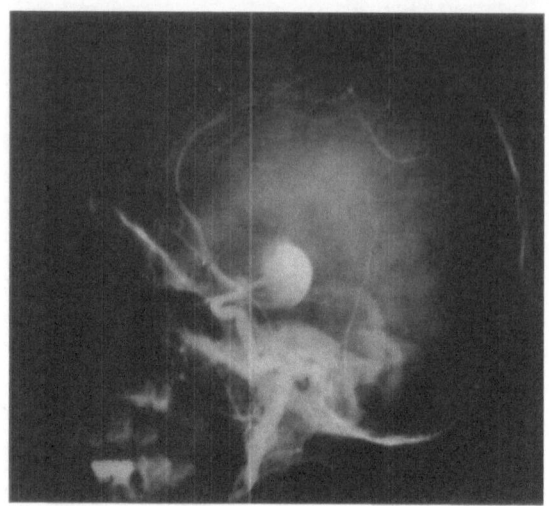

Figure 10.4. In an 8-year-old girl, severely handicapped, a rupture of a giant aneurysm of the middle cerebral artery was found after a severe head trauma.

aneurysms may be very large. Ventureyra et al.[53] reported one of the largest, 8 × 9 cm in size, in a 6-month-old infant, at the level of the posterior cerebral artery. Macrocephalus and anemia were the main clinical signs.

The surgical management of giant aneurysms remains variable because many procedures are described, such as clipping [especially for aneurysms of the MCA and PCA (posterior carotid artery)], ligature of the CA (for aneurysms of the infraclinoidal ICA), and occlusive balloon. We must note that in the literature, clipping of the neck represents only 29.5% of the cases.

In this report of the literature the results are totally different in relation to the surgical or the nonsurgical groups. In the surgical group, which represents 37 children, 73% had an excellent result, 2 were severely disabled, 3 moderately disabled, and 5 died (14%). In the nonsurgical group of 12 children, 11 (who were high risk cases) died.

Traumatic Aneurysms

Traumatic aneurysms represent a small percentage in all the series of aneurysms. We have collected 32 cases of traumatic aneurysms in children among 102 cases in the literature. Approximately 10% of pediatric aneurysms are of traumatic origin.

Histology. Histologically, there are two types:
1. In *true traumatic aneurysms* the normal structures of the arterial wall are disrupted, leaving only an intact layer of adventia.
2. In *false traumatic aneurysms* there is a fibrous organization of a hematoma that forms the aneurysm.

Pathogenesis. The pathogenesis of these aneurysms is controversial. In closed head injury (78%) the arterial wall is damaged by the mass movement of the brain, the edge of the falx to the ACA (anterior carotid artery) or their branches,[54] the free edge of the tentorium to the PCA,[55] the sphenoidal edge to the MCA. In cases of depressed fractures, bone fragments may injure the arterial wall directly. In penetrating wounds,[54] the damage of the wall results from direct injury, as aneurysms developing after puncture of a subdural hematoma.[56]

In one personal case, a 3-year-old boy presented with a large parietal fracture after a mild head trauma. A CT scan showed a vascular lesion on the convexity and an angiogram visualized a small aneurysm of a branch of the middle cerebral artery, underlying the fracture (Fig. 10.5).

Age. Age distribution does not show a significant peak of frequency, but it is interesting to note that 28% of cases in the literature concern children under the age of 2 years. Boys are much more of a concern than girls (78%).

Topographical Distribution. Considering now the topographical distribution, 90.5% are on the anterior system and mainly on the ACAs or their branches. Only four cases were on the ICA (two cases are giant aneurysms) and one case was on the intracavernous portion of ICA.

Treatment. Although spontaneous disappearance of a posttraumatic aneurysm has been reported,[57] surgical treatment seems logical. Burton et al.[55] report a mortality of 54% and Asari et al.[54] report of 32%. In most of the series the mortality and morbidity were closely related to the severity of the underlying cerebral lesions.

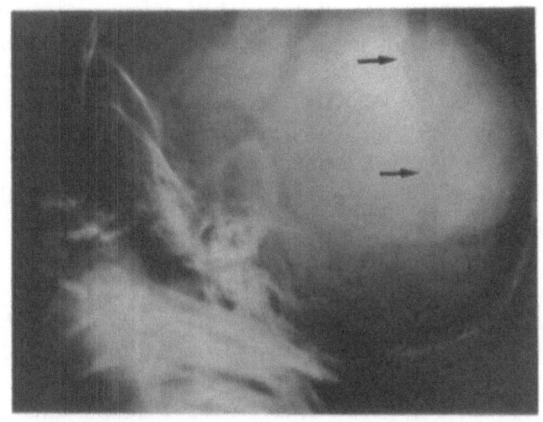

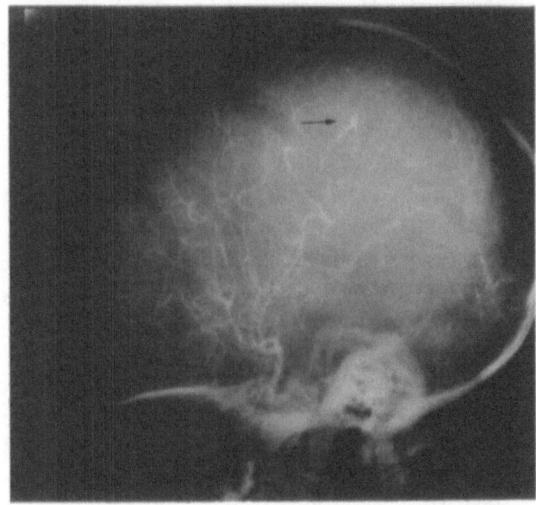

Figure 10.5. In a 3-year-old boy, after a mild head trauma, X-rays (top) show a large parietal diastatic fracture. Secondary manifestations of meningeal hemorrhage led to an angiogram (bottom) that visualized a small traumatic aneurysm of a branch of the middle cerebral artery (arrow).

Infectious Aneurysms

The frequency of these type of aneurysms is the most variable, from 4 to 34%, of all intracranial aneurysms. Though much more frequent in the older literature, their frequency in more recent publications is between 2.5 and 6%.[58]

Pathogenesis. Infectious aneurysms must be further separated into *bacterial aneurysms*, which result from bacterial infection, and true *mycotic aneurysms*, which originate from fungal infection.[58] This last type is exceptional. We reviewed 49 infectious aneurysms in the literature, but only 25 may be studied in detail.

Age and Sex. The age distribution is variable: 3 cases up to 2 years old, 7 between 2 and 5 years, 12 between 5 and 10 years, and 4 up to 15 years; 60% concern boys.

Organism. Staphylococcus (11 cases) has been the commonest organism isolated. The other organisms encountered were as follows: one *Streptococcus*, one collibacillus, one *Diplococcus pneumoniae*, and one candidiasis. No organism was detected in the remaining 11 cases.

Localization. Thirty-one aneurysms were found in 26 patients, (multiple aneurysms in 4 patients). Aneurysms were on the branches of the MCA in five cases and on the branches of the ACA in two cases. We have found 14 aneurysms on the iCaCA (intracavernous carotid artery); 2 were bilateral. Rarely they were located on the posterior system.

Treatment. Conservative treatment with prolonged antibiotic therapy has been used in 15 cases. Three aneurysms disappeared on sequential angiography. A secondary thrombosis of the ICA was observed in four cases with one death. Five children died without angiographic control.

Carotid ligation (four cases) or progressive clamp (one case) for aneurysms on the iCaCA or the ICA gave four excellent results and one child was disabled. Three direct approaches with bad results have been carried out.

Conclusion

Cerebral aneurysms in children are very rare lesions. They represent 0.5 to 2.5% of all aneurysms. In neuropediatric practice one sees one aneurysm for every five or six arteriovenous malformations. Although these aneurysms re more commonly seen in children older than 10 years, they may be observed in infancy in nearly 18% of the cases. The association with other disorders or congenital malformations is not rare in children. In contrast with what is described in adults, aneurysms in childhood are slightly more commonly located in the posterior system in nearly 15% of the cases. Giant aneurysms represent around 20%, and among them 20% are seen in infants. Vasospasm appears earlier than in adults and has a better prognosis. On average the results of surgery in children are better than in adults.

References

1. Patel AN, Richardson AE: Ruptured intracranial aneurysms in the first two decades of life. A study of 58 patients. J. Neurosurg 35:571–576, 1971.
2. Ostergaard, JR, Voldby B: Intracranial aneurysms in children and adolescents. J Neurosurg 58:832–837, 1983.
3. Locksley HB: Natural history of subarachnoid hemorrhage in intracranial aneurysms and arteriovenous malformations, based on 6,368 cases. J Neurosurg 25:219–239, 1966.
4. Pasqualin A, Mazza C, Cavazzani P, Scienza R, Da Pian R: Intracranial aneurysms and subarachnoid hemorrhage in children and adolescents. Child's Nerv Syst 2:185–190, 1986.
5. Meyer FB, Sundt TM Jr, Node NC: Cerebral aneurysms in childhood and adolescence. J Neurosurg 70:420–425, 1989.
6. Heiskanen O: Ruptured intracranial arterial aneurysms of children and adolescents. Surgical and total management results. Child's Nerv Syst 5:66–70, 1989.
7. Matson DD: Intracranial arterial aneurysms in childhood. J Neurosurg 23:567–583, 1965.
8. McDonald CA, Korb M: Intracranial aneurysms. Arch Neurol Psychiatr 42:298–328, 1939.
9. Krayenbuhl H, Yasargil MG: L'anèvrysme cérébral. Doc Geigy Ser Chir 1959.
10. Laitinen L: Arterielle aneurysm and subarachnoidal blodning hos barn. Nord Med 71:329–333, 1964.
11. Taveras JM, Wood EH: Diagnostic Neuroradiology, Williams & Wilkins, Baltimore, 1964.
12. Lapras C, Goutelle A, Brunat M, Dechaume JP: Les anévrysmes intracrâniens chez l'enfant. A propos de 4 observations. Neurochirurgie 14:891–900, 1968.
13. Suwanwela C, Suwanwela N, Charuchinda S, Honsaprabhas C: Intracranial mycotic aneurysms of extravascular origin. J Neurosurg 36:552–559, 1972.
14. Sedzimir CB, Robinson J: Intracranial hemorrhage in children and adolescents. J Neurosurg 38:269–281, 1973.
15. Thompson RA, Pribam HFW: Infantile cerebral aneurysm associated with ophthalmoplegia and quadriparesis. Neurology 19:785–798, 1969.
16. Kunk Z: Anévrysme sacculaire chez l'enfant. Cesk Neurol Neurochem 37:340–344, 1974.
17. Almeida GM, Pindaro J, Bianco E, Shibata MK: Intracranial arterial aneurysms in infancy and childhood. Child's Brain 3:193–199, 1977.
18. Sano K, Ueda Y, Saito I: Subarachnoid hemorrhage in children. Child's Brain 4:38–46, 1978.
19. Becker DH, Silversberg GD, Nelson EH, Hanbery W: Saccular aneurysm of infancy and early childhood. Neurosurgery 2:1–7, 1978.
20. Amacher AL, Drake CG: Cerebral artery aneurysms in infancy, childhood and adolescence. Child's Brain, 1:72–80, 1975.
21. Arseni C, Horwath L, Ciurea AV: Patologie Neurochirurgicala Infantila, Vol. 1. Editura Academiei Romania, 1980.
22. Gerosa M, Licata C, Fiore DL, Iraci G: Intracranial aneurysms of childhood. Child's Brain 6:295–302, 1980.
23. Visudhipian P, Chiemchanya S, Somburanasin R, Dheandhanoo D: Cause of spontaneous subarachnoid hemorrhage in Thai infants and children. A study of 56 patients. J Neurosurg 53:185–187, 1980.
24. Granieri U, Maiuri F, Colantuono C, Ceccotti C: Gli anevrismi delle arterie cerebrali in eta infantile. Riv Neurol 50:285–292, 1980.
25. Storrs BB, Humphreys RP, Hendrick EB, Hoffman HJ: Intracranial aneurysms in the pediatric age-group. Child's Brain 9:358–361, 1982.
26. Schauseil-Zipf U, Thun F, Kellerman NK, Mandlkramer S: Intracranial arteriovenous malformations and aneurysms in childhood and adolescence. Eur J Pediatr 140:260–267, 1983.
27. Hourihan M, Gates PC, McAllister VL: Subarachnoid hemorrhage in childhood and adolescence. J Neurosurg 60:1163–1166, 1984.
28. Gutierez FA, Bailes J, McLone DG: Intracranial aneurysms and pseudo-aneurysm occurring during infancy and childhood: diagnosis and surgical results. Concepts Pediatr Neurosurg 7:153–168, 1987.
29. Lipper S, Morgan D, Krigman MR: Congenital saccular aneurysm in a 19 day old neonate: case report and review of the literature. Surg Neurol 10:161–165, 1978.
30. Newcomb AL, Munns GF: Rupture of aneurysm of the circle of Willis in the newborn. Pediatrics 3:769–772, 1949.

31. Vapalahti PM, Schugk P, Tarkkaren L, Bjork-esten G: Intracranial arterial aneurysm in a three month old infant: case report. J Neurosurg 30:169–171, 1969.

32. Bremer JL: Congenital aneurysms of the cerebral arteries; an embryonic study. Arch Pathol 35:819–831, 1943.

33. Roche JL, Choux M, Czorny A, Dhellemes P, Fast M, Frerebeau P, Lapras C, Sautreaux JL: L'Anévrysme artèriel intra-crânien chez l'enfant. Etude coopérative. A propos de 43 observations. Neurochirurgie 34:243–251, 1988.

34. Shucart WA, Wolpert SM: An aneurysm in infancy presenting with diabetes insipidus. J Neurosurg 38:368–370, 1972.

35. Sherman DG, Salmon JH: Ocular bobbing with superior cerebellar artery aneurysm. Case report. J Neurosurg 47:596–598, 1977.

36. Forster FM, Alpers BJ: Aneurysm of circle of Willis associated with congenital polycystic disease of the kidneys. Arch Neurol Psychiatr 50:669–676, 1943.

37. Garcia-Chavez C, Moossy J: Cerebral artery aneurysm in infancy: association with agenesis of corpus callosum. J Neuropathol 24:492–501, 1965.

38. Sengupta RM, Lassman LP, De Moraes AA, Garvan N: Treatment of internal carotid bifurcation aneurysms by direct surgery. J Neurosurg 43:343–351, 1975.

39. Fee H, McGough E: Idiopathic multiple systemic aneurysms in a child. Am J Dis Child 137:1101–1102, 1983.

40. Finney JL, Roberts TS, Anderson RE: Giant intracranial aneurysm associated with Marfan's syndrome. Case report. J Neurosurg 45:342–347, 1976.

41. Gum GK, Nadell JA, Numaguchi Y: Giant aneurysm of bilateral internal carotid arteries in a child. Child's Nerv Syst 4:161–168, 1988.

42. Waga S, Tochio H: Intracranial aneurysm associated with moyamoya disease in childhood. Surg Neurol 23:237–243, 1985.

43. Wakabayashi T, Fujita S, Ohbora Y: Polycystic kidney disease and intracranial aneurysms. J Neurosurg 58:488–491, 1983.

44. Sindou M, Keravel Y: Les anévrysmes géants intracraniens. Approche thérapeutique. Neurochirurgie 30 (suppl 1):1984.

45. Kojima T, Waga S: More than one aneurysm on the same artery. Surg Neurol 22:403–408, 1984.

46. Cedzich C, Schramm J, Röckelein G: Multiple middle cerebral artery aneurysms in an infant. Case report. J Neurosurg 72:806–809, 1990.

47. Arai H, Sugiyama Y, Miyazawa N: Multiple intracranial aneurysms and vascular malformations in an infant: case report. J Neurosurg 37:357–360, 1972.

48. Humphreys RP, Hendrick EB, Hoffman HJ, Storrs BB: Childhood aneurysms, atypical features, atypical management. Concepts Pediat Neurosurg 6:213–229, 1985.

49. Wittle IR, Dorsch NW, Besser M: Giant intracranial aneurysms: diagnosis; management and outcome. Surg Neurol 21:218–230, 1984.

50. Sundt TM, Piepgras DG: Surgical approach to giant intracranial aneurysms. Operative experience with 80 cases. J Neurosurg 51:731–742, 1979.

51. Hacker RJ: Intracranial aneurysms of childhood: a statistical analysis of 500 cases from the world literature. Neurosurgery 10:775, 1982.

52. Lena G, Choux M: Giant intracranial aneurysms in children 15 years old or under. Case reports and literature review. J Pediatr Neurosci 1:84–93, 1985.

53. Ventureyra EC, Choo SH, Benoit BC: Super giant globoid intracranial aneurysm in an infant. Case report. J Neurosurg 53:411–416, 1980.

54. Asari S, Nakamura S, Yamada D, Beck H, Sugatani H, Higashi T: Traumatic aneurysm of peripheral cerebral arteries. Report of two cases. J Neurosurg 46:795–803, 1977.

55. Burton C, Velasco FC, Dorman J: Traumatic aneurysm of a peripheral cerebral artery. Review and case report. J Neurosurg 28:468–474, 1968.

56. Scharfetter F, Fodisch HJ, Menardi G, Twerdy K: Faux anevrysme de l'artère du gyrus angulaire, causépar une lésion au cours d'une ponction. Acta Neurochir 33:123–132, 1976.

57. Tsubokawa T, Kotani A, Sugawara T: Treatment for traumatic aneurysm of the cerebral artery. Identification between deteriorating type and spontaneously disappearing type. Neurol Surg 3:663–672, 1975.

58. Rout D, Snarma A, Mohan PK, Rao VRK: Bacterial aneurysms of the intracavernous carotid artery. J Neurosurg 60:1236–1242, 1984.

CHAPTER 11

Endovascular Treatment of Cerebrovascular Pathology

A. Beltramello

Since the introduction of noninvasive imaging techniques (computed tomography, ultrasound, magnetic resonance imaging), superselective cerebrospinal angiography has been playing a major role as well as a therapeutic procedure prior to surgery or as an alternative. Surgical neuroangiography is now also a well-established therapeutic technique.

In many centers selective and superselective angiography is becoming a sophisticated procedure both in diagnostics and prior to embolization. At present, embolization plays the most important role in interventional angiography, but other endovascular approaches, such as "in situ" chemotherapy or chemoembolization with drug-charged microspheres, are worthy of mention. In the field of neuropediatrics, the value of therapeutic angiography has slowly gained general acceptance owing to the special nature of pediatric patients. Today there are no reasons to prevent its widespread diffusion, provided that it is performed by experienced and skilled teams under the correct indications.[1]

There is a wide range of possible indications: head and neck pathologies; intracranial, spinal, and spinal cord lesions. When dealing with infants and children, it is mandatory in the author's opinion never to undertake an irreversible type of treatment without the certainty that it is actually curative as well, in order to let the young patient completely recover from his/her disease. For these reasons, it is advisable to avoid radiotherapy and surgical ligatures on vessels feeding vascular malformations or tumors. These procedures are harmful and of no use, as they do not prevent the development of collateral pathological networks, but hinder a possible endovascular approach, which would permit the parent vessel to be spared and allow

for any subsequent endovascular approaches. The use of fluids, such as nonresorbable embolic agents like IBCA (isobutylcyanoacrylate), which are characterized by rapid and irreversible polymerization, is usually not indicated because of the risk of complications from the possible embolization of external carotid to the ophthalmic artery and intracranial anastomoses, as well as possible embolization of the external carotid supply to the cranial nerves in lesions located near the skull base. IBCA, in particular is suspected to have teratogenic activity;[2] therefore, it is our opinion that it must not be used in young patients with a long life expectancy.

Intracranial Vascular Lesions

These lesions represent a therapeutic challenge both for the neuroradiologist and the neurosurgeon: actually, this pathology is not very prevalent in pediatric patients and, apart from the problem of general anesthesia, the technical features are not very different from the procedures used for adults. Whenever possible, it is advisable to keep the young patient alert in order to detect any neurological complications linked to the embolization treatment as soon as possible.

Materials and Methods

Embolization procedures are performed under general anesthesia or systemic sedation. The femoral route is generally preferred because it is more comfortable for the patient and more versatile and can thus accommodate itself to any special circumstances in the examination. Nevertheless, special caution must be taken in infants and small children because of their known tendency to have arterial spasms.

When repeated examinations are performed, the contralateral femoral artery may be used to avoid any significant damage to the arterial walls that could interfere with the normal growth of the lower limb. Three- to 5-French catheters are used, introduced into the femoral artery after an arterial puncture with 22- to 18-gauge needles. If possible, the catheter is inserted gradually, beginning with the smallest needle. The puncture site is dilated and then the chosen catheter is inserted. Frequent flushing with heparinized solution is advisable because of the small size of the catheters used. Before embolization, it is of paramount importance to obtain a complete vascular map of the lesion. Selective and superselective injections are mandatory.

Nonionic, water-soluble contrast media are preferable at the lowest concentration and dosage. Because embolizations are relatively long procedures, up to 6–8 mg/kg of contrast material can be safely used if the cardiac pump and renal function are normal. The child must be protected with adequate anti-X-ray protection, and optimal collimation of the X-ray beams must be adopted.

Imaging subtraction is necessary for the most important films. Digital subtraction angiography (DSA) is a formidable technical device, which significantly shortens the overall time required and is associated with a marked decrease in the concentration and amount of contrast medium needed. It gives the neuroradiologist the opportunity to make "real time" decisions, and therefore its use in therapeutic angiography is of paramount importance.[3,4]

Brain Arteriovenous Malformations (AVMs)

Brain AVMs in pediatric patients represent 12% of all treated cerebral angiomas in our department. Like our treatment plan for adults, we use our own technique based on the wing microcatheter for intravascular navigation and embolization with Polylene threads[5,6] in order to obliterate the nidus of the malformation and devascularize the arterial feeders, usually as a presurgical procedure. In our experience, embolization alone is curative only in a few cases, and

surgery is required for complete cure of the lesion. Even if only small portions of the arteriovenous malformation are left in place, the patient with this residual angioma is still at risk of hemorrhaging.

Embolization Technique

Our technique is a modification of the Debrun balloon catheter system,[7] with the distal end of the Silastic microcatheter completely open and exposed. To prepare this catheter a No. 17 latex balloon is put on a 2.5-French Silastic microcatheter. The tip of the balloon is then cut so that the tips of the microcatheter and balloon are aligned and the distal end of the Silastic microcatheter is completely exposed. With fine microsurgery forceps, five vertical cuts are made on the walls of the balloon surrounding the catheter as far as its neck. At the end of the procedure, five small latex wings have been created around the tip of the catheter (Fig. 11.1). These "floating" wings increase the area exposed to the bloodstream, and consequently the traction of the microcatheter along the direction of blood flow is strengthened.

Intravascular navigation is flow dependent and is obtained by a propulsion chamber. The microcatheter is slipped into an outer 6-French polyethylene coaxial catheter. Once the microcatheter has reached the desired position, superselective angiograms of the vascular feeders are obtained without blocking the blood flow. Manual injections of 1 to 2 ml of contrast medium are adequate, with digital subtraction angiographic equipment, to obtain reliable maps of the AVM and its feeders. As embolic agents, both fluids and particles can be used with our multipurpose microcatheter; therefore, it is suitable both for AVM embolization and for injection of chemotherapeutic agent. We have used the wing microcatheter for isobutyl 2-cyanoacrylate (IBCA) delivery, but our experience is based mainly on the use of threads, which can be injected through this catheter as well as through other ones commercially available.[8,9] Polyfilament Polylene-3-0 threads (0.2 mm in diameter) cut 1.5 to 2 mm long are fitted into 22-gauge catheter needles loaded (five emboli each) before the embolization procedure and ready for use. The loaded catheter needle is connected to a 2.5-ml syringe and inserted into

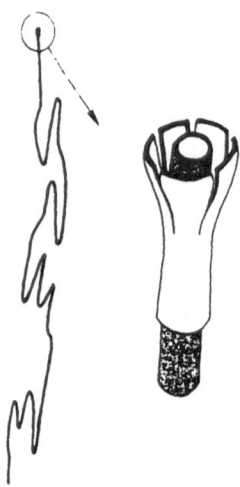

Figure 11.1. Drawing of wing microcatheter; magnified circle shows small latex wings surrounding tip of Silastic microcatheter, in which distal end of catheter is completely exposed.

the proximal end of the microcatheter. Emboli are then discharged into the artery by 1.5 to 2 ml of saline. The great majority of threads reach the nidus of the AVM, and a progressive embolization is achieved under continuous angiographic control and neurologic observation in the alert patient. Because this technique results in a progressive embolization, the higher flow shunts are the first to close, followed by the slower flow ones. Only when shunt flow is markedly reduced, at the very end of the procedure, can a few threads be deposited on the walls of the arterial pedicles, very close to the AVM. At the end of each procedure, superselective angiography of the embolized feeder is carried out by means of the same microcatheter.

Once one feeder is embolized, the same microcatheter can be moved to other feeders, without the need for complete withdrawal; in this way, many pedicles can be embolized in the same session. Control angiograms with the outer coaxial polyethylene catheter are obtained at the end of each embolization, and, if necessary, angiography during various phases of the procedure can be performed without removing the microcatheter (Fig. 11.2).

Embolization by means of our microcatheter system with polylene threads proved to be a useful and reliable tool to achieve, in conjunction with surgery, complete cure in a significant number of critical AVMs.

Morbidity and technical failures are both so low as to justify the embolization as the first step in the treatment plan of the majority of critical AVMs. Pathologic studies of brain AVMs resected after embolization have demonstrated the absence of angionecrosis. A moderate inflammatory response can be seen that tends to be alleviated by the fourth week.

The immunologic response to thread emboli is cell mediated, not humoral. It gives origin to a self-maintaining granulomatous–fibrotic process, which begins after the first month and peaks at the third month. The threads used in our procedures are nonreabsorbable, biocompatible, nontoxic, and useful as embolizing agents for brain AVMs.

Arteriovenous Fistula and Giant Aneurysms

Balloon technology has greatly improved the therapeutic possibilities in this area of pathology. Nowadays, the endovascular approach is the method of choice in the treatment of intracranial arteriovenous fistulas, both congenital and posttraumatic. In the majority of cases closure of the fistula along with preservation of the parent vessel can be obtained.[10]

This goal can be achieved both with detachable balloons and with particulate embolization after intracranial navigation of the arterial feeder.

Detachable balloons are the best embolizing materials for fistulas fed by the large intracranial arteries proximal to the circle of Willis (Fig. 11.3) while, in our experience, embolization with very long (4 to 5 cm) pieces of Polylene 3-0 threads (0.2 mm in diameter) delivered by microcatheters selectively placed in the feeding arteries is a reliable and effective treatment for fistulas fed by middle-sized arteries[11] (Fig. 11.4). Particularly interesting was the case of a young patient, aged 17 years, who was suffering with a long-lasting untreatable left trigeminal neuralgia. Magnetic resonance imaging (MRI) revealed a significant direct compression of the proximal portion of the left trigeminal nerve by a vascular loop of the elongated left vertebral artery, secondary to the presence of an angiographically demonstrated direct intracranial "straight-line" AV fistula between the left

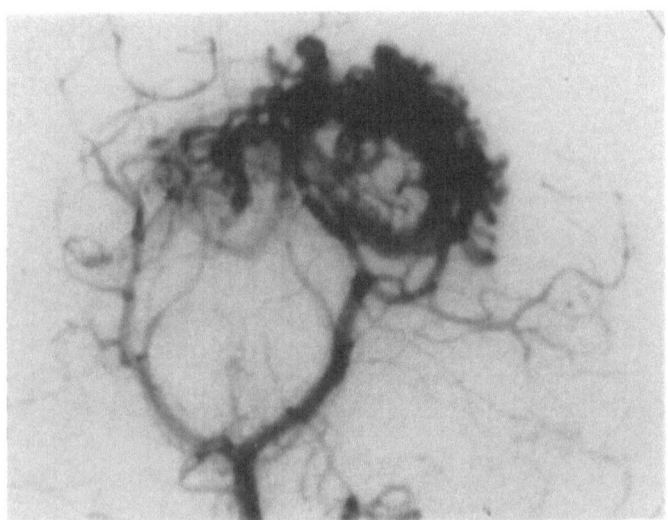

Figure 11.2A

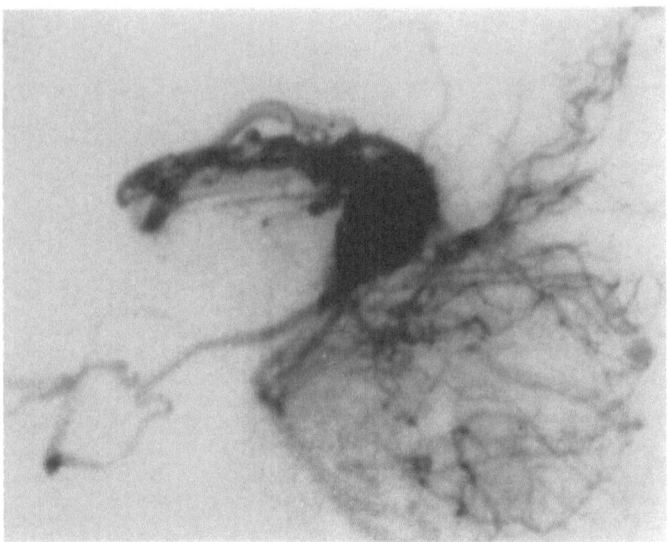

Figure 11.2B

Figure 11.2. Brain AVM of the choroidal system in a 9-year-old child who bled twice. (**A** and **B**) Preembolization angiograms. (**C** and **D**) Super-selective angiograms of the medial (**C**) and lateral (**D**) posterior choroidal arteries using a wing micro-catheter. (**E** and **F**) Angiographic control after embolization with Polylene threads.

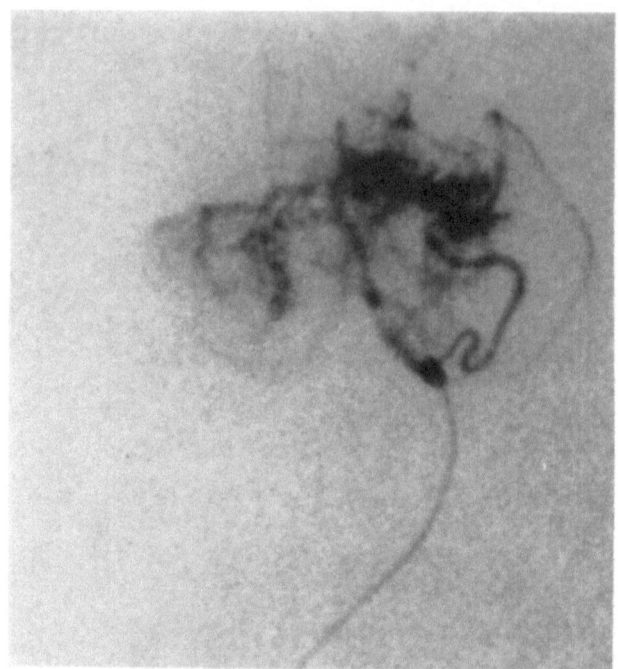

Figure 11.2C

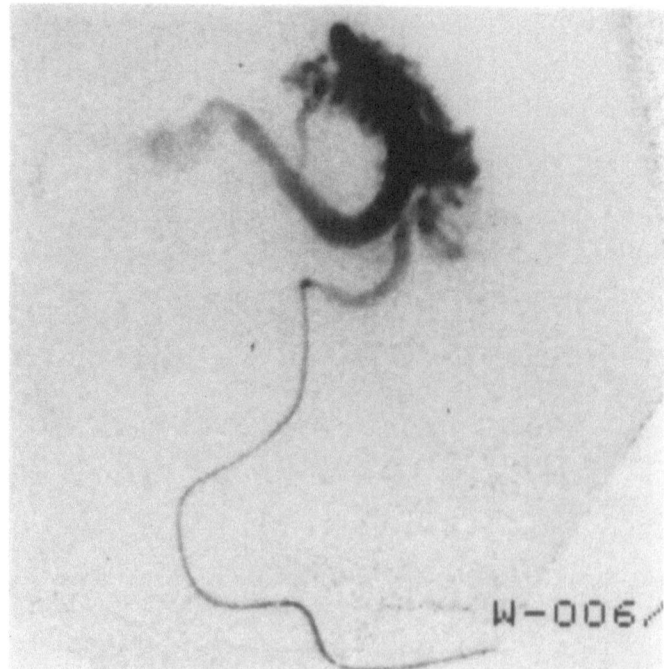

Figure 11.2D

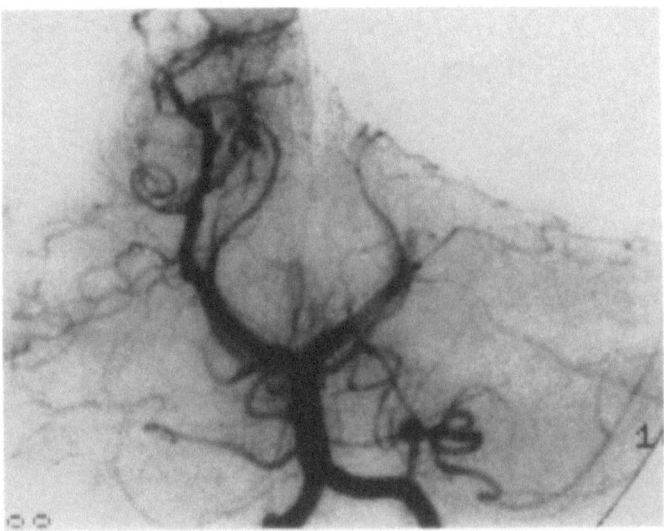

Figure 11.2E

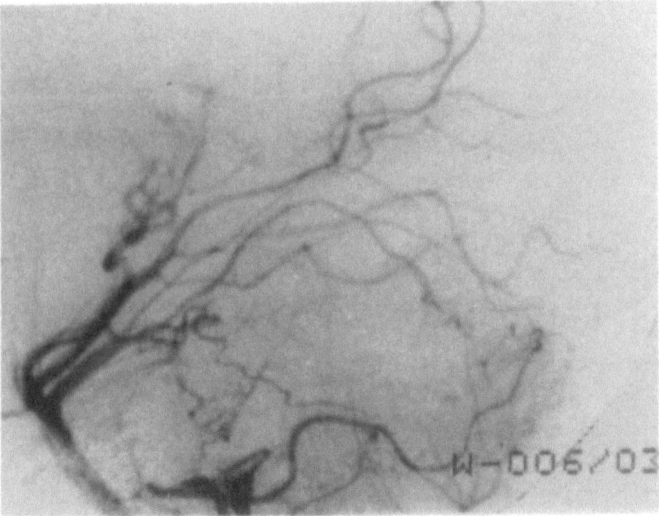

Figure 11.2F

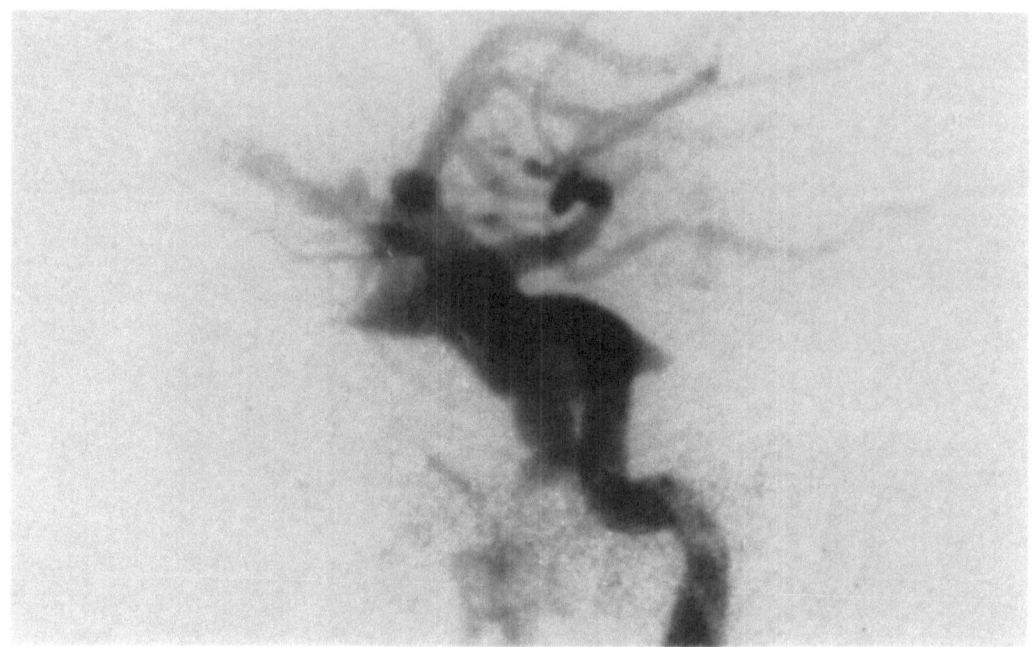

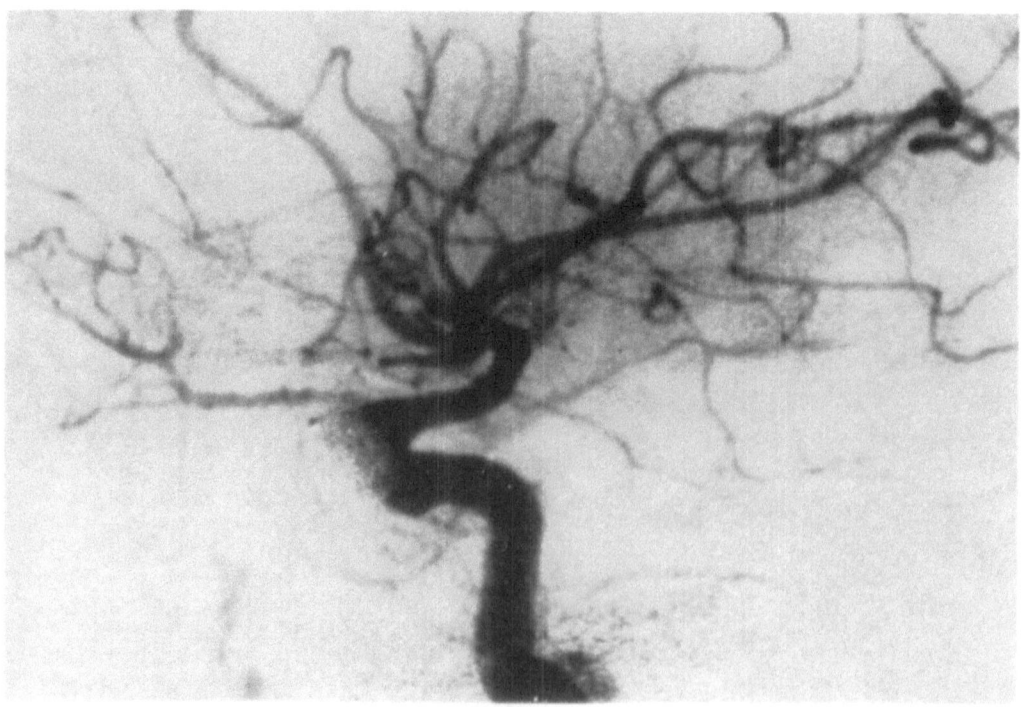

Figure 11.3. Posttraumatic caroticocavernous fistula in a 13-year old boy before (**A**) and after (**B**) embolization with one Debrun detachable balloon.

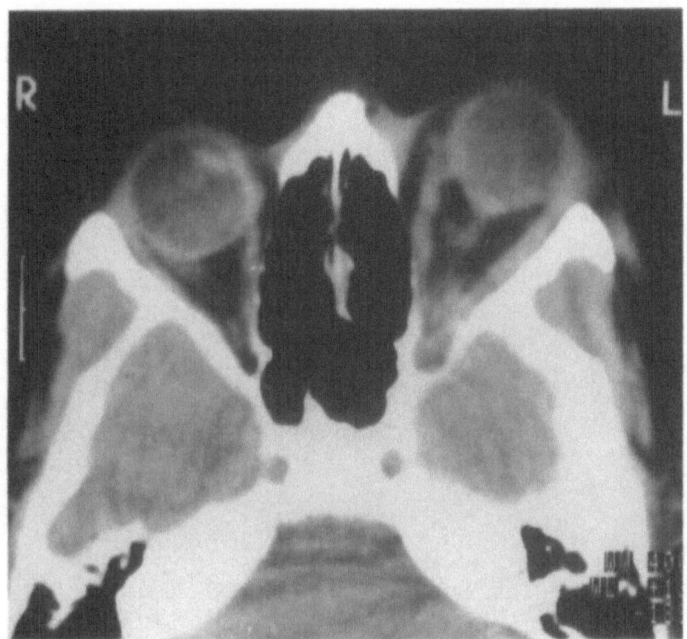

Figure 11.4A

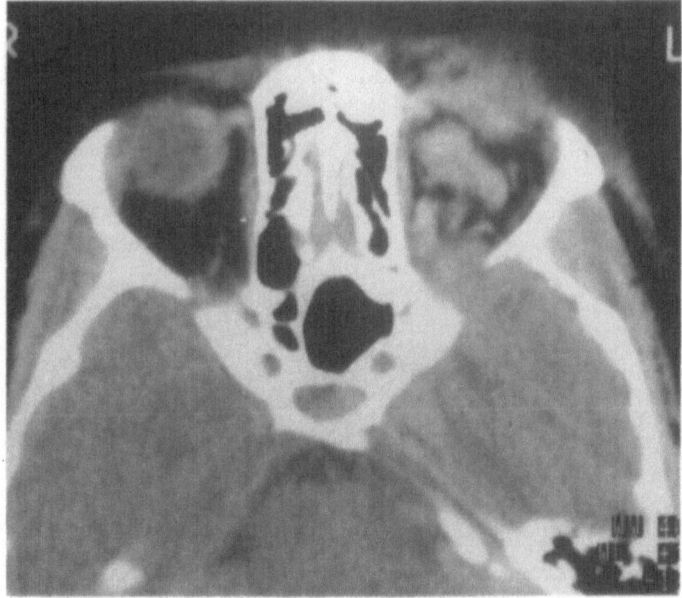

Figure 11.4B

Figure 11.4. Congenital caroticocavernous fistula in a 15-year-old girl. Left proptosis and amaurosis since birth; recent onset of intracranial bruit and worsening exophthalmos. (**A** and **B**) CT scan shows left exophthalmos with serpiginous vascular structures in the left orbit associated to an enlargement of the superior orbital fissure. Common left carotid angiogram (**C**) reveals a caroticocavernous fistula fed both by the meningeal branches of the external carotid artery [(**D**) before, (**E**) after polyvinil alcohol (PVA) embolization] and by branches of the ophthalmic artery (**F**). Ophthalmic artery was navigated (**G**) and embolized with polylene threads (**H**). (**I** and **J**) Angiographic control after embolization reveals the complete closure of the fistula.

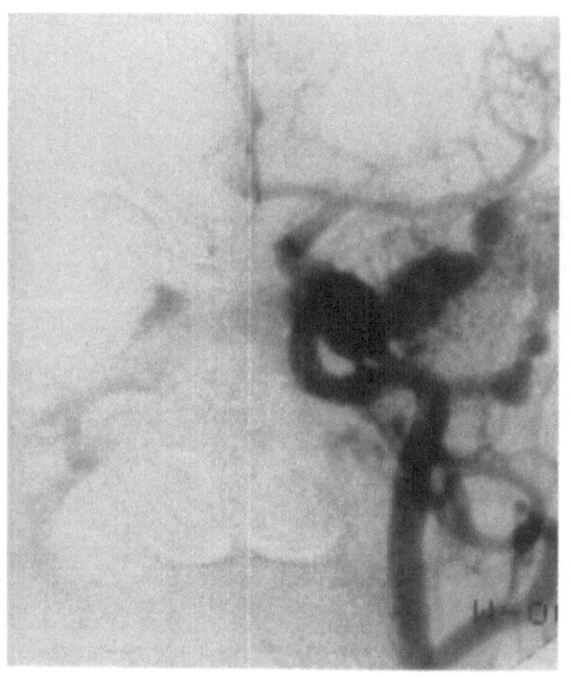

Figure 11.4C

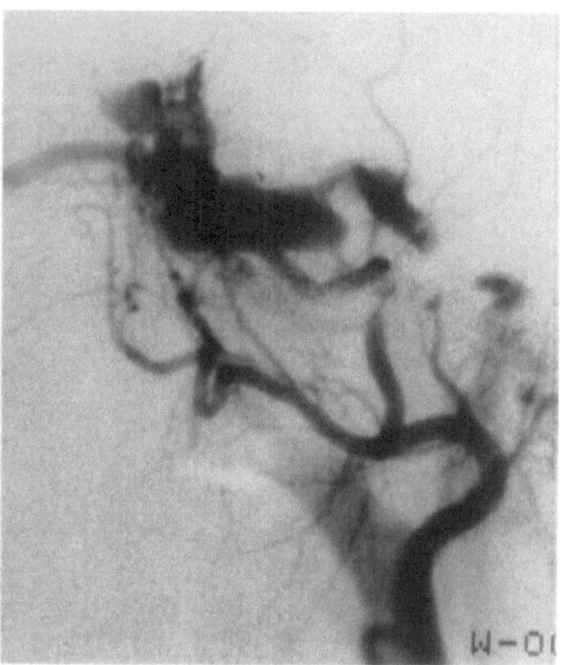

Figure 11.4D

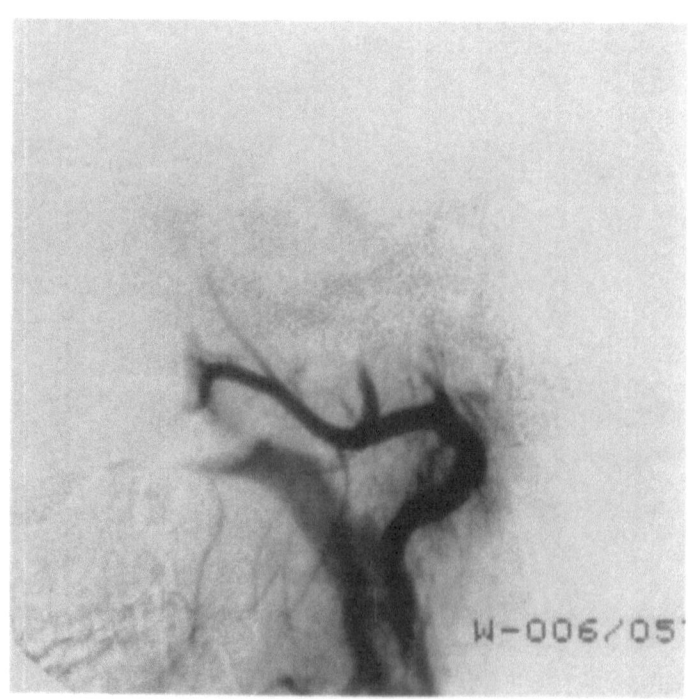

Figure 11.4E

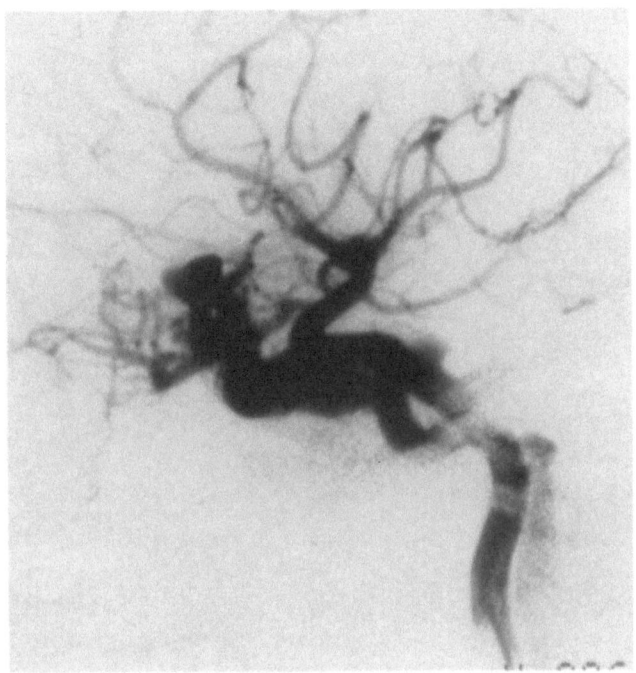

Figure 11.4F

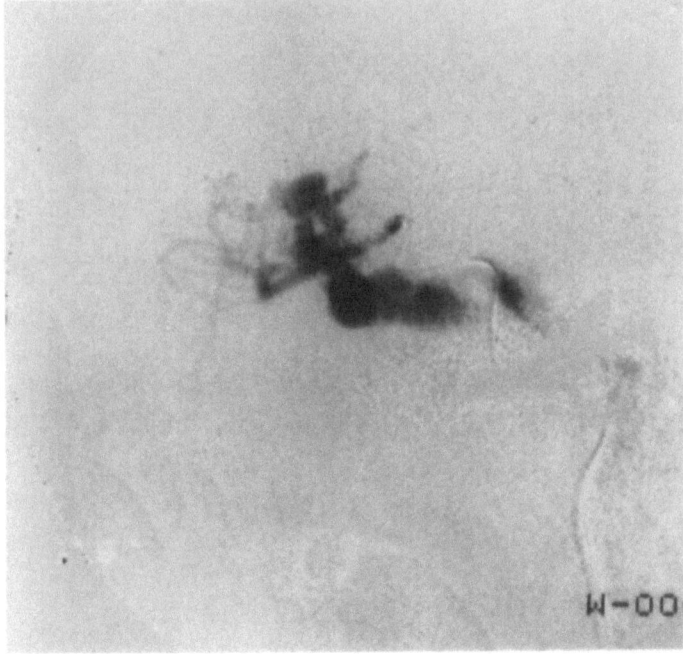

Figure 11.4G

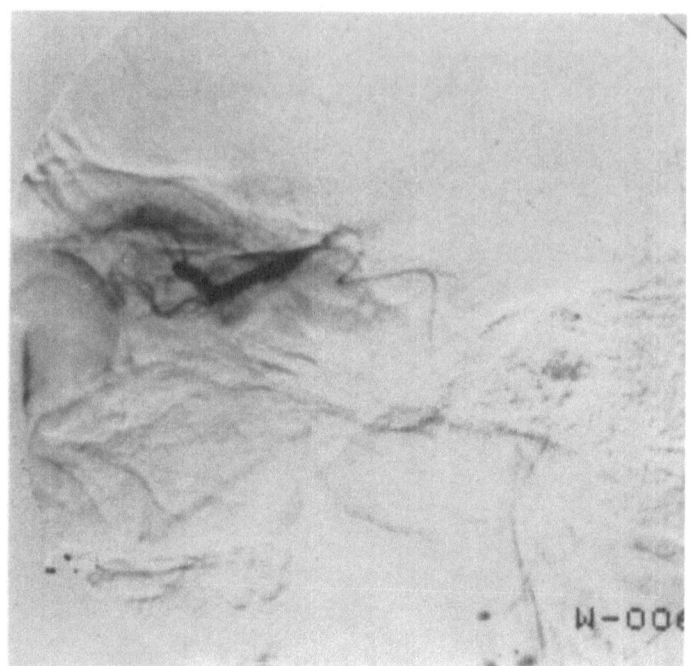

Figure 11.4H

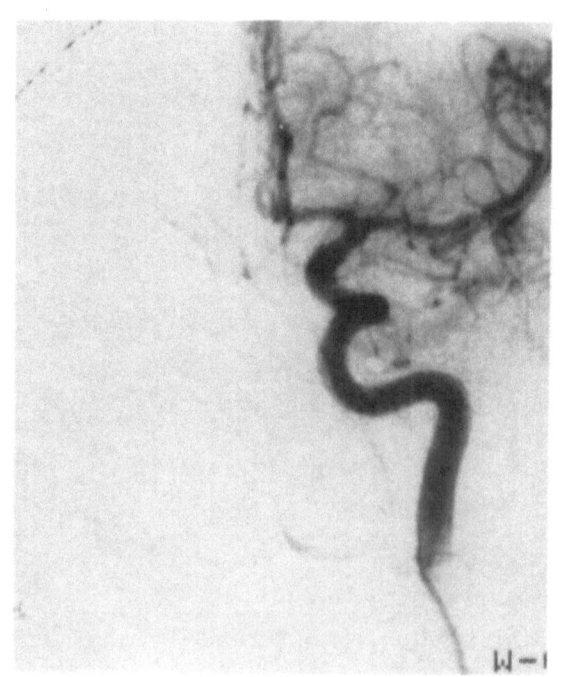

Figure 11.4I

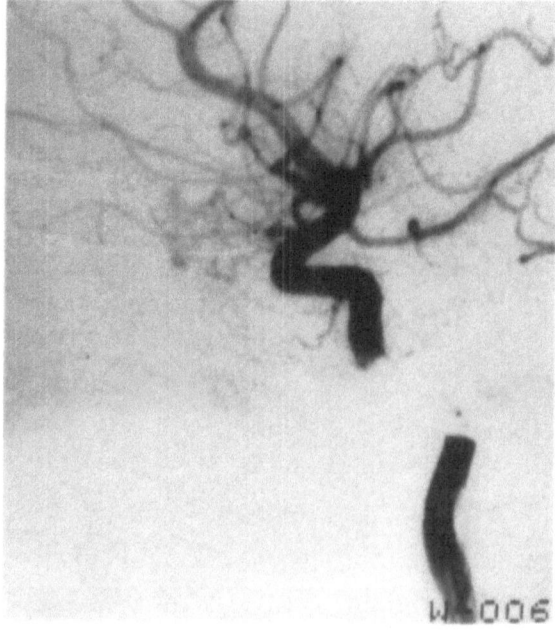

Figure 11.4J

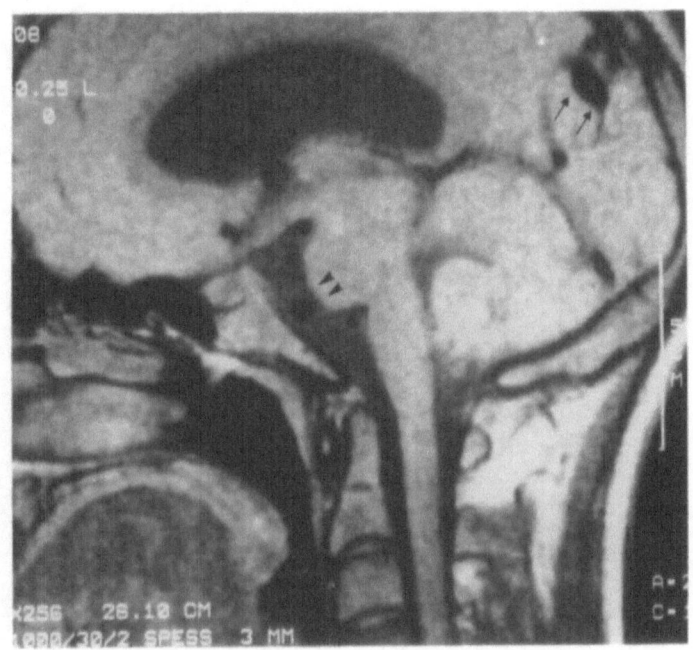

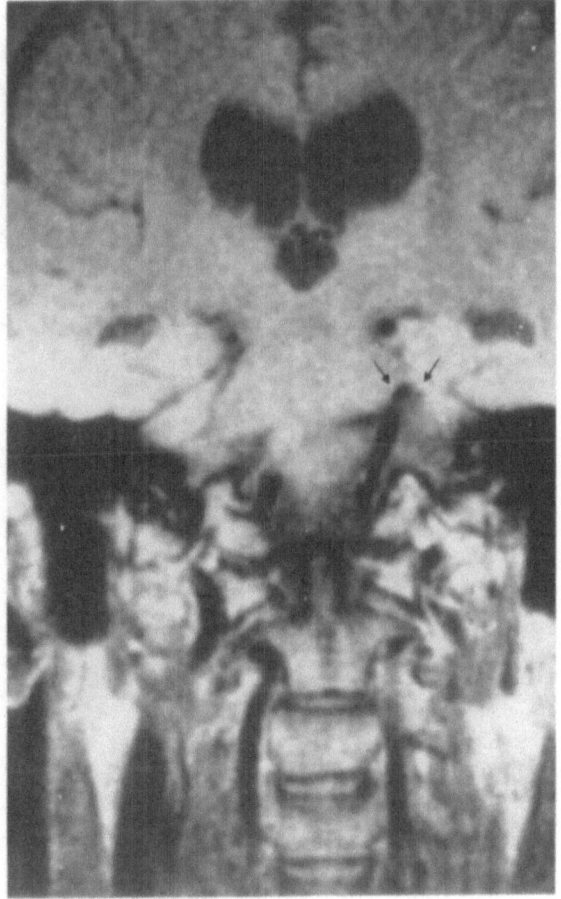

Figure 11.5. Intracranial arteriovenous fistula in a 17-year-old boy suffering a long-lasting, untreatable left trigeminal neuralgia. MRI in the sagittal plane (**A**) reveals an area void of signal in the occipital region characteristic of vascular structure (arrows) and another vascular structure anterior to the pons just in front of the emergence of the fifth cranial nerve (arrowheads). MRI in the coronal plane clearly shows an elongated left vertebral artery (**B**, arrows) with a vascular loop directly compressing and displacing the left fifth cranial nerve at its emergence from the brainstem (**C**, arrowheads). (**D** and **E**) Left vertebral angiogram reveals a direct "straight-line" AV fistula between the left posterior cerebral artery and a large vein draining into the superior longitudinal sinus. Posterior cerebral artery was navigated (**F**) and embolized (**G**) with long fragments of polylene threads. (**H** and **I**) Postembolization angiograms show the complete closure of the fistula.

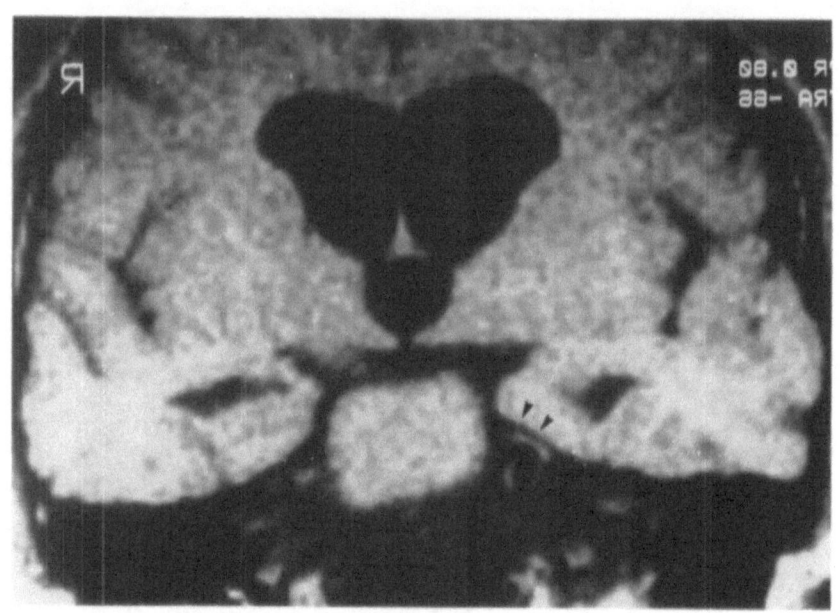

Figure 11.5C

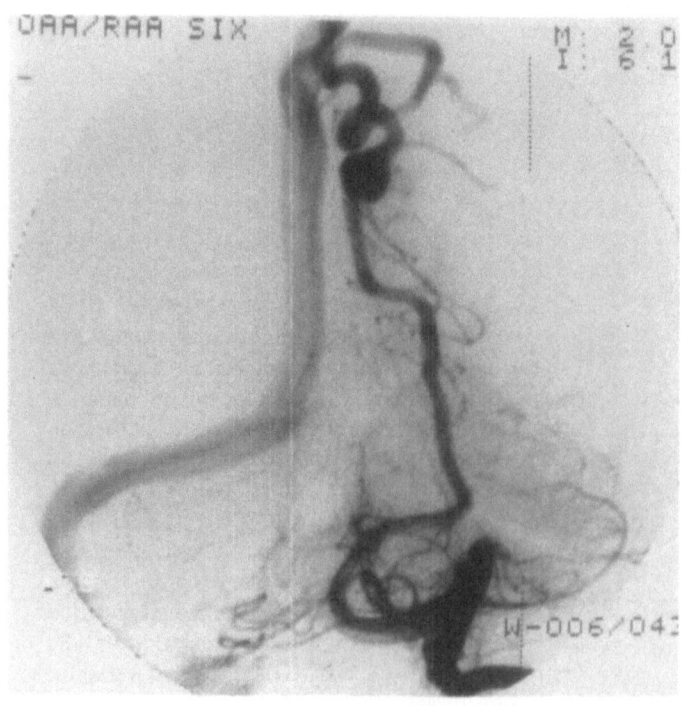

Figure 11.5D

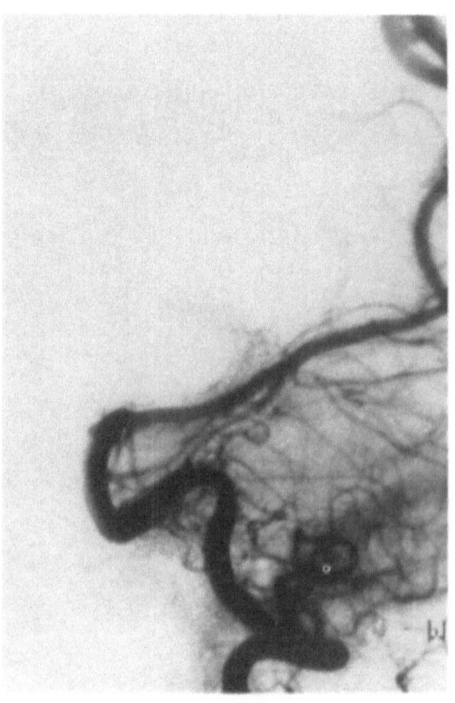

Figure 11.5E

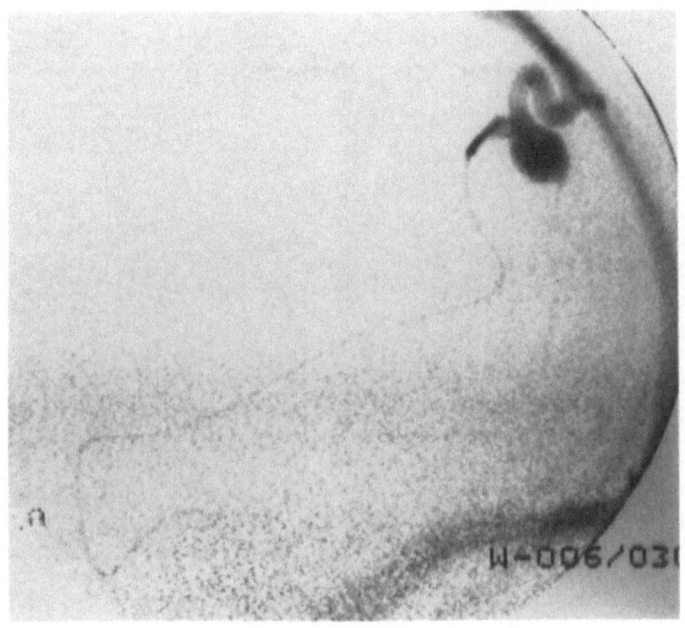

Figure 11.5F

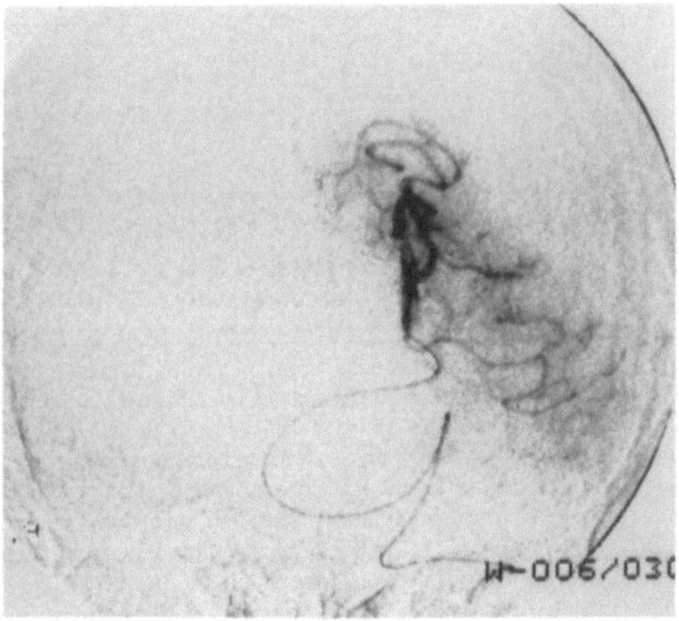

Figure 11.5G

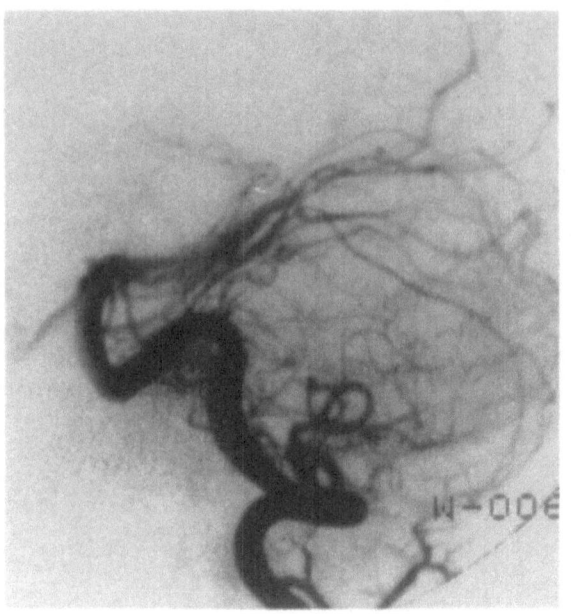

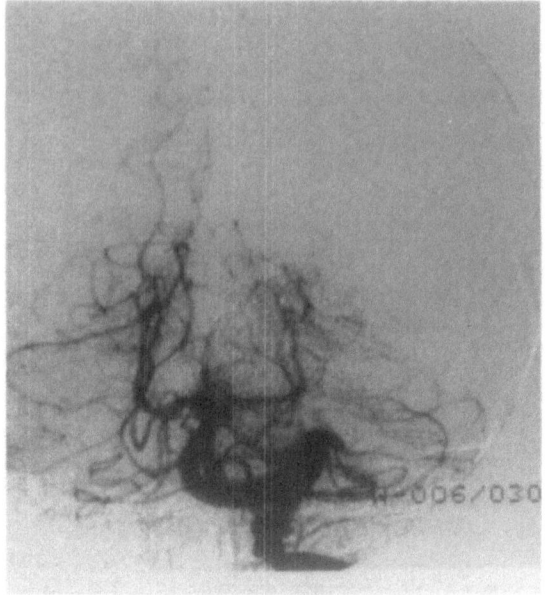

Figure 11.5H   **Figure 11.5I**

Figure 11.6. Giant dysplasic aneurysm of the internal carotid artery in a 13-year-old boy. (**A**) CT scan after contrast medium administration. (**B** and **C**) Pre-embolization angiogram. (**D**) Postembolization angiogram reveals that the internal carotid artery is closed by the balloon (arrows); aneurysm can no longer be seen; external carotid artery is well opacified. (**E**) Contralateral carotid artery injection shows good cross-filling associated to a significant displacement of both precommunicating segments of anterior cerebral arteries, due to the mass effect exerted by the giant aneurysm. (**F**) With standard X-rays, the three detached balloons are evident: the first at the level of the neck of the aneurysm, the second just below, the third at the origin of the internal carotid artery (arrows). (**G**) at CT scan of the skull base, the two balloons in the carotid canal are evident (arrows). (**H** and **I**) Control CT scan after contrast medium (c.m.) administration 3 months later shows significant endoluminal thrombosis and calcification of the walls of the aneurysm; the dome of the aneurysm is still patent. (**J** and **K**) MRI in the coronal and axial planes performed 10 months later reveals that the upper portion of the aneurysm is void of signal, thus indicating persistence of blood from inside (**J** and **K**, arrows) associated to an image consistent with a hypertrophied left posterior communicating artery (**K**, arrowheads). (**L** and **M**) Control angiography on the same date shows no evidence of the aneurysm from the contralateral carotid injection; displacement of A1 segments is no longer recognizable. The dome of the aneurysm is opacified (**M**, arrows) via a huge posterior communicating artery (**M**, arrowheads) injected from the basilar trunk.

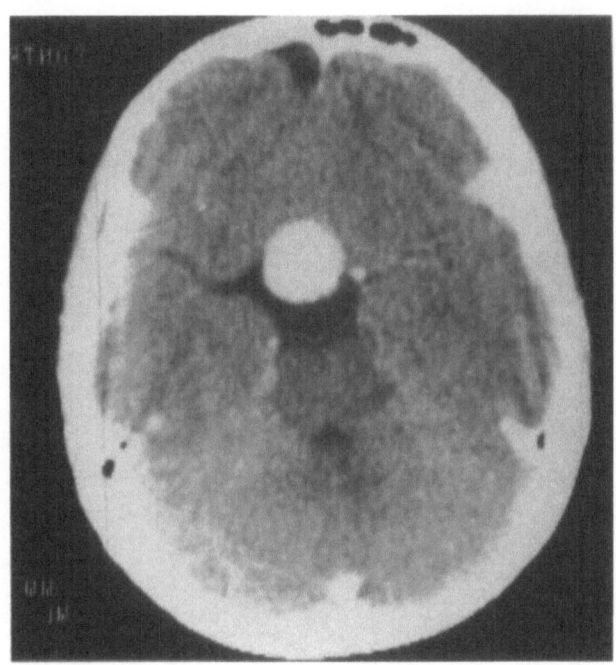

Figure 11.6A

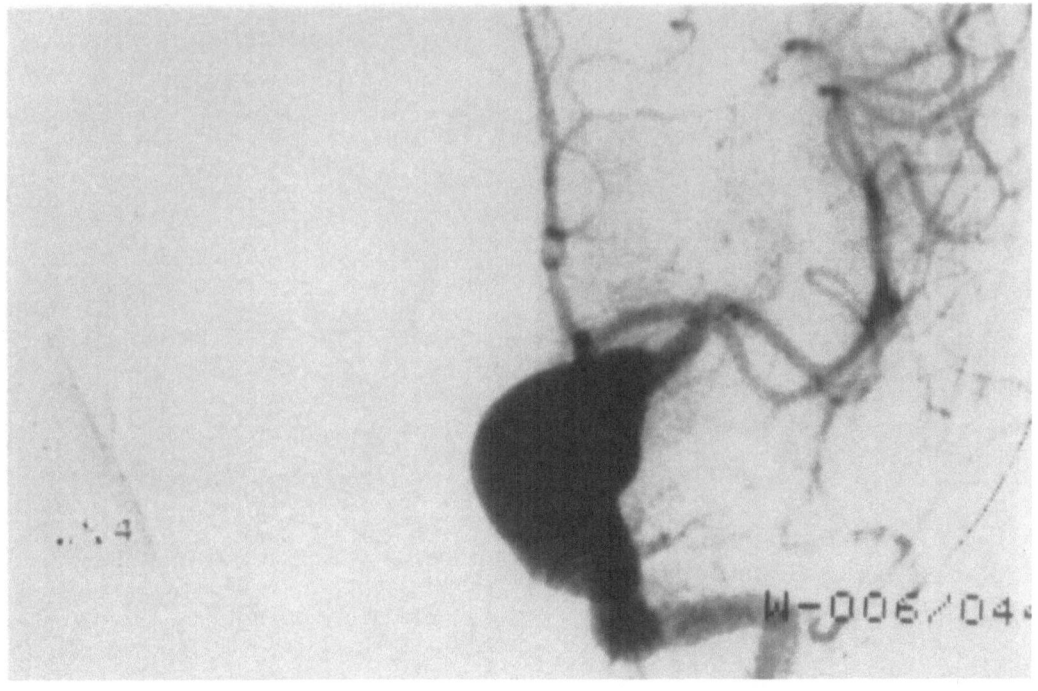

Figure 11.6B

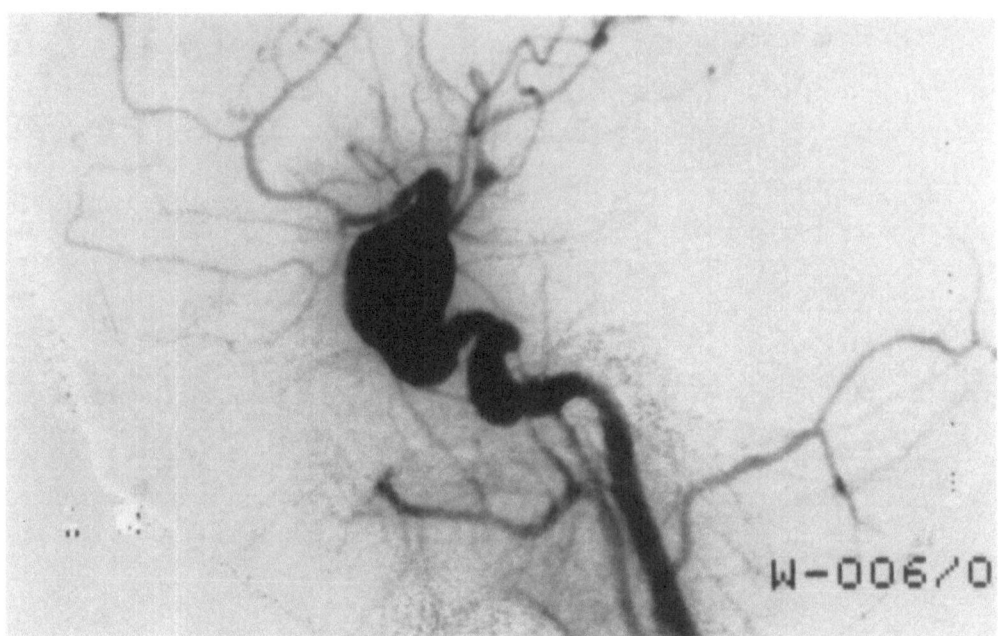

Figure 11.6C

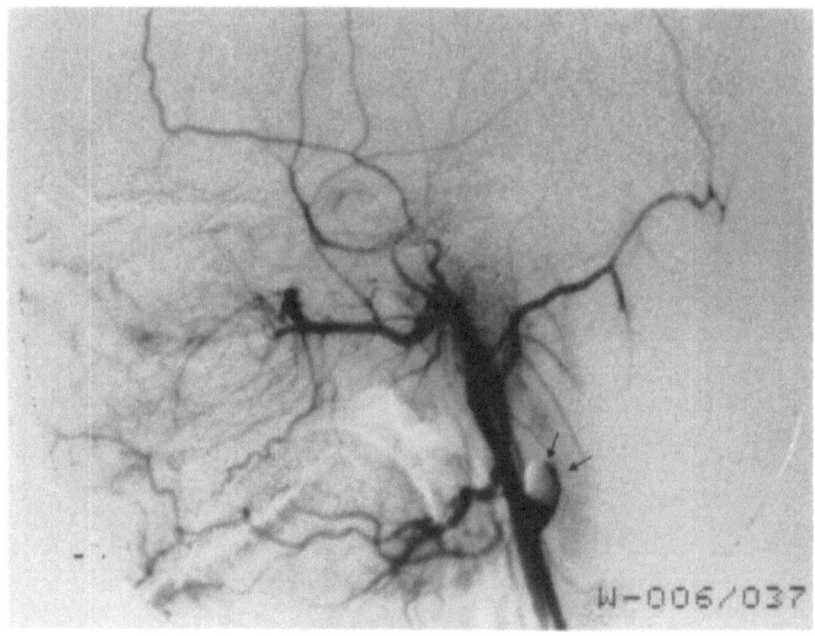

Figure 11.6D

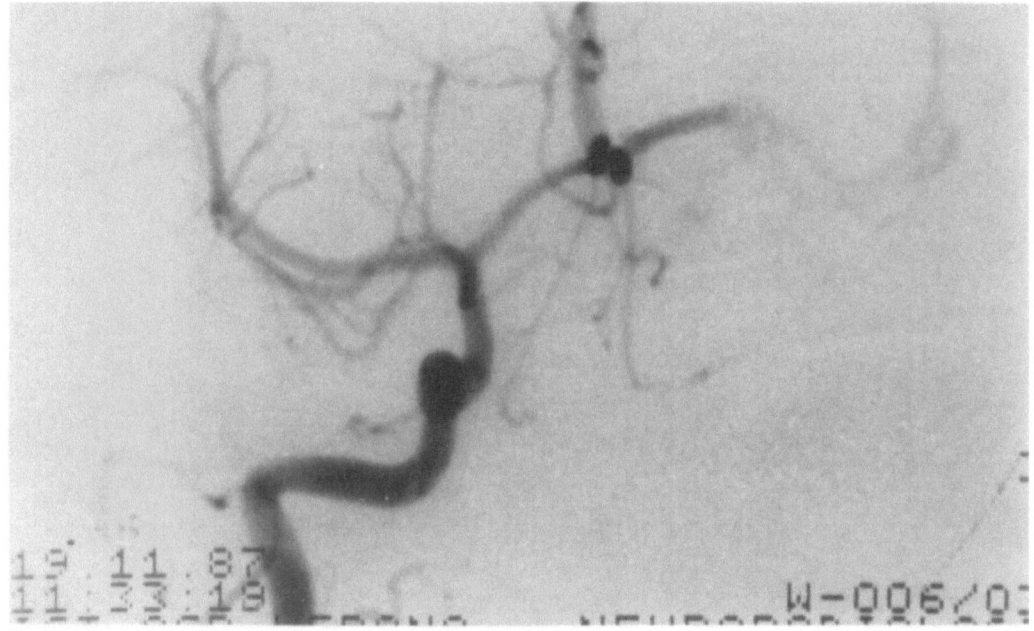

Figure 11.6E

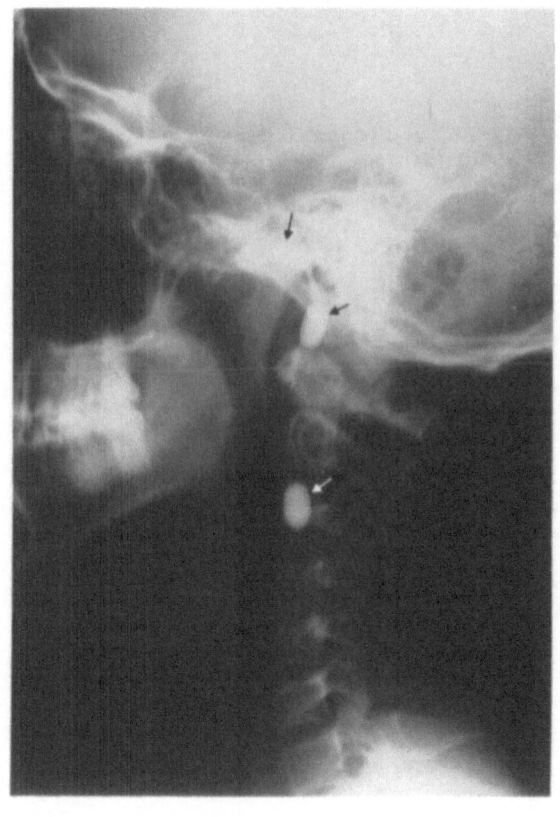

Figure 11.6F

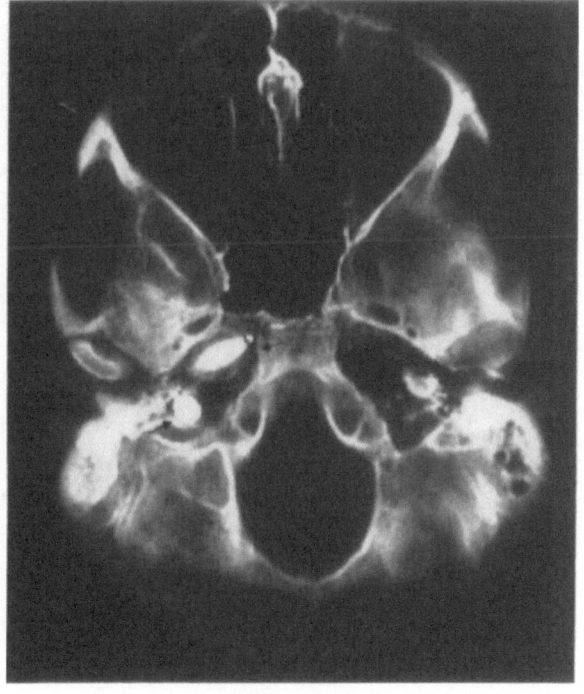

Figure 11.6G

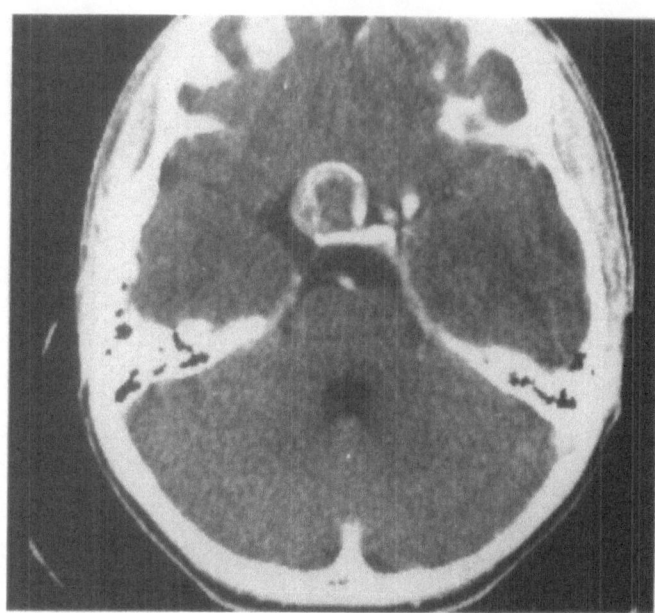

Figure 11.6H

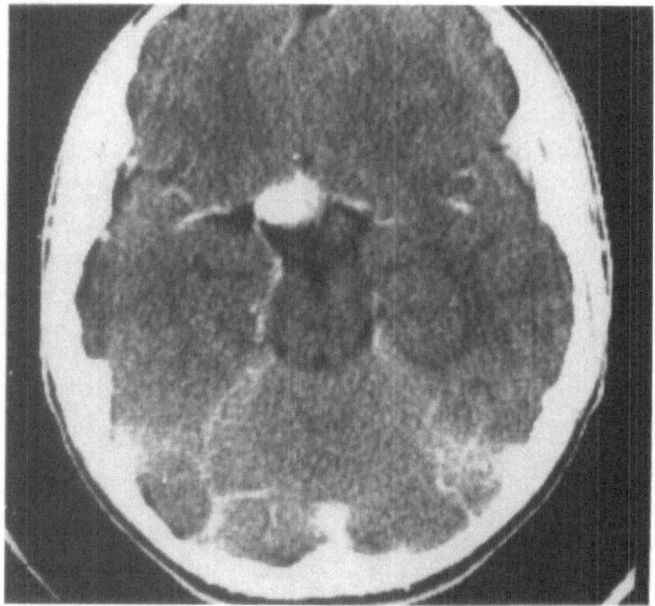

Figure 11.6I

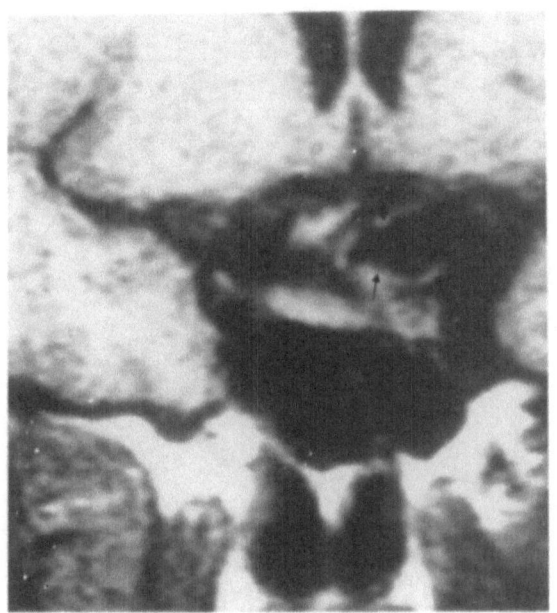

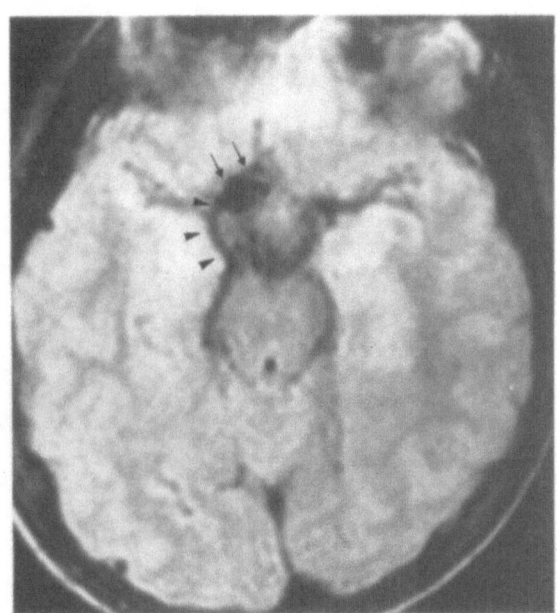

Figure 11.6J   **Figure 11.6K**

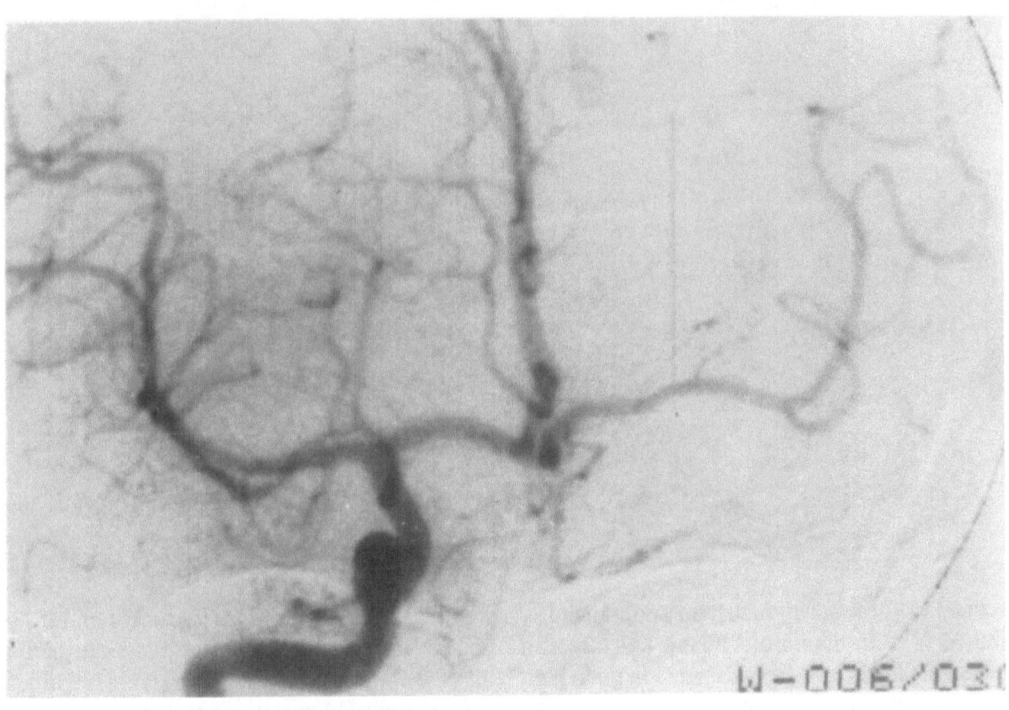

Figure 11.6L

Figure 11.6M

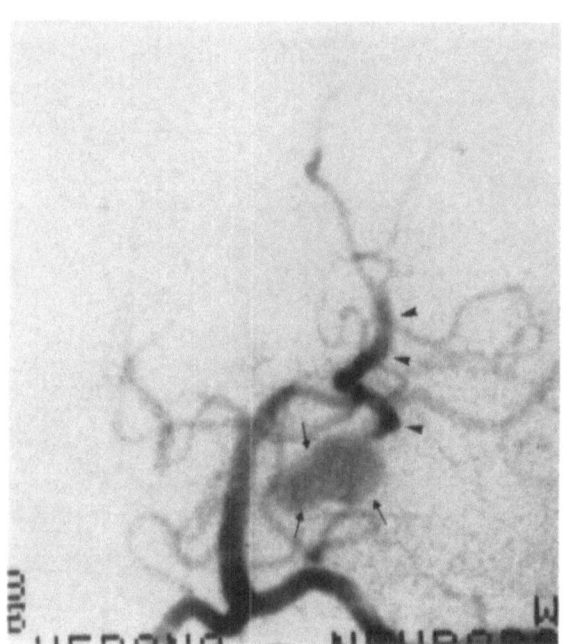

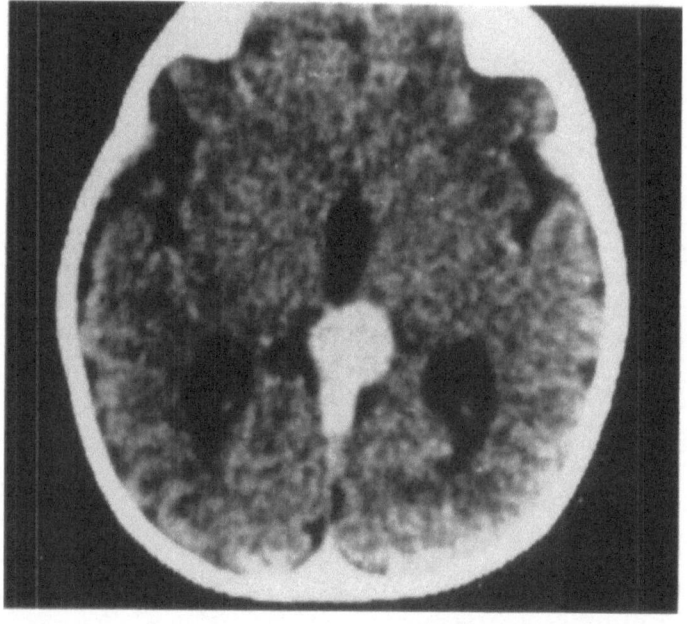

Figure 11.7A

Figure 11.7. Vein of Galen aneurysm spontaneously thrombosed in a 14-month-old infant. (**A**) CT scan (twelfth day of life) reveals spherical mass in the region of the vein of Galen. (**B–E**) Three-vessels angiography (thirty-second day of life) shows a vein of Galen aneurysm fed by the choroidal, lenticulostriate, and posterior cerebral arteries of both sides with drainage toward the superior sagittal sinus via the falcine sinus. (**F**) Control CT scan (8 months of age): a significant decrease in size, both of the malformation and the ventricles, is evident. (**G**) CT scan (14 months of age): mild ventricular dilation; no lesion can be found at the level of the vein of Galen. (**H–M**) Three-vessels angiography (14 months of age): disappearance of the vein of Galen aneurysm; absence of opacification of the deep venous galenic system. Rerouting of the venous outflow via prominent cortical veins draining into superior sagittal and lateral sinuses (**K**, arrowheads).

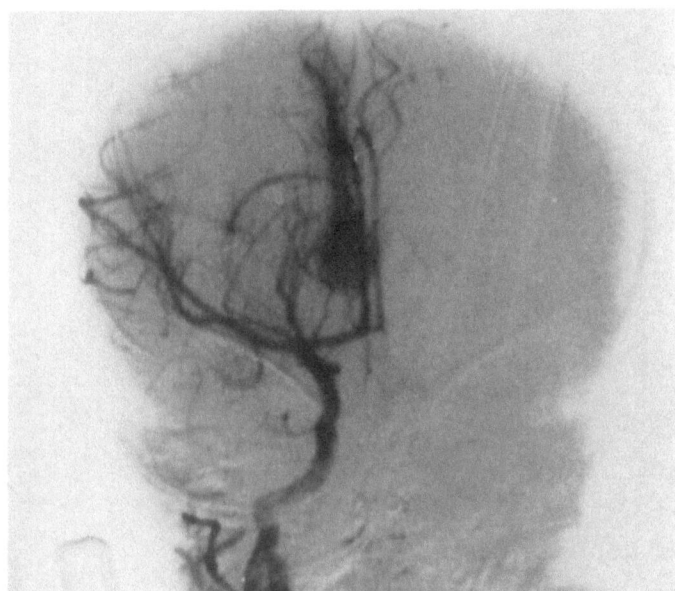

Figure 11.7B

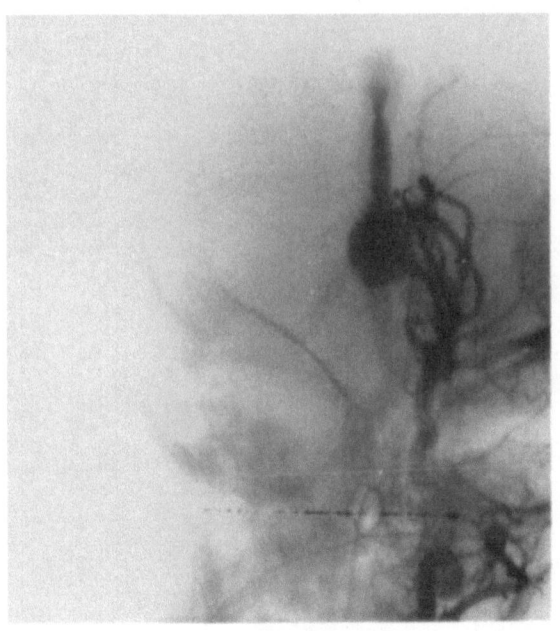

Figure 11.7C

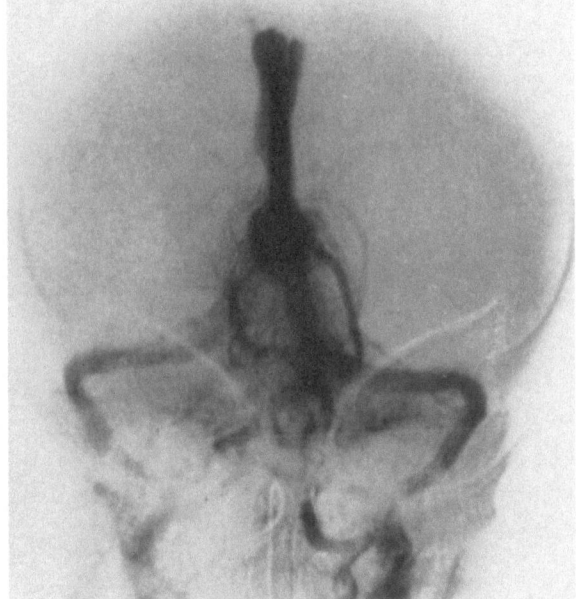

Figure 11.7D

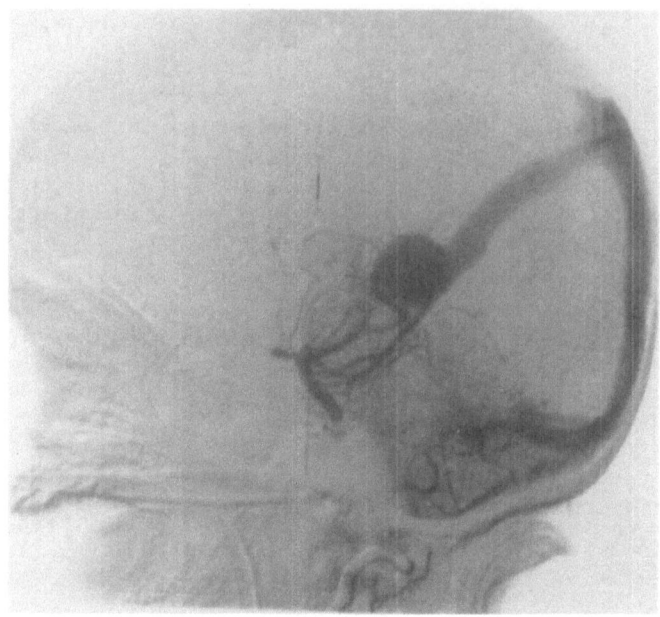

Figure 11.7E

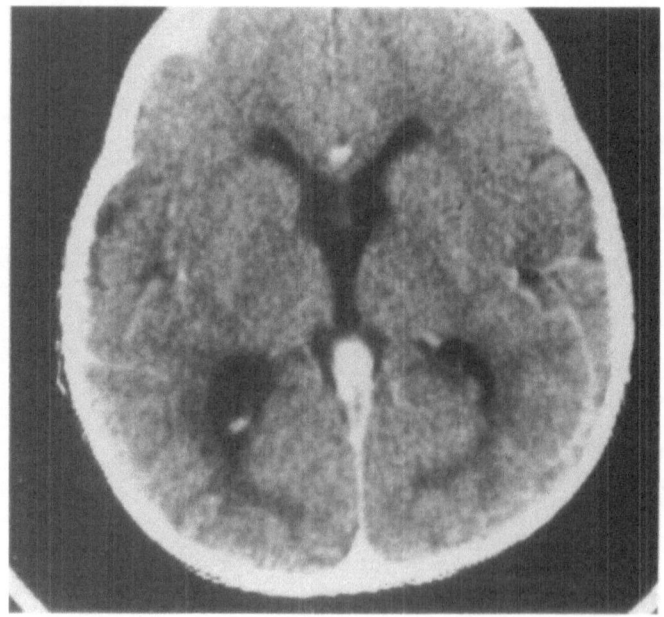

Figure 11.7F

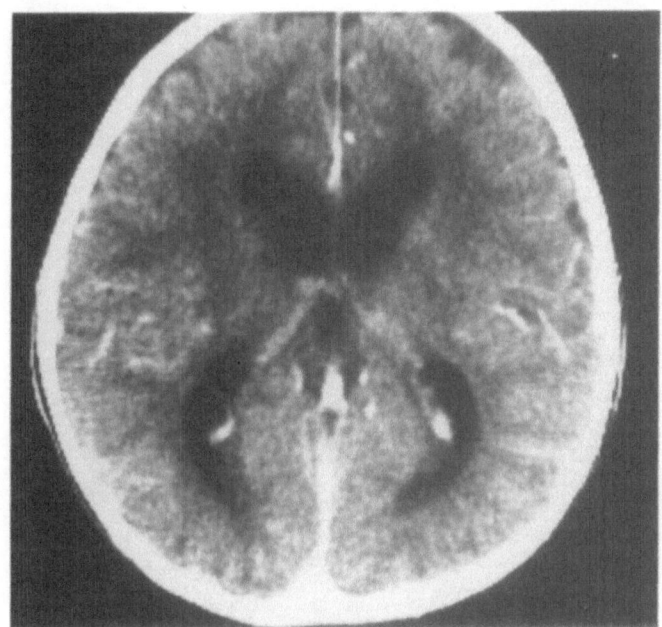

Figure 11.7G

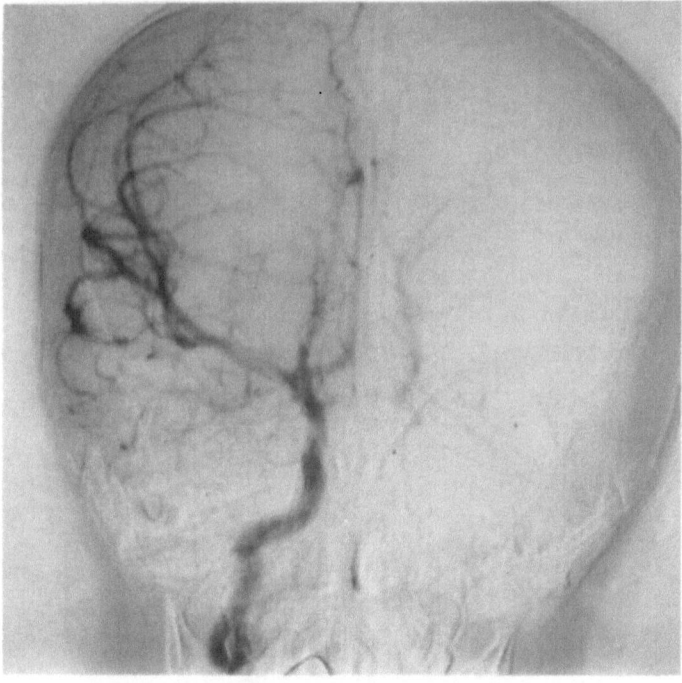

Figure 11.7H

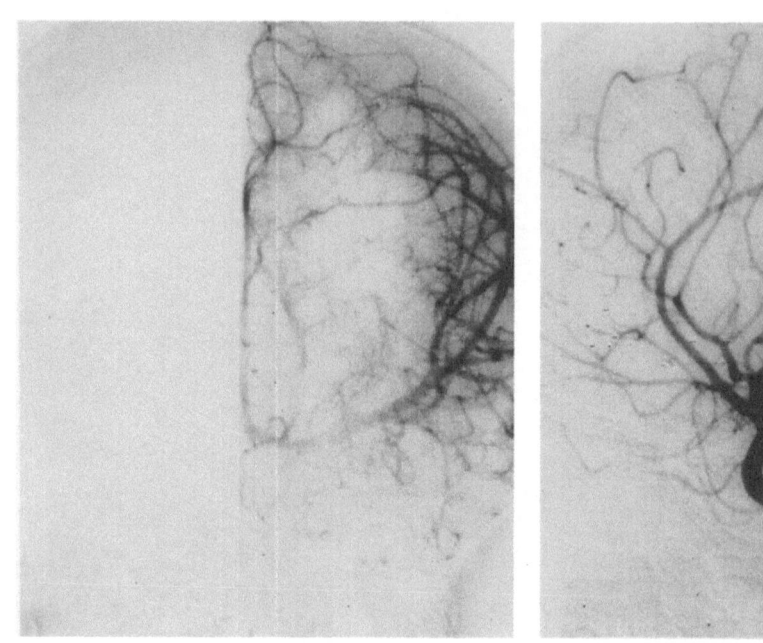

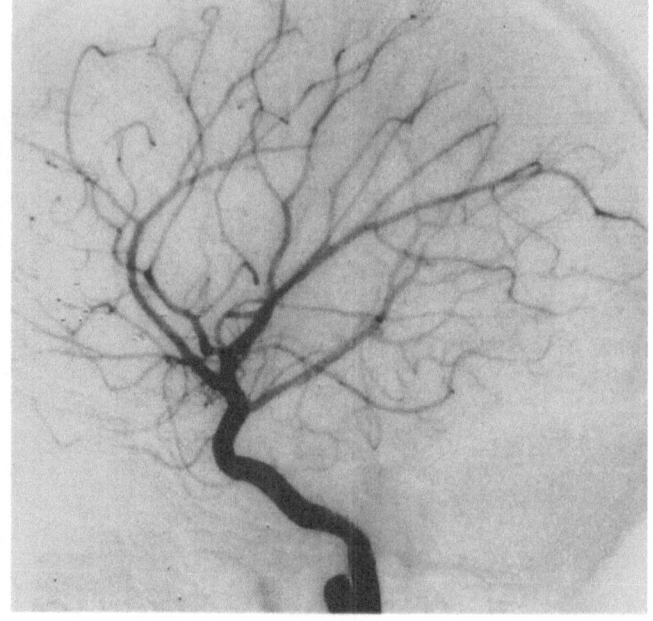

Figure 11.7I

Figure 11.7J

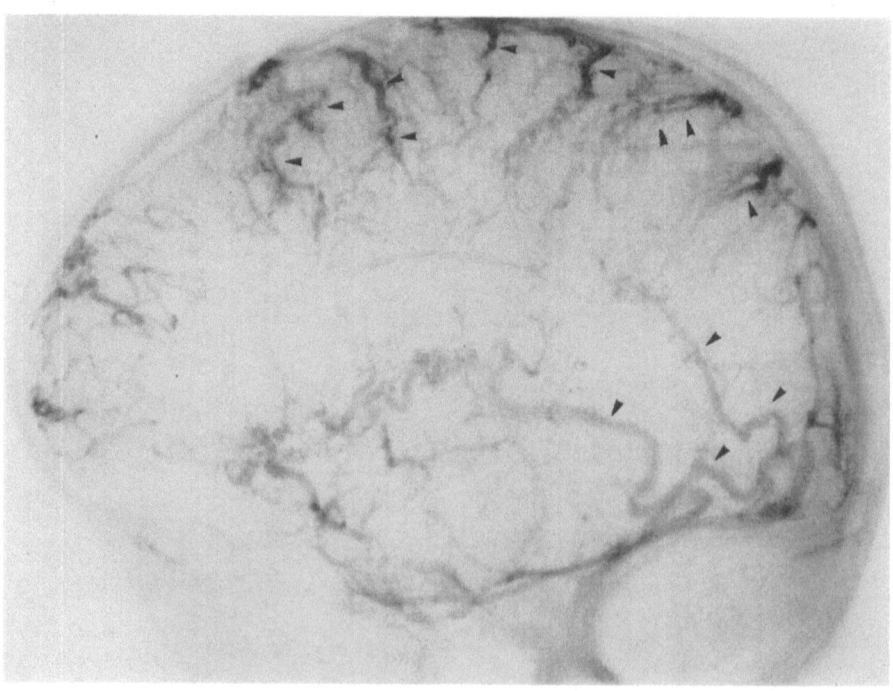

Figure 11.7K

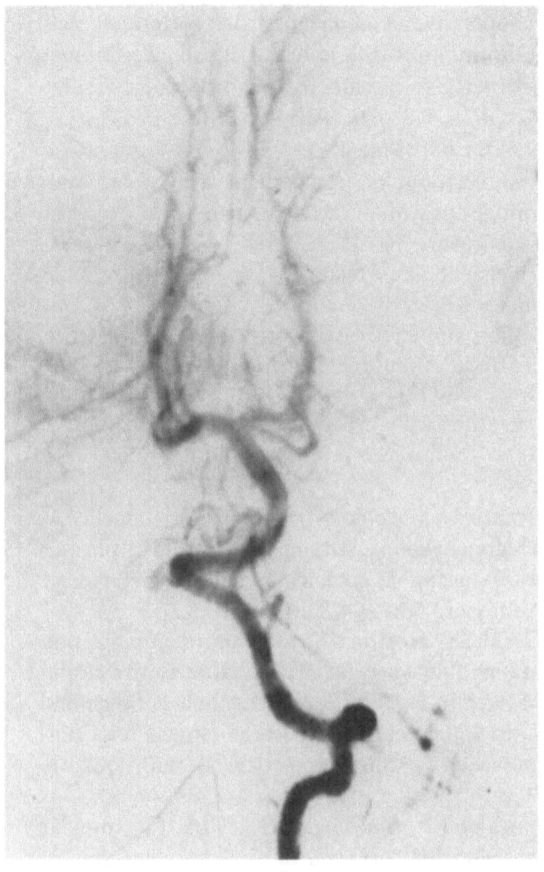

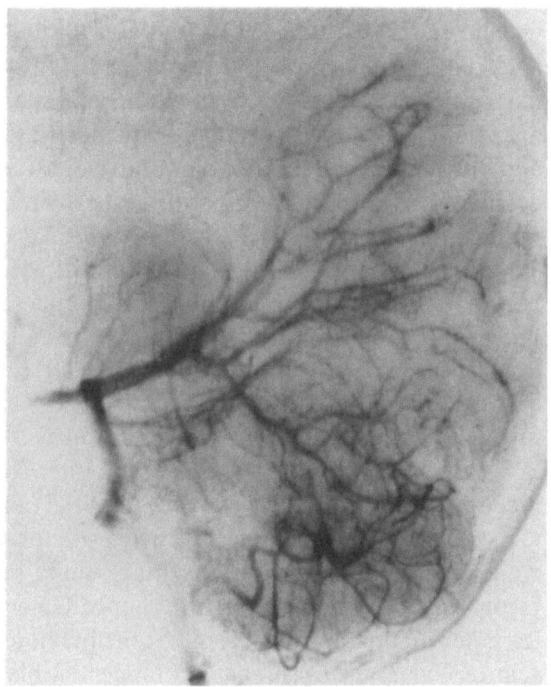

Figure 11.7M

Figure 11.7L

posterior cerebral artery and a large vein draining into the superior longitudinal sinus.

Embolization by the means of wing microcatheter and long pieces of Polylene threads resulted in the complete closure of the fistula (Fig. 11.5).

Trigeminal neuralgia immediately decreased and 1 month later the patient was completely symptom-free.

Six months later follow-up angiography demonstrated that closure of the fistula was stable, without recanalization.

On the other hand, closure of the main arterial axis must be considered a safe, stable cure of most intracranial giant aneurysms (Fig. 11.6). Nevertheless, with recent technical advances it is now possible to treat some intracranial aneurysms by detachable balloon embolization and spare the parent vessel.

Vein of Galen aneurysmal malformations deserve special care: the extremely high morbidity and mortality associated with all forms of management continues to pose a tremendous challenge. Recent advances in endovascular embolization techniques can offer significant advantages alone or in conjunction with surgery.[12-15]

Finally, it must be remembered that spontaneous thrombosis of brain arteriovenous malformations is a rare, but possible, event;[16] furthermore, in the paediatric age, it would seem more prone to occur, especially for peculiar localization.

More than 20 cases of spontaneously thrombosed vein of Galen aneurysms can be found in the literature, thus confirming the complex spectrum of this malformation which, on fortuitous occasions, can benefit from a natural cure so that in the series of Lasjaunias et al. up to 10% of arteriovenous galenic malformations spontaneously thrombosed.[17] In our experience, two cases of spontaneous thrombosis of vein of Galen aneurysms occurred: one of these is worthy of mention. A girl, born by cesarian delivery at the fortieth week for hydrocephalus, was submitted in another institution to CT scan on the twelfth day of life; CT scan showed the presence of a spherical enhancing mass in the region of the vein of

Galen, draining into an enlarged dural sinus (Fig. 11.7). Angiography (thirty-second day of life) confirmed the presence of a vein of Galen aneurysm fed by the choroidal, lenticulostriate, and posterior cerebral arteries of both sides; the drainage was toward the superior sagittal sinus via the median prosencephalic vein and falcine sinus. The baby at the age of 8 months was referred to us for consultation concerning a possible endovascular management of the lesion: neurological examination was normal and no signs of intracranial hypertension were found. CT scan revealed a significant decrease in size both of the ventricles and the malformation. When the girl was 14 months old, CT scan disclosed only mild ventricular dilation while neither masses nor calcifications could be recognizable in the region of the vein of Galen. Repeated angiography showed that the previous vein of Galen aneurysm was no longer visible; the deep venous galenic system was not opacified. The venous outflow rerouted via prominent and tortuous collateral pathways to cortical veins draining into superior sagittal and lateral sinuses.

References

1. Lasjaunias P, Doyon D: Angiographie dia-gnostique et thérapeutique en neuropédiatrie. Revue de 32 cas de lesions maxillo-faciales et cervicales entre 1977 et 1981. Ann Otol Laryngol 98:625–628, 1981.
2. Vinters JV, Galil KA, Lundic MJ, Kaufmann JCE: The histotoxicity of cyanoacrylates. A selective review. Neuroradiology 27:279–291, 1985.
3. Beltramello A, Benati, A, Maschio A, Perini S: Therapeutic angiography in infants and children. Pediatr Neurosci 3:79–91, 1987.
4. Beltramello A, Benati A, Perini S, Maschio A: Interventional angiography in neuropediatrics. Child's Nerv Syst 5:87–93, 1989.
5. Benati A, Beltramello A, Maschio A, Perini S, Rosta L, Piovan E: Endovascular treatment of intracranial AVMs. Combined embolization with a multipurpose mobile wing microcatheter system. J Neuroradiol 14:99–113, 1987.
6. Benati A, Beltramello A, Colombari R, Maschio A, Perini S, Da Pian R, Pasqualin A, Scienza R, Rosta L, Piovan E, Scarpa A, Zamboni G:

Preoperative embolization of arterio-venous malformations with polylene threads. Techniques with wing microcatheter and pathologic results. AJNR 10:579–586, 1989.
7. Debrun G, Vineula F, Fox AJ, Drake CG: Embolization of cerebral arteriovenous mal-formations with bucrylate. Experience of 46 cases. J Neurosurg 56:615–627, 1982.
8. Rufenacht D, Merland JJ: A new and original microcatheter system for hyperselective catheter-ization and endovascular treatment without risk of arterial rupture. J Neuroradiol 13:44–54, 1986.
9. Rufenacht D, Merland JJ: Superselective cathe-terization using very flexible, formed catheters. Acta Radiol Suppl (Stockholm) 369:600–602, 1987.
10. Benati A, Maschio A, Perini S, Beltramello A: Treatment of posttraumatic carotid-cavernous fistula using a detachable balloon catheter. J Neurosurg 53:784–786, 1980.
11. Hecht ST, Horton JA: Silk suture embolization of high flow vascular malformations. In: Nadjmi M (ed.), Imaging of Brain Metabolism Spine and Cord Interventional Neuroradiology Free Com-munications. Springer-Verlag, Berlin, 1989, p. 303.
12. Nuckle JP, Quisling RG: The transtorcular embolization of vein of Galen aneurysms. J Neurosurg 64:731–735, 1986.
13. Berenstein A, Epstein F: Vein of Galen malformations: combined neurosurgical and neuroradiologic intervention. In: American Asso-ciation of Neurological Surgeons, (eds.), Pediatric Neurosurgery. Surgery of the Developing Ner-vous System. Grune & Stratten, New York, 1982, pp. 637–647.
14. King WA, Wackym PA, Vinuela F, Peacock WJ: Management of vein of Galen aneurysms. Combined surgical and endovascular approach. Child's Nerv Syst 5:208–211, 1989.
15. Lasjaunias P, Rodesch G, Pruvost Ph, Grillot Laroche F, Landrieu P: Treatment of vein of Galen aneurysmal malformation. J Neurosurg 70:746–750, 1981.
16. Pasqualin A, Vivenza C, Rosta L, Scienza R, Da Pian R, Colangeli M: Spontaneous disappearance of intracranial arterio-venous malformations. Acta Neurochir 76:50–57, 1985.
17. Lasjaunias P, Terbugge K, Piske R, Lopez Ibor L, Manelfe C: Dilatation de la veine de Galien. Formes anatomo-cliniques et traitement en-dovasculaire à propos de 14 cas explorés et ou traités entre 1983 et 1986. Neurochirurgie 33:315–333, 1987.

CHAPTER 12

Linear Accelerator Radiosurgery of Cerebral Arteriovenous Malformations in the Pediatric Age Group

Federico Colombo

Introduction

In Leksell's definition, *radiosurgery* means the destruction of intracranial targets, defined by a stereotactic procedure, by focusing radiation energy from external sources.[1] In this new surgical method, the radiation beam was thought to replace the surgeon's instrument in "open" procedures, mainly in the field of functional neurosurgery (Parkinsonism, intractable pain, psychiatric disorders), with the aim of avoiding the otherwise rare operative complications such as hemorrhage or infections. The first apparatuses employed in clinical practice were based on the principle of arc irradiation. After the very early operations performed either with the aid of particulated beams or low-energy X-ray beams,[2] Leksell proposed the first multicobalt radiosurgical unit (the gamma unit)[1,3] with the aim of giving nothing more than another surgical instrument to be manipulated by the neurosurgeon's hand. In this apparatus, from 179 to 201 shielded ^{60}Co sources, arrayed on a spherical sector (70 to $110 \times 140°$), the collimated beams are directed toward the target point, localized by the stereotactic procedure.

With increasing clinical experience, the first application field (functional neurosurgery) proved to be barren, so new fields were explored. Backlund et al.[4] started to irradiate tumors in the pineal region and craniopharyngiomas. Leksell[5] proposed stereotactic irradiation of acoustic neuromas. Rahn et al.[6] employed radiosurgical treatment for pituitary adenomas. In 1972, Steiner et al. performed the first radiosurgical operation in a patient with a cerebral arteriovenous malformation (AVM).[7] Since that early report, in his hands, radiosurgery has gained wide acceptance as a safe and efficient method for cure of this life-threatening disease.[8-10]

Other authors pioneered different forms of radiosurgery. Kjellberg et al.[11] and Kjellberg[12] developed a radiosurgical procedure employing a stereotactically focalized Bragg-peak proton beam from a 186-MeV cyclotron at Harvard. Similarly, Fabrikant et al.[13] gained experience with a radiosurgical procedure based on the helium ion beam from a 230-MeV cyclotron. Both these techniques, however efficient, shared with Leksell's gamma unit the drawback of being expensive and exclusively dedicated to neurosurgical work.

In recent years, under the compelling influence of radiosurgery achievements, other radiosurgical techniques, employing the more widely available standard cobalt unit[14] or linear accelerators have been tested[15-21] and employed in clinical practice.[22-27]

Our original procedure—introduced in 1982—has proven safe and reliable in a series of 213 patients affected by a variety of intracranial lesions unsuitable to open surgery.[23-25] From November 1984 until October 1989 we have treated 120 patients affected by cerebral arteriovenous malformations. Among them, 24 were under 15 years of age. The aim of this chapter is to present our technique, and the results obtained in the pediatric group.

The Principle

Dose concentration inside target volume is obtained by multiple, noncoplanar, arc irradiations.[17] The stereotactically defined target is made to coincide with the linear accelerator isocenter, the virtual point around which the X-ray source rotates. A single arc irradiation is performed on a 100 to 160° arc. Then the target is rotated around a vertical axis passing through the isocenter, and arc irradiations are repeated in different angular positions, distributed through a 160° cylindrical sector.

Physical and Dosimetric Considerations

Because steepness of dose gradient and uniformity of dose volume distribution are dependent on the width of the spherical sector through which the radiation is administered, the first step was to try to optimize the angular amplitude of arc irradiations and their spatial distribution around the target.

With regard to a single arc, the highest concentration is obtained by arc irradiation as wide as possible (180°). In practice, angle values up to 180° do not provide improvement in dose distribution, owing to the overlap of parallel opposite fields. Moreover, taking into account the relationship of nearby arc irradiations, beams of adjacent arcs come close or overlap near the extremities of the arcs. For the sake of a more uniform dose distribution, a reduction of arc amplitude is advisable. We decided to employ 9 to 17 arc irradiations, 140 to 160° wide, equally distributed (each 10 to 20° in a 160° cylindrical sector). The irradiation spherical sector is 140 × 160°.

The second step was to determine the dose emitted by the radiation machine.[28] Measurements were performed with the aid of an ionization chamber connected to Ionex 2500/3 equipment (Nuclear Enterprise, Reading, England) in a polyethylene phantom. The variation of the emitted dose with field size was determined by film dosimetry. The choice among different available radiotherapy machines (a ^{60}Co unit, and 4- and 18-MV linear

accelerators) was made by comparing isodose distributions in phantoms. A 4-MV energy level has been selected as the most suitable in terms of sparing effect to healthy tissues.

In a third step, the complete irradiation procedure was simulated and tested, with the aid of Anderson Rando,[27a] and using polyethylene phantoms fixed to the stereotactic frame. Mechanical tests have demonstrated that during rotation of both linear accelerator and stereotactic frame, the distance between isocenter and the target is always less than 1.5 mm.

Dose distribution was calculated by an AECL TP 11 computer system, and was verified by film dosimetry. Also, with normal, built-in, square collimators a number of arcs equal or superior to 5, regularly interspaced on a 160° solid angle, is able to provide an approximately spherical inner isodose pattern. Isodoses obtained by standard square collimators were compared to those obtained by adjunctive, round-shaped collimators such as those employed by Betti and Derechinsky[4] and Hartmann et al.[18] No significant improvement of dose gradient has been obtained by adjunctive collimators.[28] Finally, the dose absorbed by critical organs was measured. While treating intracranial targets of 15-mm diameter, absorbed doses were found to be 0.17% at the thyroid gland, 0.08% at the lens, and 0.02% at the gonads.[17,28]

As a result of the preliminary physical evaluation, we obtained a working sheet plotting diameter of percentage isodoses in sagittal, axial, and frontal planes for collimator surface area openings from 5 × 5 to 50 × 50 mm.

Operative Technique

Target coordinates were always calculated by stereotactic angiography. Angiography is necessary not only to localize the arteriolar part of the pathologic vessel tangles—the selected target—but also to identify nearby vessels that can still feed functional areas and, consequently, must be spared by an obliterating radiation dose.

In a first step, the patient is fixed to a base ring in the operating room and stereoradiographies are taken in both antero-posterior (AP) and latero-lateral (LL) views. Since in our stereotactic unit radiological parameters such as focus-to-target and focus-to-film distance can be varied, X-ray magnification can be made to coincide with that of preoperative angiography: at that moment, bony profiles of stereo X-rays are superimposed upon preoperative angiograms and target coordinates are calculated in a first approximation ($\pm$ 5 mm).[29] The patient is fixed to the angiographic table by means of head frame holder. Because of the short focus-to-film distance, radiological distortion must be taken into account. After the centering procedure, a millimetric ruler is positioned in the plane where the target lies, according to calculations made in the stereotactic suite. AP and LL X-rays are taken and radiological distortion in the target plane is extrapolated. Selective, high-speed angiography is performed, usually by catheterization via a transfemoral route. Recently, a similar procedure has been employed in combination with digital subtraction angiography. With the aid of the working sheet, collimator openings are determined so as to have the selected isodose encompassing the nidus of the arteriovenous malformation.

We usually define TI as the isodose surface inside which an adequate dose is absorbed so as to obtain a therapeutic effect (arteriolar obliteration). We consider a dose from 15 to 30 Gy, depending on target volume, safe and effective for TI in AVMs.

Also, for each particular case a risk isodose (RI) is defined as the isodose outside which any radiosensitive structure absorbs less than the dose entailing a significant risk of radionecrosis. RI depends on biological factors—radiosensitivity of adjacent healthy tissues—but also on "criticity" of nearby functional structures, such as visual pathways, brainstem, etc. Also if our experience seems to confirm that a radiosurgical single dose of 10 Gy is tolerated by silent brain, the dose that can be safely delivered to a functional structure can be lower, reaching 8 to 6 Gy and even less if the structure is suffering ischemia or compression.

Two other important factors may influence the choice of dose: observation interval and target volume.[30] Observation interval is the time period in which we may observe radiosurgery

clinical effects: higher doses produce earlier effects than lower ones. Early therapeutic effects could be the goal in patients with a higher bleeding risk. The same consideration holds true for untoward effects: a very long observation interval must be anticipated in young patients with AVMs. In Kjellberg's experience, isoeffect lines (log-dose versus log-time) have a slope of -0.27.[30]

According to this statement, we prefer to give those patients with more than a 30-year life expectancy and low bleeding risk a dose as low as 70% of that employed in elderly patients, with a high bleeding risk. This fact, together with the reported higher radiation sensitivity of the child's nervous system structures, explains the lower doses employed in patients under 10 years of age.

The volume of the target seems to be very important in determining the risk of potential adverse effects. While for small targets (up to 15-mm diameter) 125 to 35 Gy was considered practicable, for AVMs larger than 20 mm we took into consideration the relation log-dose versus log-radius.[25] Once these evaluations were completed, ideal dose and diameter are stated for both TI and RI. With the aid of the working sheet, collimator dimensions are stated. Very often TI is selected as the 80% isodose—where dose gradient is steeper—but also other percentage isodoses can be selected.

Not in every situation may the choice of collimator be ideally satisfying. Since dimensional relation between different percentage isodoses obtainable with a single collimator is fixed, there is the possibility that the most favorable situation (having all the target volume inside TI and all radiosensitive structures outside RI) may not be possible. This situation is more probable in AVMs with highly radiosensitive structures—cranial nerves II and V, and brainstem—located right on their surface or directly encased in them. Also, with our smaller fields the difference in diameter between the 80 and 20% isodose is 10 mm. Consequently, one must choose between two alternatives, either to reduce the diameter of TI and to have the outer shell of the target volume exposed to a radiation dose insufficient for obtaining therapeutic effect, or to expose a radiosensitive structure to a significant risk of radionecrosis. In this situation, we prefer to elect RI as the most important factor for determining collimator dimensions.

Once target coordinates have been calculated and collimators selected, the patient, always fastened to the base ring, is fixed to the tool holder of our original stereotactic apparatus.[31] This apparatus works with a spherical system: when stereotactic coordinates are set, a tool as long as the radius of a characteristic ideal sphere reaches the target from any direction. In radiosurgical procedures, the surgical tool is replaced by a millimetric ruler. The aim of this ruler is to materialize the radiation beam for procedure simulation and for calculation of the depth of tissues through which the beams must pass before reaching the target (depth of the tissue equals length of the radius minus length of the extracranial ruler). The ruler is moved around the target, following a trajectory identical to movements of the linear accelerator beam, and the tissue depth is recorded each 30°. The lengths of various depths recorded are utilized for reconstructing, on the dose-planning computer drawing board, the head profile along preset planes of irradiation. The total amount of dose emitted by the linear accelerator (in monitor units [MU] is determined to obtain the prescribed dose into target volume.

The patient is moved to the linear accelerator room. A holder allowing the fixation of either the base ring or the base-ring phantom is fixed to the treatment couch of a Varian 4-MV linear accelerator (Varian Associates, Inc., Palo Alto, CA). Target coordinates are set on phantom rulers. The phantom is fixed to the holder and the target is made to coincide to the linear accelerator isocenter, marked by the front pointer, by controlled movements of the treatment couch. Specially designed brakes are tightened to avoid uncontrolled movements of the treatment couch. The phantom is removed, and in its place is fixed the base ring with the patient (Fig. 12.1). A first arc irradiation is undertaken. After the completion of the first arc, the couch is rotated a preselected number of degrees around a vertical axis passing through the isocenter and arc irradiations are repeated in 9 to 17 planes, equally distributed along a solid angle of 160°.[16,17,23,24,29]

Results

Our series consists of 120 patients, treated from November 1984 to October 1989. Patients were evaluated on a regular follow-up basis. Cerebral angiography was performed at 12-month intervals until the AVM was completely obliterated

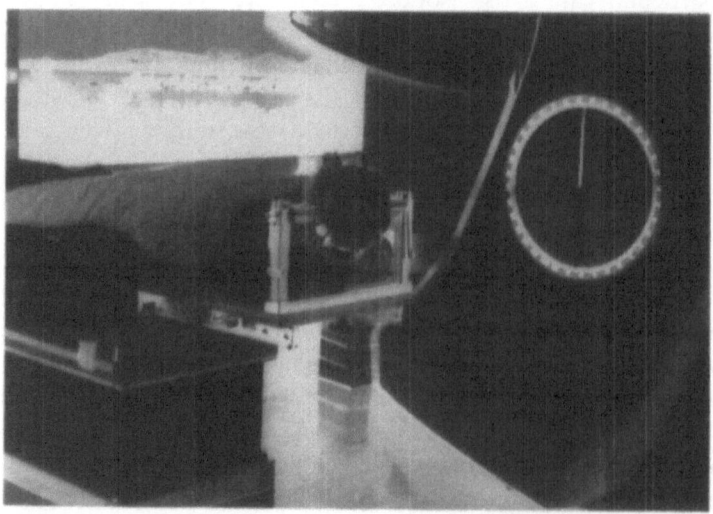

Figure 12.1. The patient, fixed to treatment couch, is ready for multiple arc irradiations.

or had stabilized. Computerized tomography (CT) scan was performed at 6-month intervals for the first 3 years.

We herein present results obtained in 24 patients under 15 years of age. Nine were male and 15 female. At the moment of treatment, age ranged from 6 to 15 years. Seven patients had the AVM located in or involving significantly the basal ganglia. Two patients harbored lesions involving the corpus callosum. The remaining patients harbored hemispheric lesions, located either in the temporal (four cases), frontoparietal (rolandic) (seven cases), occipital (three cases), or frontal (one case) lobes. Thirteen AVMs involved the left side, 9 the right, and 2 occupied the midline. Presenting symptoms were bleeding in 22 cases and epilepsy in 2 cases. Two patients harbored multiple intracranial angiomas. A 6-year-old boy had two arteriovenous malformations and three cavernous angiomas. A 15-year-old girl had three arteriovenous malformations of the corpus callosum and basal ganglia.

Eight patients had previous treatment for their AVMs. Seven patients underwent incomplete removal by open surgery. In one patient, four repeated attempts to embolize were performed.

AVM dimensions varied from 8 to 40 mm in maximal dimension.

All our pediatric patients were treated with a single field. This option is always technically feasible owing to the availability of an infinite number of field dimensions, obtained by modifying the aperture of collimators. Radiation dose varied from 15 to 34 Gy at the target point, administered in a single session. The entire tangle of pathologic arteriolar vessels could be covered with a dose considered adequate for obliteration in 18 patients. In the remaining group (six patients) only a part of the arteriovenous malformation was treated. None of our patients were treated by multiple small fields aimed at feeding arteries.

The mean follow-up is 21.3 months (ranging from 1 to 42 months). To date, clinical information is available from all patients. No rebleeding was observed after treatment. Out of 19 patients with more than 1-year follow-up, 17 (89.4%) underwent 12-month control angio-

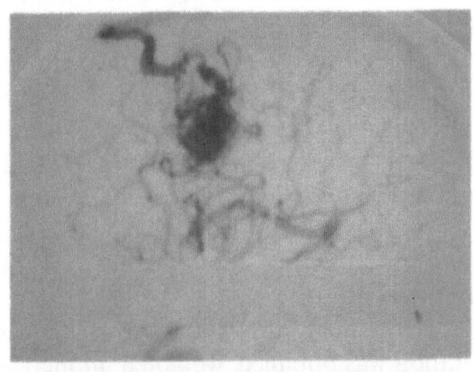

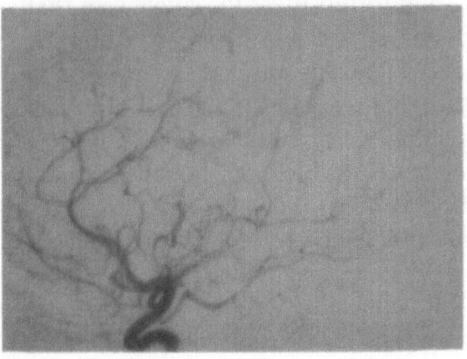

Figure 12.2. Case 13: an 11-year-old female. Serious bleeding episode 2 months before admission. Large (25 × 27 × 30 mm) deep fronto-parietal AVM fed by left middle cerebral artery. Treatment: 20 × 20 mm field, 30 Gy at target point, TI 80% (24 Gy). Left carotid angiogram (**A**) before treatment; (**B**) 12 months after treatment.

graphy. Two patients, both in good clinical condition, refused angiographic control. In 9 patients, complete obliteration of the malformation was demonstrated (52.9%) (Fig. 12.2). In two other cases, total obliteration was demonstrated only at 24-month follow-up angiography, raising the complete obliteration rate to 71.4% at 2 years (five out of seven patients followed for more than 24 months). In seven patients the obliteration was evident but not complete. In those patients in which only a part of the malformation was obliterated, isodose distribution was superimposed upon follow-up angiographies. In these cases, the volume of the obliterated part was encompassed by isodose surfaces indicating absorbed doses from 15 to 29 Gy. Other features were prominent in follow-up angiographies of incompletely obliterated cases. A narrowing of arterial feeders, together with a diameter reduction and straightening of venous drainages, was observed in six of seven cases. In these cases a marked slowing of blood flow velocity through the malformation was also evident. In one patient, harboring a huge basal ganglia malformation fed by perforating vessels from the middle cerebral artery, we noted a regression of classical steal phenomenon affecting the adjacent anterior cerebral territory.

In one patient in whom a significant obliteration was obtained, we noted an increase in size and tortuosity of the single vein that was still patent after radiosurgery. We think that in this case there was an increase in intraluminal pressure due to bloodstream rerouting, caused by the obliteration of the other draining veins.

In cases in which epilepsy was the most prominent sign (two cases) no significant influence of irradiation on seizure frequency or type was ascertained. In one patient we observed untoward clinical syndromes after radiosurgery. A 15-year-old boy with a deep parietal AVM (15 mm in diameter, 33.7 Gy of radiation) suffered marked worsening of a preirradiation contralateral motor syndrome. Time of appearance (from month 9) and an *ex adjuvantibus* criterion seem to relate this worsening to radiosurgery. CT examination revealed a contrast-enhanced area corresponding to the treated volume, together with a large hypodense area around it. In three cases, CT examination at 6 or 12 months disclosed a significant hypodense area encircling the treated AVM, in one case with an extension into the territory of a tributary vessel. No evident clinical symptoms appeared.

Discussion

Arteriovenous malformations represent the most frequent source of intracranial bleeding during infancy and childhood. About 15% of patients treated for a cerebral angioma are under 16 years of age.[32]

Radiosurgery is an effective method for treating AVMs, a potentially life-threatening disease. However, the probability of cure must be carefully balanced with the risk of adverse effects, particularly dangerous in young patients. Controversy exists among different authors with respect to optimal dose to be delivered. Steiner recently stated that a dose of at least 25 Gy should be given to the entire malformation.[9,10] AVMs up to 25 to 30 mm in diameter can be covered with one or more fields, in this case requiring a dose reduction.[8] Treatment of feeders with multiple small fields seems to afford a lesser chance to be effective.[7,9,10] No dose reduction is suggested for younger patients.

Kjellberg's procedures for determining the doses for AVM treatment are based on an empirical nomogram relating log-dose to log-diameter. Age is considered only as a factor influencing the observation interval. While a small malformation requires, in Kjellberg's opinion, at least 35 Gy, a large (up to 50 to 100 mm in diameter) AVM should be successfully irradiated by protons with no more than 10 or 5 Gy.[30,33]

Fabrikant moved from 45 Gy, used early in his experience, to the present 15 to 25 Gy delivered to the center of the target volume.[13,34]

The only published series of patients treated by a linear accelerator-based radiosurgical technique belongs to Betti et al.[22] In these patients, doses are delivered from 20 to 70 Gy, the large majority varying from 30 to 50 Gy. Also, in this material, no difference in dose planning is reported in pediatric patients.

Our approach to the choice of the dose has been flexible. In our opinion AVMs up to 20 mm in diameter can be treated by a dose from 25 to 35 Gy, according to previously described factors (age, bleeding risk, observation interval, nearby radiosensitive structures). For AVMs larger than 20 mm in diameter, our policy to reduce the dose according to a log-dose versus log-diameter nomogram. The starting point of this algorithm for deciding treatment doses in large AVMs was the Kjellberg nomogram log-dose versus log-diameter (Kjellberg, personal communication). With increasing experience the line relating these two parameters has been modified by us, taking into account data obtained in incompletely obliterated cases. Follow-up angiography of these cases has been examined. Isodose distribution was superimposed on the obliterated part and the dose absorbed at the edge of the

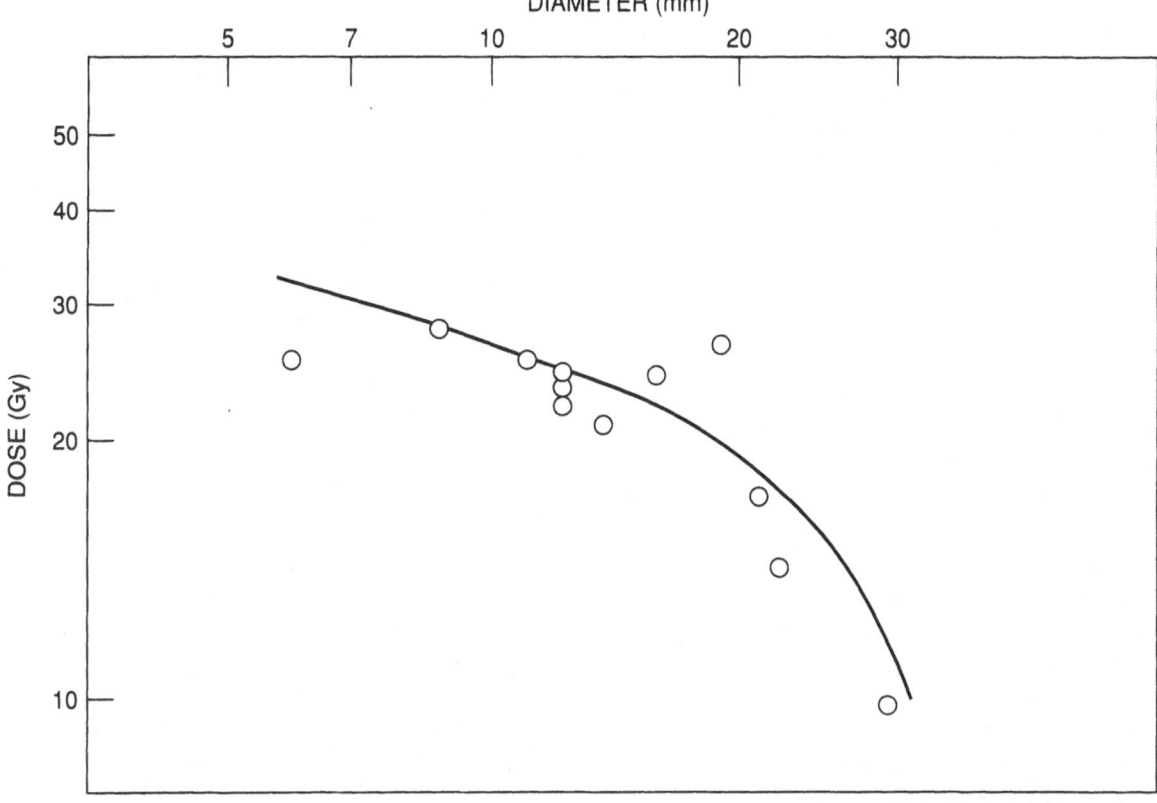

Figure 12.3. Log-dose versus log-diameter plot relative to 13 cases of incomplete therapeutic effect. Dose has been evaluated at the edge of the obliterated volume. Isoeffective line has been extrapolated.

obliterated volume was calculated. We have obtained a series of points relating the amount of dose absorbed at the edge of obliteration to the diameter of the volume in which positive obliteration has taken place. These experimental data have been inserted in the log-dose versus log-radius diameter (Fig. 12.3). The resulting isoeffective line may be taken as the rule for treatment dose planning.

In major published series, results are not interpreted with respect to patient's age and only rough obliteration data in the entire population of treated patients are reported. Steiner achieves total obliteration in 33.7% after 1 year and 86% after 2 years. Undue effects—usually transient —appear in 2 to 3%. Rebleeding occurred in only 12 patients—all incompletely obliterated cases—among 450.[9,10]

A large series is reported by Kjellberg, including 717 patients. Follow-up angiography was performed in 57% of his material. Total (22%) and subtotal (29%) obliteration was obtained at the 2-year follow-up. Two cases of

radionecrosis were observed but the real percentage of undue effects seems to be higher, 2%.[33]

Fabrikant and co-workers report on 316 cases of AVMs, in 80% of whom total obliteration was obtained. The treated patient rebleed rate was 6.5%, most hemorrhages occurring in the first 12 months after irradiation. Persistent neurological deficits were observed in 5 to 6% of patients.[34]

Betti and co-workers report on 41 patients with angiographic follow-up. This series does not represent the results obtained in the entire group of patients because angiographic control was performed only in patients in whom a significant modification of the CT picture was demonstrated after radiosurgery. Results are strongly influenced by the diameter of treated lesions, varying from 81.3% complete obliteration in AVMs under 12 mm of diameter to 12% in AVMs over 25 mm.[22]

Our results seem to confirm the efficacy and safety of radiosurgical treatment, also in the pediatric age group. A 43% total obliteration rate—in our 120-patient series—for 1 year is very close to the percentages reported by Steiner[9] and Steiner and Lindquist.[10] Furthermore, the results obtained in the restricted series of pediatric patients are even better (50%) in short-term follow-up. Also, even though our cases with a follow-up longer than 24 months are few (only seven patients under 15 years), the total obliteration rate at 2 years seems to be significantly lower. The higher 12-month obliteration rate may be explained by a shorter latency time for therapeutic effect in infancy and childhood, whereas the lower 24-month obliteration rate could be the consequence of the lower doses employed. We have no explanation for the lower rebleed rate after treatment we observed in our series of pediatric patients. Also, in our experience radiosurgical treatment is more effective in small AVMs that can be completely encompassed by an adequate dose, although there are a few significant exceptions. In two patients complete obliteration was induced by treating only a part of the AVM with a dose supposed adequate, leaving other parts relatively underdosed (6 and 5 Gy absorbed at the far edge of the malformation). In these cases we aimed at the part where feeding arteries converged and from which venous drainage departed. These cases seem to support the theory of the existence of a *nidus*, defined as the site of pathologic arteriovenous shunt, the selective occlusion or removal of which entails complete AVM obliteration.[35] A possible location of the nidus is, in our opinion, the arteriolar part immediately adjacent to the source of the draining vein. In monocompartmental AVMs with a single draining vein, there should be only one nidus, while in large, multicompartimental AVMs more than one target—one for each vein—should be irradiated to achieve obliteration.

In radiosurgical treatment planning there are three alternatives:

1. Treatment of the entire tangle of arteriolar shunt vessels (the best alternative, when feasible)
2. Treatment of all the arterial feeders (as in Steiner's early experience)
3. Irradiation of the arteriolar part of the AVM, proximal to the source of draining vein or veins

The confirmation of the existence of this "Achille's heel" would be of great interest, allowing the reduction of the volume of the target to be treated. The real impact of this possibility, whenever verified, in patients in whom there is considerable concern about late, untoward radiation effects—such as those in the pediatric age groups—need not be emphasized here.

References

1. Leksell L: Stereotaxis and Radiosurgery: An Operative System. Charles C Thomas, Springfield, IL, 1971.
2. Leksell L: Stereotaxis radiosurgery in trigeminal neuralgia. Acta Chir Scand 137:311–314, 1971.
3. Arndt J, Backlund EO, Larsson B, Leksell L, Noren G, Rosander K, Rahn T, Sarby B, Steiner L, Wennerstrand J: Stereotactic irradiation of intracranial structures: physical and biological considerations. In Szikla G (ed.), Stereotactic Cerebral Irradiations. Elsevier, Amsterdam, 1979, pp. 81–92.
4. Backlund EO, Rhan T, Sarby B: Treatment of pinealomas by stereotactic radiation surgery. Acta Radiol 13:368–376, 1974.
5. Leksell L: Stereotactic radiosurgery. J Neurol Neurosurg Psychiat 46:797–803, 1983.
6. Rahn T, Thoren M, Hall K, Backlund EO: Stereotactic radiosurgery in Cushing's syndrome: acute radiation effects. Surg Neurol 14:85–92, 1980.
7. Steiner L, Leksell L, Greitz T, Forster DMC, Backlund EO: Stereotactic radiosurgery for cerebral arteriovenous malformations. Report of a case. Acta Chir Scand 138:459–462, 1972.
8. Steiner L, Greitz T, Backlund EO, Leksell L, Noren G, Rahn T: Radiosurgery in arteriovenous malformations of the brain. Undue effects. In: Szikla G (ed.), Stereotactic Cerebral Irradiations. Elsevier, Amsterdam, 1979, pp. 257–269.
9. Steiner L: Radiochirurgia delle malformazioni arterovenose cerebrali. In: Da Pian R, Pasqualin A, Scienza R (eds.), Aneurismi e Angiomi Cerebrali. Cortina, Verona, 1986, pp. 307–329.
10. Steiner L, Lindquist C: Radiosurgery in cerebral arteriovenous malformation. In: Tasker RR (ed.), Neurosurgery: State of the Art Review. Hanley & Belfus, Philadelphia, 1987, pp. 329–336.

11. Kjellberg RN, Koehler AM, Preston WM, Sweet WH: Stereotaxic instrument for use with the Bragg peak of a proton beam. Confin Neurol 22:183–189, 1962.

12. Kjellberg RN: Stereotactic Bragg peak proton radiosurgery method. In: Szikla G (ed.), Stereotactic Cerebral irradiations. Elsevier, Amsterdam, 1979, pp. 93–100.

13. Fabrikant JI, Lyman JT, Hosobuchi Y: Stereotactic heavy ion Bragg peak radiosurgery for intracranial vascular disorders: method for treatment of deep arteriovenous malformations. Br J Radiat 57:479–490, 1984.

14. Barcia Salorio JL, Hernandez G, Broseta J, Gonzales Darder J, Ciudad J: Radiosurgical treatment of carotid-cavernous fistula. Appl Neurphysiol 45:520–522, 1982.

15. Betti O, Derechinsky V: Irradiation stéréotaxique multifasceaux. Neurochirurgie 29:295–298, 1983.

16. Colombo F, Benedetti A, Pozza F, Zanardo A, Avanzo RC, Chierego G, Marchetti C: New technique of external stereotactic irradiation by means of linear accelerator for treatment of intracranial tumors not surgically amenable. Acta Neurochir 73:80, 1984.

17. Colombo F, Benedetti A, Pozza F, Avanzo RC, Marchetti C, Chierego G, Zanardo A: External stereotactic irradiation by linear accelerator. Neurosurgery 16:154–160, 1985.

18. Hartmann G, Schlegel W, Sturm V, Kober B, Pastyr O, Lorentz WJ: Cerebral radiation surgery using moving field irradiation at a linear accelerator facility. Int J Radiat Oncol Biol Phys 2:1185–1192, 1985.

19. Heifetz MD, Wexler M, Thompson R: Single beam radiotherapy knife: a practical theoretical model. J Neurosurg 60:814–818, 1984.

20. Lutz W, Winston KR, Maleki N: A system for stereotactic radiosurgery with a linear accelerator. Med Phys 13:611–617, 1986.

21. Olivier A, Lotbinière A: Stereotactic techniques in epilepsy. In: Tasker RR (ed.), Neurosurgery: State of the Art Review. Hanley & Belfus, Philadelphia, 1987, pp. 257–287.

22. Betti O, Munari C, Rosler R: Stereotactic radiosurgery with the linear accelerator: treatment of arteriovenous malformations. Neurosurgery 24:311–321, 1989.

23. Colombo F, Benedetti A, Pozza F, Zanardo A, Avanzo RC, Chierego G, Marchetti C: Stereotactic radiosurgery utilizing a linear accelerator. Appl Neurophysiol 48:133–145, 1985.

24. Colombo F, Benedetti A, Pozza F, Avanzo RC, Chierego G, Marchetti C, Dettori P, Bernardi L, Pinna V: Radiosurgery using a 4 MV linear accelerator. Technique and radiobiological implications. Acta Radiol Suppl 369:603–607, 1986.

25. Colombo F, Benedetti A, Casentini L, Zanusso M, Pozza F: Linear accelerator radiosurgery of arteriovenous malformations. Neurosurgery 24:833–840, 1989.

26. Sturm V, Kober B, Hover K, Schlegel W, Boesecke R, Pastyr O, Hartmann G, Schabbert S, Winkel K, Kunze S, Lorentz W: Stereotactic percutaneous single dose irradiation of brain metastases with linear accelerator. Int J Radiat Oncol Biol Phys 13:279–282, 1987.

27. Valentino V: Stereotactic radiation therapy in arteriovenous malformations and brain tumors using the Fixter system. Acta Radiol Suppl 369:608–609, 1986.

27a. Alderson SW, Lanzl L, Rollins M, Spira J: An instrumented phantom system for analog computation of treatment plans. AJR 87:185–195, 1962.

28. Chierego G, Marchetti C, Avanzo RC, Pozza F, Colombo F: Dosimetric considerations on multiple arc stereotactic radiotherapy. Radiother Oncol 12:141–152, 1988.

29. Colombo F, Benedetti A, Pozza F, Zanardo A, Avanzo RC, Chierego G, Marchetti C: Linear accelerator radiosurgery: technical note. In: Pluchino P, Broggi G (eds.), Advanced Technology in Neurosurgery. Springer-Verlag, Heidelberg, 1987, pp. 170–177.

30. Kjellberg RN: Isoeffective dose parameters for brain necrosis in relation to proton radiosurgical dosimetry. In: Szikla G (ed.), Stereotactic Cerebral Irradiations. Elsevier, Amsterdam, 1979, pp. 157–166.

31. Colombo F, Zanardo A: Clinical application of an original stereotactic apparatus. Acta Neurochir (Suppl) 33:569–573, 1984.

32. Mazza C, Pasqualin A, Da Pian R: Angiomi cerebrali in età pediatrica. In: Da Pian R, Pasqualin A, Scienza R (eds.), Aneurismi e Angiomi Cerebrali. Cortina, Verona, 1986, pp. 209–216.

33. Kjellberg RN: Stereotactic Bragg peak proton beam radiosurgery for cerebral arteriovenous malformations. Ann Clin Res 18 (Suppl 47) :17–19, 1986.

34. Fabrikant JI, Levy RP, Frankel KA, Philips MH, Lyman JT, Chuang FY, Steinberg GK, Marks MP: Stereotactic helium ion radiosurgery for the treatment of intracranial arteriovenous malformations. In: Heikkinen H, Kiviniitty K (eds.), International Workshop on Proton and Narrow Photon Beam Therapy. Oulu University Printing Center, Oulu, Finland, 1989, pp. 33–37.

35. Doppman JL: The nidus concept of spinal cord arteriovenous malformations. Br J Radiat 44:758–763, 1971.

CHAPTER 13

Sturge–Weber Disease

Concezio Di Rocco

Introduction

Neural cutaneous syndromes constitute a rather heterogeneous group from a clinical standpoint. They include several distinct forms that have in common developmental anomalies of neural and other ectodermal structures; in particular, the brain, the skin, and the retina. In many of these syndromes, also known as phakomatoses and ectodermal dysplasias, visceral abnormalities are associated as well.[1]

Owing to their relatively higher incidence, five main syndromes are distinguished, namely tuberous sclerosis (Bourneville–Pringle disease), neurofibromatosis (von Recklinghausen disease), retinocerebellar angiomatosis (Hippel–Lindau disease), ataxia-telangiectasia (Louis–Bar or Border–Sedgwick disease), and encephalofacial angiomatosis (Sturge–Weber disease). Cerebrovascular disorders, due to congenital anatomical abnormalities (segmental ectasia, stenosis, tortuosity) or acquired lesions (neurofibromatous involvement of the cerebral arterial tree, calcifications of the vascular wall), have been documented in these syndromes.[2–4] Sturge–Weber disease differs from other neurocutaneous syndromes such as Hippel–Lindau, von Recklinghausen, and the Bourneville–Pringle disease because it is not inherited and is not associated with intracranial neoplasms. However, in this syndrome an extensive capillary–venous malformation affecting one, and occasionally both, cerebral hemispheres may be associated with intractable epilepsy and progressive mental retardation, which may eventually require extensive surgery, such as lobectomy or hemispherectomy.

Historical Background

In 1860 Schirmer[5] was the first to describe the coexistence of facial nevus flammeus and buphthalmos in a man aged 36. He did not mention a seizure disorder or mental symptoms.

In 1879, at the meeting of the Clinical Society of London, Sturge[6] reported on the case of a 6½-year-old girl who had an extensive teleangiectatic nevus of the right side of the face and head, a right-sided buphthalmos, as well as epileptic fits beginning in the left hand. In contrast with leading medical colleagues of the London Clinical Society, Sturge inferred that the right side of the brain was also involved in the nevoid condition. In subsequent years, postmortem studies of other patients by Kalischer,[7] as in 1897 a child who died at 1½ years, as well as in vivo observations by Cushing[8] in 1906 of two children, aged, respectively, 4 and 5 years, provided indirect confirmation of Sturge's prediction. Cushing pointed out the tendency of the facial nevi to follow the distribution of one or more branches of the trigeminal nerve and described the abnormal vascularity of the dura mater covering the affected cerebral hemisphere ("in all probability representing a naevoid condition similar to that present on the skin"), as well as the adhesions of this structure to the leptomeninges.

The atrophy of the affected cerebral hemisphere was first suggested in vivo by Weber[9] in 1922 by using simple X-ray examinations of the skull. The author noted a great difference between the two sides of the brain ["The left cerebral hemisphere appeared sclerosed; at all events, it was more opaque and gave a somewhat deeper shadow than the right hemisphere. It seemed to occupy only about two-thirds of the left half of the cranial cavity and to be surrounded by cerebrospinal fluid (external hydrocephalus)"].

Six years later, Weber provided accurate skiagrams of the same patients, demonstrating that "the whole of the left side, excluding the cerebellum" appeared to be small, "as if sclerosed or bound down by thickened or partially calcified leptomeninges." He also described calcareous deposits "in the walls of angiectatic vessels or in their thrombosed channels," or "extravascular" as a result of hemorrhages or thrombotic necroses.

Similar radiographic findings had been presented at the meeting of the Radiological Society of Copenhagen in 1921 by Ove Wissing, who showed a roentgenogram of the skull of a young man with a sinous "shadow" in the right occipital lobe, corresponding to the outline of the pia mater. The report was not published; however, subsequent information on the same patient, and in particular the observation of the substantial staticity of the radiological "shadow," may be found in reports published some years later by the same author and Krabbe.[10,11]

Table 13.1. Definitions and eponyms of Sturge–Weber disease.

Eponyms
    Parkes, Weber, Kalischer, Krabbe, Sturge, and Dimitri in nearly every possible combination

Definitions
    Encephalotrigeminal angiomatosis
    Encephalofacial angiomatosis
    Angiomatosis capillare et venosum calcificante
    Intracranial teleangiectasia
    Cerebrocutaneous angiomatosis
    Calcified pseudoangioma of the brain
    Benign subcortical calcification
    Nevoid amentia
    Extensive capillary–venous malformation
        affecting one hemisphere of the brain
    Benign subcortical calcification
    Nevoid amentia
    Extensive capillary–venous malformation affecting one hemisphere of the brain
    Associated facial and intracranial hemangioma
    Facial and meningeal angiomatosis
    Encephalofacial neuroangiomatosis
    Neuro–ophthalmo–cutaneous syndrome

Demonstrations of the radiological abnormalities were also provided by Dimitri[12] in 1923, who presented a case before the Neurological Society of Argentina, and in 1927 by Marque,[13] as well as by Brushfield and Wyatt.[14]

In 1934, Krabbe[10] published an accurate study on the radiological and anatomopathological anomalies occurring in encephalotrigeminal angiomatosis. The author pointed out the presence of fine granules of lime salts in the "outer layer of the cortex, and not in the pia mater" ("the pia mater did not contain any calcification either in the connective tissue or in the vessels") as well as the decreased number of neurons in the calcified areas of the brain.

In 1936, Bergstrand et al.[15] published an extensive monography on Sturge–Weber disease, illustrating the pathological characteristics, the clinical manifestations of the condition, as well as the surgical indications.

Definition

Before Krabbe[10] suggested the name of Weber–Dimitri disease in 1934 and Bergstrand[14] coined the currently accepted eponym Sturge–Weber disease in 1935, the encephalotrigeminal angiomatosis was associated to the names of Kalischer,[7] Weber,[9] Krabbe,[10] and Dimitri[12] in nearly every possible combination. Similarly, the condition was described under a large variety of anatomopathological definitions[17] (Table 13.1).

Sturge–Weber disease or encephalotrigeminal syndrome consists of the following pathological elements:

1. Cutaneous angiomatosis (nevus flammeus, capillary nevus, *port-wine* stain nevus) in the territory of distribution of the trigeminal nerve, usually the first and the second branch
2. Dural and leptomeningeal angiomatosis of the cerebral hemisphere corresponding to the affected side of the face
3. Abnormal calcifications of the cortical vessels and cortical parenchyma underlying the leptomeningeal angiomatosis
4. Varying degrees of atrophy of the involved cerebral hemisphere
5. Buphthalmos or glaucoma of the eye on the affected side

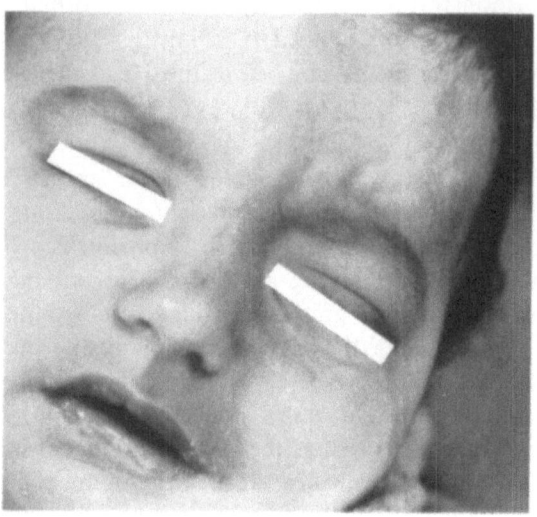

Figure 13.1. Child with Sturge–Weber disease. The facial nevus follows the distribution of the upper divisions of the left trigeminal nerve.

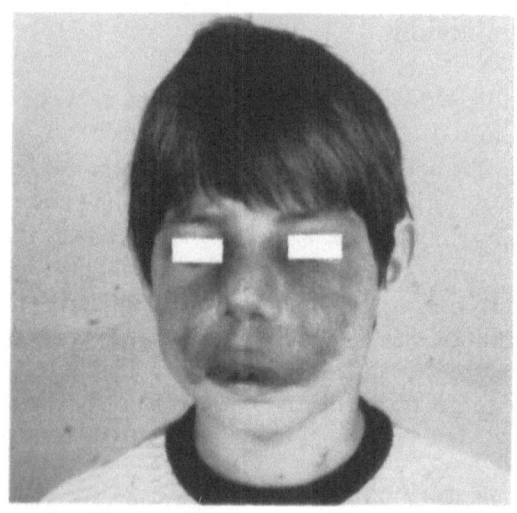

Figure 13.2. Bilateral facial nevus in a 10-year-old boy with Sturge–Weber disease.

The typical clinical manifestations of the disease include:

1. Epileptic seizures, usually beginning in early infancy, and often of the Jacksonian type
2. Contralateral hemiparesis or hemiplegia
3. Homonymous hemianopsia
4. Varying degrees of mental retardation and behavior disturbance

Pathological Manifestations

Vascular Changes

Facial Nevus

The typical cutaneous lesion of Sturge–Weber disease is the dermal capillary–venous nevus, or port-wine nevus, of the face. The color of the lesion may range from pink to deep purple, but at times it may be relatively pale or barely distinguishable from the adjacent normal skin. Usually, the nevus is flat (nevus planus) and blanches under pressure; in very rare cases it may assume a tuberous aspect. The color of the angioma may vary under the influence of factors such as thermal changes, strains, respiratory activity, and fever. Generally, however, the vasoconstrictive and vasodilatative reactivity of the lesion is diminished compared to the normal adjacent skin.[4]

The nevus is present at birth and characteristically follows the distribution of one trigeminal nerve. The area of the upper divisions of the nerve is more commonly involved, while the lower division is usually spared.[18] Although more frequently unilateral and rarely crossing the midline (Fig. 13.1), the nevus may be observed to extend bilaterally (Fig. 13.2). The bilateral form has been evaluated to account for about 10% of the cases,[19] though it may reach a proportion as high as 20% of the subjects in some series reported in the literature.[20,21]

Incomplete cases of Sturge–Weber disease with meningeal angiomatosis and without the facial nevus have also been described,[22–28] with a frequency varying from 5 to 15% in the different series.[21,25]

The topographical extent of the facial nevus varies from a few centimeters to relatively large lesions, which may involve the head, face, and neck, the conjunctival, oropharyngeal, lingual, and nasal mucosae, as well as other parts of the body.

It is worth noting, however, that the distribution of the facial nevus, although not confined to one side of the body in all the cases, does not always strictly follow the limits of the skin metameres. In fact, an overlapping over several segments can be noticed in some patients. This has been correlated by some authors[4,29] to the possibility of an involvement of the sympathetic fibres rather than to the results of a true metameric anomaly of the embryos.

The extent of the facial nevus is not proportional to the degree of severity of the neurological symptoms, neither is its location a reliable indicator of the topography of the cerebral lesion,[30] as was incorrectly suggested in the past.[31]

Cerebromeningeal Angiomatosis

The vascular changes that affect the central nervous system as well as its meningeal coverings are the most important anomalies of the encephalotrigeminal syndrome, as they account for its principal clinical manifestations.

Although some authors have denied the primary involvement of the brain[24] and regarded the parenchymal lesions as secondary to the vascular malformation of the meninges, others have demonstrated angiomatous changes both in the gray and white matter vessels.[17]

The involvement of the dura mater, leptomeninges, and the scalp has suggested[8] that the angiomatous changes in Sturge–Weber disease could be correlated with Streeter's third stage of embryonal vascular differentiation,[32,33] during which "a general cleavage of the veins around the brain (the future pial vessels) from those belonging to the membranous skull (the dural and diploic vessels) and its integument (the scalp veins)" takes place.[34] The process results in the subdivision of the vascular system into three laminae that form the circulation of the scalp, dura, and pia mater. The common derivation of the meningeal, choroidal, and facial vessels would thus explain the vascular malformations of three anatomical areas in Sturge–Weber disease and their metameric distribution. However, when considering the

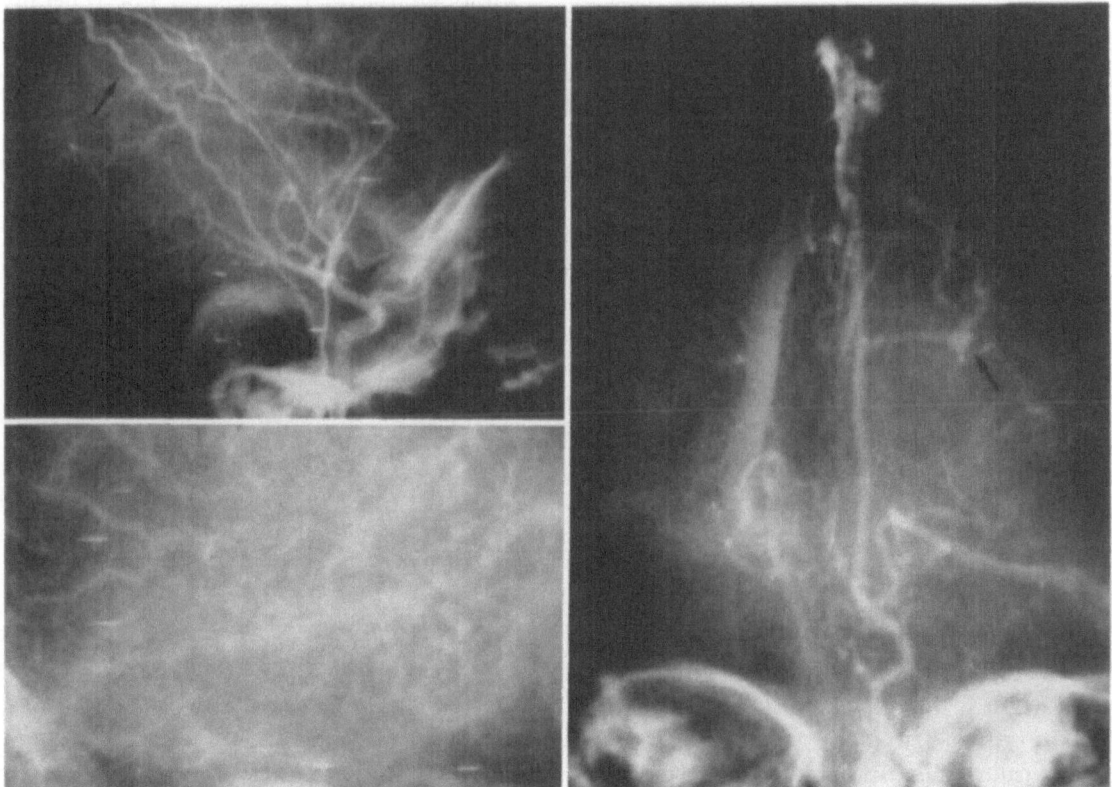

Figure 13.3. Sturge–Weber disease. Cerebral angiography demonstrates the hyperplasia of the vessels originating from the external carotid artery (upper left), diffuse blushing in the capillary phase (lower left), and abnormal veins and venous sinuses (right).

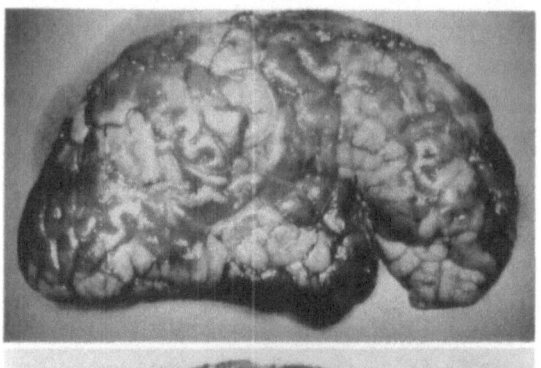

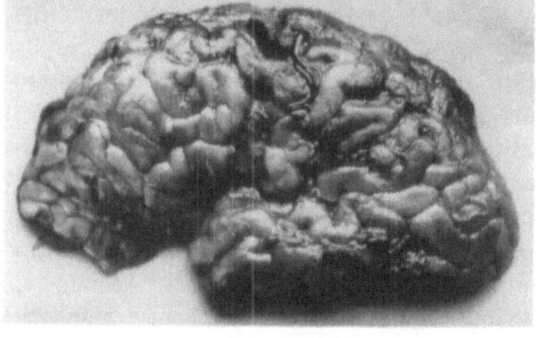

Figure 13.4. Surgical specimens of two cases of Sturge–Weber disease: left cerebral hemisphere (above), right cerebral hemisphere (below). In both cases the leptomeningeal angiomatosis is irregularly distributed on the entire cortical surface; only a few cortical gyri appear to be spared.

simultaneous involvement of the vessels of both the gray and white matter of the brain, a more complex series of events apt to interfere with the early process of vascular development (formation of primitive plexus and successive resolution of some vessels or a group of vessels functioning as a transitory or temporary vascular system) should be taken into account. Thus, the vascular anomalies observed in Sturge–Weber disease could be regarded as an incomplete developmental metamorphosis, with remnants of the primitive plexiform connections or abnormal persistence of the transitory system.[35] In favor of this hypothesis could be the observation of vascular abnormalities found in other parts of the body[4,35] as well as the polymorphism that characterizes the histopathological vascular anomalies in subjects with Sturge–Weber syndrome. Besides the angiomatous changes, patients with this syndrome may, in fact, present anomalies of the venous

sinuses, arteriovenous malformations, and arterial thrombosis[26] (Fig. 13.3).

At the gross examination, the angiomatosis of the dura is manifested by irregular and deeply pigmented areas containing enlarged blood vessels, which generally correspond to underlying focal thickenings of the leptomeninges with numerous congested and irregularly dilated small-caliber vessels. Generally, the dura is not adherent to the leptomeninges and the leptomeningeal angiomatosis is prevalently found in the occipital pole, although the lesion can be located in all the cerebral lobes (Fig. 13.4). Even if arteries and capillaries can participate in the formation of the angioma, the vessels composing it are mostly veins, so that the leptomeninges may assume a dark blue color in some areas.

The pial vessels are markedly injected and may show an abnormal proliferation over the cortex (Fig. 13.5), in some cases completely covering the cerebral parenchyma in the form of a thick, mushy, purplish-red mass (Fig. 13.6).

Although the pial vessels do not generally penetrate the underlying cortical gyri, they may be anatomically connected to a rich capillary network of the subjacent cortex by means of

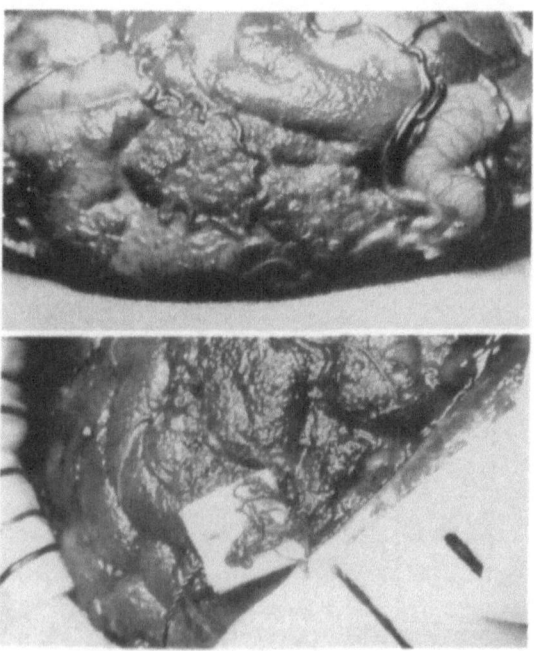

Figure 13.5. Localized abnormal proliferation of the pial vessels over the cerebral cortex in two patients with Sturge–Weber disease.

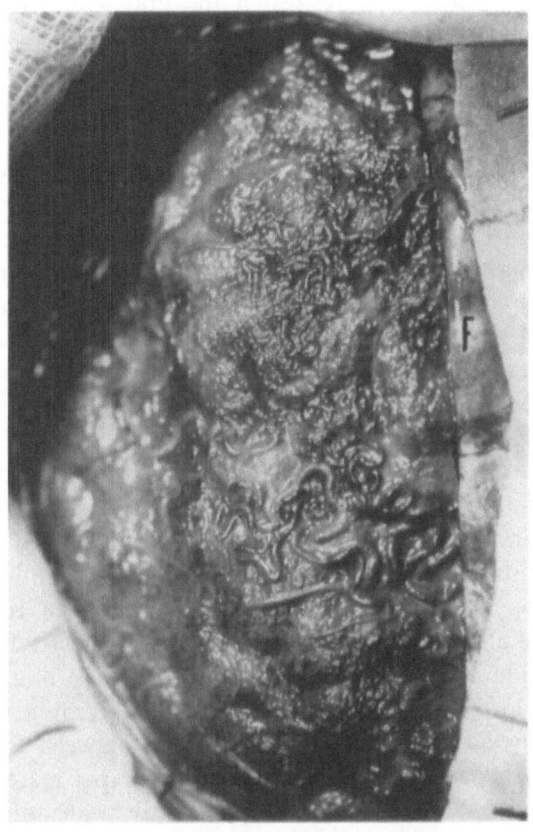

Figure 13.6. Abnormal proliferation of the pial vessels completely covering the left cerebral hemisphere of an infant with Sturge–Weber disease. Note also the anomalous and dilated veins discharging into the superior sagittal sinus. F, Falx cerebri.

numerous piercing feeder vessels. Close to these capillaries fine calcification deposits can invariably be noticed at the microscopic examination, and it is therefore conceivable that these structures also participate in the disease as pial angiomatosis.

Choroid Angiomatosis

Vascular abnormality in Sturge–Weber disease commonly affects the bulbar conjunctiva and the conjunctiva of the lower lid. The iris may show abnormality in pigmentation, becoming darker on the affected side. The choroid vessels also exhibit angiomatous changes; the angioma has a honeycomb pattern and as rule is not pigmented, usually varying in color from gray to yellow, thus appearing lighter than its surroundings when transilluminated.[36] In some cases, the angioma may show dark red areas, for which the retina has been compared to a sea of tomato sauce surrounding the optic disk. Most authors have stressed the difference in color between the normal and involved eye.[37]

The tumor appears as a localized elevation of the retina at the posterior pole of the eyeball or near the optic disk. In fact, it is usually located between the macula and the disk.

The choroid angioma, which consists of dilated vascular channels lined with endothelium and separated by a small amount of stroma, is congenital, although it may not manifest clinically until adolescence or adulthood; the congenital nature is demonstrated by its imperceptible merging with the normal choroidal vasculature and by the fact that it does not increase in size during life.[36]

Skull Angiomatosis

The skull of subjects with Sturge–Weber disease may become thicker than normal on the side corresponding to the meningeal angioma, and eventually show an accentuated diploic pattern because of the underlying hemiatrophy.[18,30,38]

Some authors, however, have raised the question of the possibility of an osseous venous angiomatosis[8,39] as a direct or indirect cause of the bone hypertrophy.[40]

Angiomatosis of Visceral Organs

The visceral organs are frequently involved in the syndrome.[4,41–44] Although secondary metabolic changes, hematemesis from gastric hemorrhage, and gangrene of the colon from circulatory insufficiency have been reported,[29,30] the abnormalities of the visceral organs in Sturge–Weber disease usually are of little clinical importance.

Neuropathological Changes

At the gross examination, the most striking features of the cerebral hemisphere involved in the encephalofacial angiomatosis are the decreased size, the firmer-than-usual consistency, and the flaming red surface in the areas covered by the meningeal angioma (Figs. 13.4 and 13.6).

The main anatomical landmarks can be easily. identified, although some gyri and convolutions may show marked sclerosis (Fig. 13.5).

Usually, the excessive vascularity of the pia mater affects mainly the occipital or parietooccipital regions, and in particular the calcarine fissure, although the frontal and temporal lobes may also be involved.

Beneath the hypervascularized meninges, the outer part of the cortex may be more resistant than normal, and may impart a "gritty" sensation[25] on sectioning, owing to its content of calcified material.

At the microscopic examination, loss of neurons and fibers, proliferation of glial cells, and the presence of calcifications are the most important changes, together with the already-mentioned angiomatous character of the dura,

leptomeninges, vessels of the gray and white matter, choroid, and iris[17,20] (Fig. 13.7). In some areas, parenchymal lesions resulting from repeated damage due to meningeal hemorrhage are evident.[8]

The *calcifications* may be regarded as the characteristic finding in Sturge–Weber disease; the phenomenon has been the subject of numerous observations and pathogenic interpretations. The deposition of calcium in the brain of patients affected by encephalofacial angiomatosis was first noticed upon gross examination in a post-mortem study by Hebold[45] in 1913. In the same year, Volland[46] demonstrated microscopically the presence of intracerebral calcifications. Weber,[9,47] in 1922 and 1928, described the characteristic wavy, double-contoured aspect of such calcifications on the roentgenographic examination of the skull (Fig. 13.8). This aspect was believed by Dimitri[12] to correspond to calcified blood vessels of the angioma. In 1934, Krabbe,[10] however, denied any relationship between the calcifications and the vessels of the pia mater, and pointed out their intracortical localization (mostly in the second and third layers of the cerebral cortex). Actually, Sturge–Weber disease calcifications, which present especially in the middle regions of the cortex, may in places spread into the deeper regions and also into the white matter.[30] Calcifications may be found within the wall of cortical vessels and within the perivascular spaces[17] (Fig. 13.9). The calcium deposits may be granular and loosely distributed or else confluent in scattered clumps of greater dimensions. The major calcifications, which can be visible macroscopically, are generally globular or irregularly lobulated; some of them are made up of concentric layers so that they seem to be conglomerated from smaller ones (Figs 13.10 and 13.11). The finest deposits are situated close to the very numerous capillaries, characteristic of this condition[21] (Fig. 13.12). Where the calcification phenomena are predominant, the normal cerebral architecture is obliterated, with secondary proliferation of glial cells and the destruction of ganglion cells. The white matter underlying areas of extensive cortical calcifications usually shows slight shrinkage. The demarcation between calcified areas and the

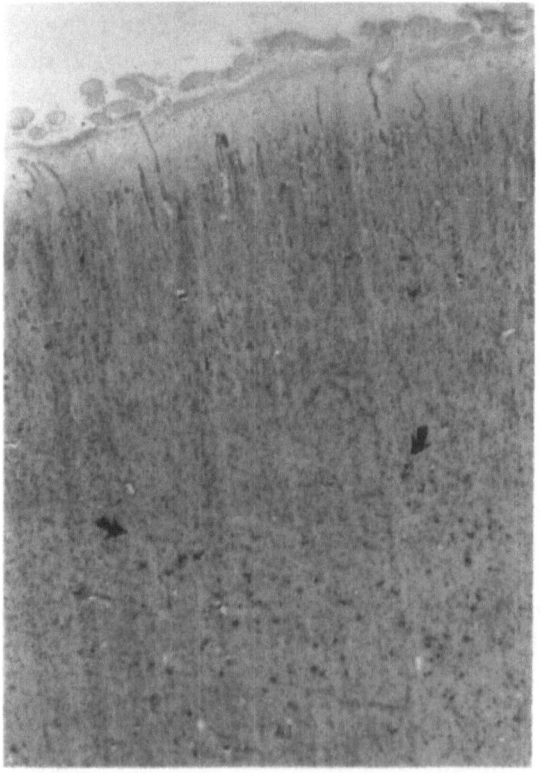

Figure 13.7. Occipital lobe section in a case of Sturge–Weber disease demonstrating the angioma over the cerebral cortex, loss of cortical neurons, and gliosis, as well as calcifications (third cortical layer and underlying white matter) (arrows). (HE; × 65.)

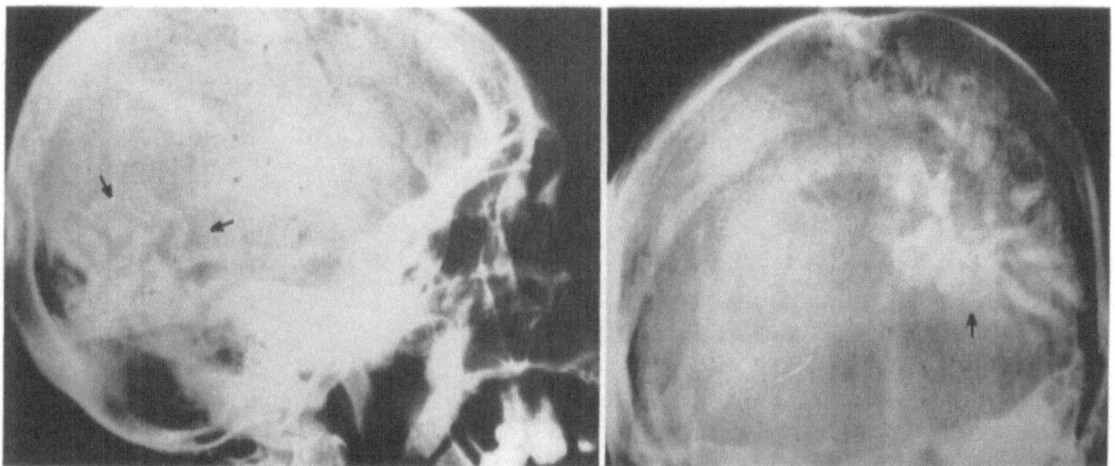

Figure 13.8. Skull X-ray examination in an 8-year-old boy with Sturge–Weber disease, showing the characteristic double-contoured calcifications in the occipital region. In the anteroposterior (AP) view (right) the asymmetry of the skull, due to the atrophy of the underlying cerebral hemisphere, is well apparent.

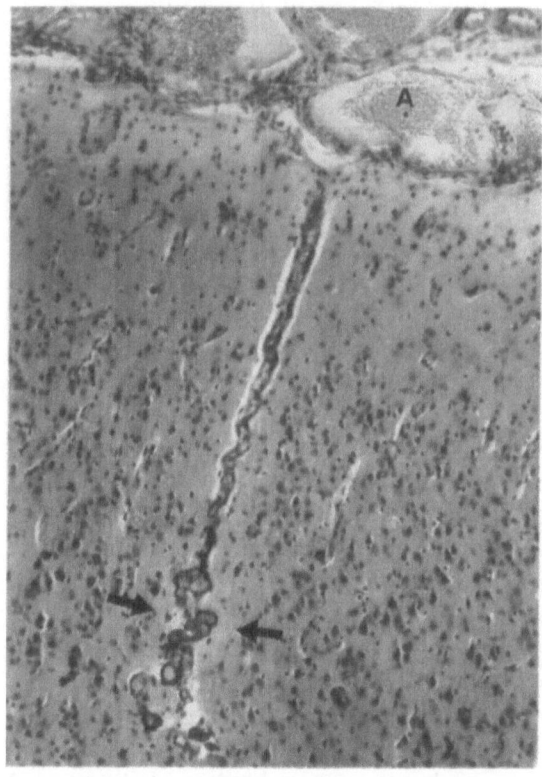

Figure 13.9. Occipital lobe section. Note the leptomeningeal angioma (A), the loss of cortical neurons with gliosis, and the perivascular calcifications, which tend to become confluent (arrows) within the third cortical layer. (HE; × 250.)

adjacent normal parenchyma of the cortex may be fairly sharp. As the number of nerve cells is reduced in the calcified areas, some authors[21] have suggested the possible correlation of mental degeneration with the progressive deposition of lime salts, and the secondary parenchymatous degeneration and gliosis. Two main groups of hypotheses have been hitherto put forth with regard to the progressive formation of the calcifications. The first of them takes into account an active role of specific vascular and/or mesenchymal factors[18]; the second considers the calcifications to be a secondary phenomenon, in all likelihood of dystrophic origin, resulting from prolonged convulsive states and repeated phasic alterations in local cortical blood flow.[48,49] Several authors have stressed the altered permeability of the vessel wall.[40,50,51] This increased permeability would account for the passage of proteins and calcium phosphate or carbonate from the vascular lumen into the perivascular space, followed by secondary crystallization within the cerebral parenchyma. Ultramicroscopic studies[35] have demonstrated a relatively complex series of events, such as the production of an acid mucopolysaccharidic substance, acting as the matrix of calcifications within the vascular wall (Fig. 13.12), the precipitation of the inorganic component of calcifications (calcium

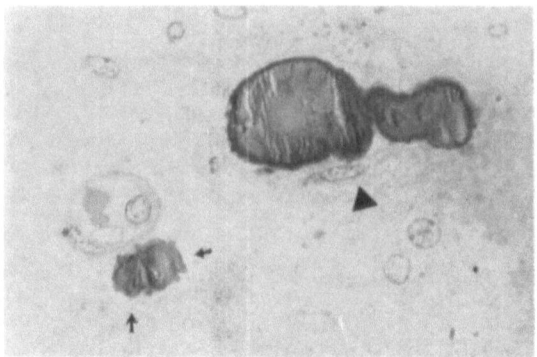

Figure 13.10. Semithin section of the occipital cortex. Irregularly lobulated calcifications of small size are anatomically related to a capillary vessel (arrows). A large calcification with a concentric lamellar structure is also shown (arrowhead). (Toluidine blue; × 1000.)

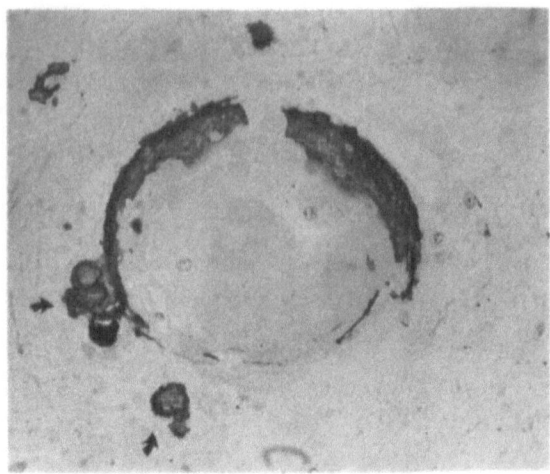

Figure 13.12. Semithin section of the occipital cortex, demonstrating periodic acid–Schiff stain (PAS)-positive material within the wall of a capillary vessel. Small calcifications are also demonstrated in the perivascular space (arrow). (PAS; × 1000.)

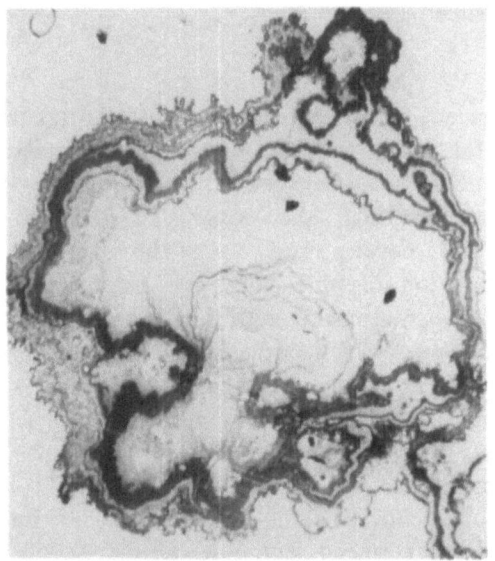

Figure 13.11. Ultrastructural study of a calcification in Sturge–Weber disease: note the lamellar organization.

phosphate) on the granular formations of the organic matrix, and their progressive increase in size, mainly outside the vessels (Fig. 13.13). Although such studies do not exclude the secondary role of other factors such as anoxia, neuronal necrosis, variations of local ions and alkalinity, they indicate the predominant importance of the vascular factor and of the increase in acid mucopolysaccharides, which pose a great affinity for binding calcium, as already observed in the past by other authors.[52,53] It is possible

that individual variations of this metabolic activity might account for the different clinical evolution that can be recorded in subjects with Sturge–Weber disease.

Ophthalmic Changes

In their monograph, in which 257 cases were collected from the literature, Alexander and Norman[18] found that *buphthalmos* (48 cases) and *glaucoma simplex* (25 cases) were the ocular changes associated with encephalofacial angiomatosis, with an incidence of approximately 30%.

Buphthalmos may be recorded as the classical ocular lesion of Sturge–Weber disease; in fact, it was described by Schirmer in the first report on the condition.[5] The lesion has already taken place in the prenatal period, when the abnormally high tension results in a distension of the immature and plastic sclera. The angioma of the choroid is often associated with glaucoma. The association is not clearly understood. Although hypersecretion has been demonstrated in several cases the coefficient of outflow has, in fact, often been found to be within normal limits.

In some cases, the condition has been explained on the grounds of an abnormality in choroidal circulation, mainly due to calcium

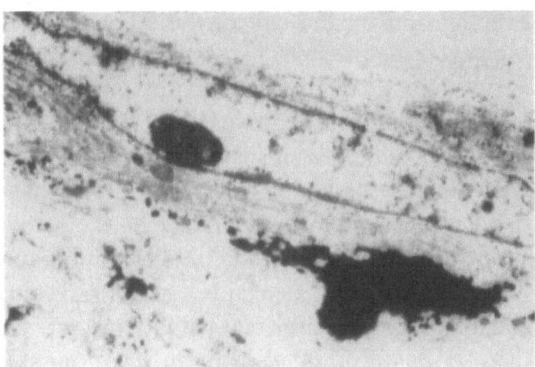 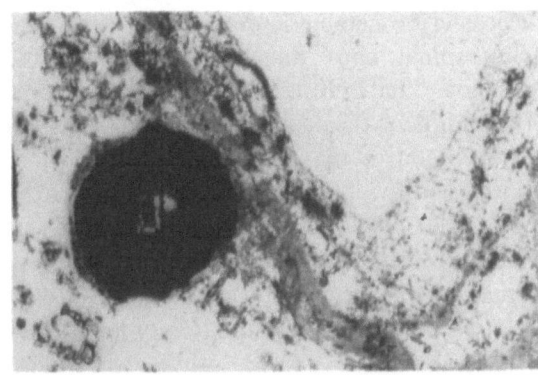

Figure 13.13. Ultramicroscopic study of the occipital cortex. On the left, an acid mucopolysaccharidic substance, which tends to diffuse outside the vessel, is seen within the wall of a cerebral capillary (× 7800); on the right, the same substance acting as matrix for the calcification process appears to have migrated outside the vessel (× 9400).

deposits throughout its structures. Four main hypotheses were propounded by Miller[36]:

1. The neural theory (congenital disorder of the sympathetic supply to the eye, accounting for the dilation of the uveal capillaries and the slowing of the blood stream, and, possibly, for the heterochromia of the iris as well)
2. The cranial theory (obstruction and secondary vascular stasis of the circulation of the eye, depending on the presence of an angioma of the meninges in the territory of tributaries draining into the cavernous sinus)
3. The mechanical theory (malformation in the angle of the anterior chamber impeding the aqueous outflow)
4. The vascular theory (venous stasis in the uvea responsible for aqueous hypersecretion and possibly interfering with outflow)

The same author, however, indicated the limits of such theories, namely the absence of heterochromia in many subjects with encephalofacial angiomatosis, the absence of glaucoma in Horner syndrome, which results from a sympathetic deficit, the occurrence of glaucoma in patients with nevus flammeus but without meningeal vascular anomalies, and the lack of demonstration of any anatomical abnormality in the angle of the anterior chamber at the gonioscopic and histological examinations.

Childhood glaucoma differs from that of the adult, as it rarely responds to medical management alone. In recent times, however, surgical control of the condition, which stresses the importance of an early recognition and management prior to the occurrence of irreversible ocular damage, has become more rewarding.[54] In children, glaucoma is rarely symptomatic, especially in the early stage. A detailed ophthalmic assessment (demonstration of increased intraocular pressure, increased corneal diameter, optic nerve cupping, glaucomatous defects of the visual field) is consequently required in young subjects with Sturge–Weber disease and even the "normal" patients should be reexamined periodically.[55]

Diagnosis

In spite of the numerous reports devoted to Sturge–Weber disease, there is no complete agreement on the specific criteria for the diagnosis of the condition. However, the association of the facial nevus with the leptomeningeal angiomatosis and/or the choroidal angioma has been indicated as the essential component of the syndrome.[56] In fact, the clinical (hemiparesis, epilepsy, mental retardation, buphthalmos, glaucoma) and the radiological (intracranial calcifications, cranial asymmetry) manifestations appear to be secondary effects of the vascular anomaly. The criterion rules out pathological conditions such as familial noncalcifying meningeal angioma, facial nevi associated with cerebellar symptoms, and facial nevi of metameric distribution accompanying spinal cord angiomas. According to Alexander and Norman,[18] the topographic distribution of the facial nevus is an essential characteristic of the syndrome, as only those subjects in whom it corresponds to the supraocular region should be regarded as affected by the condition. The existence of incomplete or atypical forms of Sturge–Weber disease[29] has emphasized the role of laboratory techniques in achieving the correct diagnosis.[28,57–59] In 1957, Poser and Taveras[26] indicated the diffuse homogeneous increase in density during the capillary and venus phases of cerebral angiography as a typical finding of the condition. The same authors also listed the relatively scarce arterial changes and the more significant venous anomalies corresponding to the presence of the intracranial angioma, telangiectesias, arteriovenous malformations, and phenomena of arterial thrombosis. They also mentioned the occurrence of vascular changes corresponding to cerebral atrophy or avascular space-occupying lesions, such as subdural hematomas. Following the studies by Huang and Wolf[60] concerning the medullary veins and the direction of the cerebral venous circulation, various authors have stressed the insufficient cortical venous drainage in patients with Sturge–Weber disease at angiographic investigations, and the main direction of the venous circulation toward the deep venous systems.[29,50,61,62] Thrombosis of the superficial veins as well as their insufficient congenital development have been suggested for interpreting the angiographic findings. Most of the radiological signs reported in the literature correspond to relatively late phases of the disease. For example, the skull asymmetry, the enlarged vascular channels of the skull, and the overdeveloped air sinuses[38] should be regarded as due to the underlying cerebral atrophy, more than as typical findings of the condition. Also, the calcifications are usually a late sign when visible on the X-ray examination of the skull. With the exception of a few reports,[21,42,63,64] these lesions have been rarely seen in the first year of life.[18,26,30,65] On the other hand, 65[21,61] to 90%[66] of the patients show the typical

intracranial calcifications at the radiographic examination by the end of the second decade. However, the presence of calcifications at a very early age has been documented by post-mortem brain radiographic examinations, as well as by autoptic studies, even in children, whose skull X-ray films had not revealed any calcium deposit when performed alive.[20] At the present time high-resolution computed tomography (CT) allows the detection of intracerebral calcifications in subjects with Sturge–Weber disease before they can been seen on skull radiographs (Figs. 13.14 and 13.15). The same examination permits the precise definition of the areas of the cerebral cortex most involved in the atrophic process resulting from the disturbance in cerebral blood flow and from calcium deposition, as well as the detection of other typical findings of the condition, such as the ipsilateral enlargement of the lateral cerebral ventricle and the decreased volume of the ipsilateral hemicranium.[61,64,67–72] In general, at CT scan examination the atrophic areas are usually larger than those of cortical calcification.[70,73] After contrast medium administration, CT provides the direct visualization of the regions corresponding to the leptomeningeal angiomatosis, the essential lesion in Sturge–Weber disease. It is not clear whether the enhanced areas following the contrast infusion correspond directly to the malformed and dilated vessels of the angioma or represent indirect proof of the lesion by demonstrating only the permeability defect of its vascular channels. The last hypothesis seems supported by the results of other investigations, such as radionuclide brain scanning,[42] which demonstrates a diffuse or patchy increase in radioactivity emanating from the affected cerebral areas, following an initial diminished perfusion "blush," a finding believed to translate as an abnormal capillary permeability.[61] Conjecturally, the extent of contrast enhancement should represent the size of the leptomeningeal angioma; however, it more probably corresponds to the minimum size of the malformation, that is, the area where the vascular abnormalities are more marked, while the angioma is possibly more extensive.[73] Magnetic resonance imaging appears to have the same effectiveness as CT in

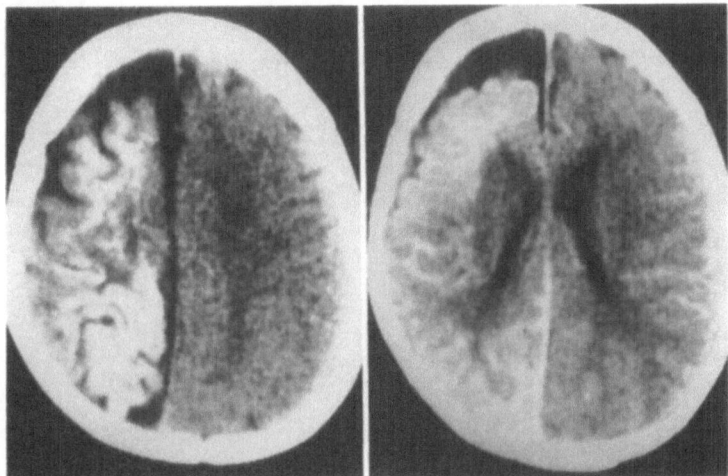

Figure 13.14. CT scan in an infant with Sturge–Weber disease, demonstrating the calcification process involving the left cerebral hemisphere, mainly at the level of the occipital lobe. The affected hemisphere is atrophic and induces a mild cranial asymmetry.

detecting the cerebral atrophy; being a relatively safer procedure, the technique may be very useful in monitoring the evolution of the disease.

The possible contribution to the diagnosis of Sturge–Weber disease by other modern techniques, such as positron emission tomography (PET) or single photon emission computed tomography (SPECT), has not yet been evaluated extensively. Hypometabolism but also hypermetabolism have been demonstrated by the former technique,[74] while the latter has shown areas of marked hypoperfusion resulting from postictal phenomena as well as from chronic ischemia.[58]

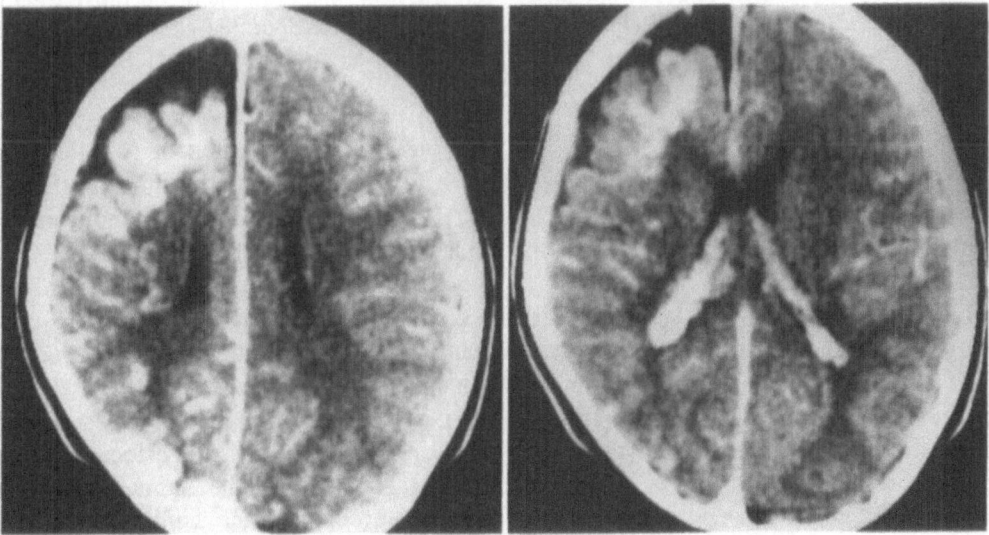

Figure 13.15. CT scan of an infant with Sturge–Weber disease, demonstrating the severe involvement of the left cerebral hemisphere. The calcium deposits prevail at the level of the frontal lobe, which is obviously atrophic. The examination also reveals the angiomatous changes of the choroid plexuses.

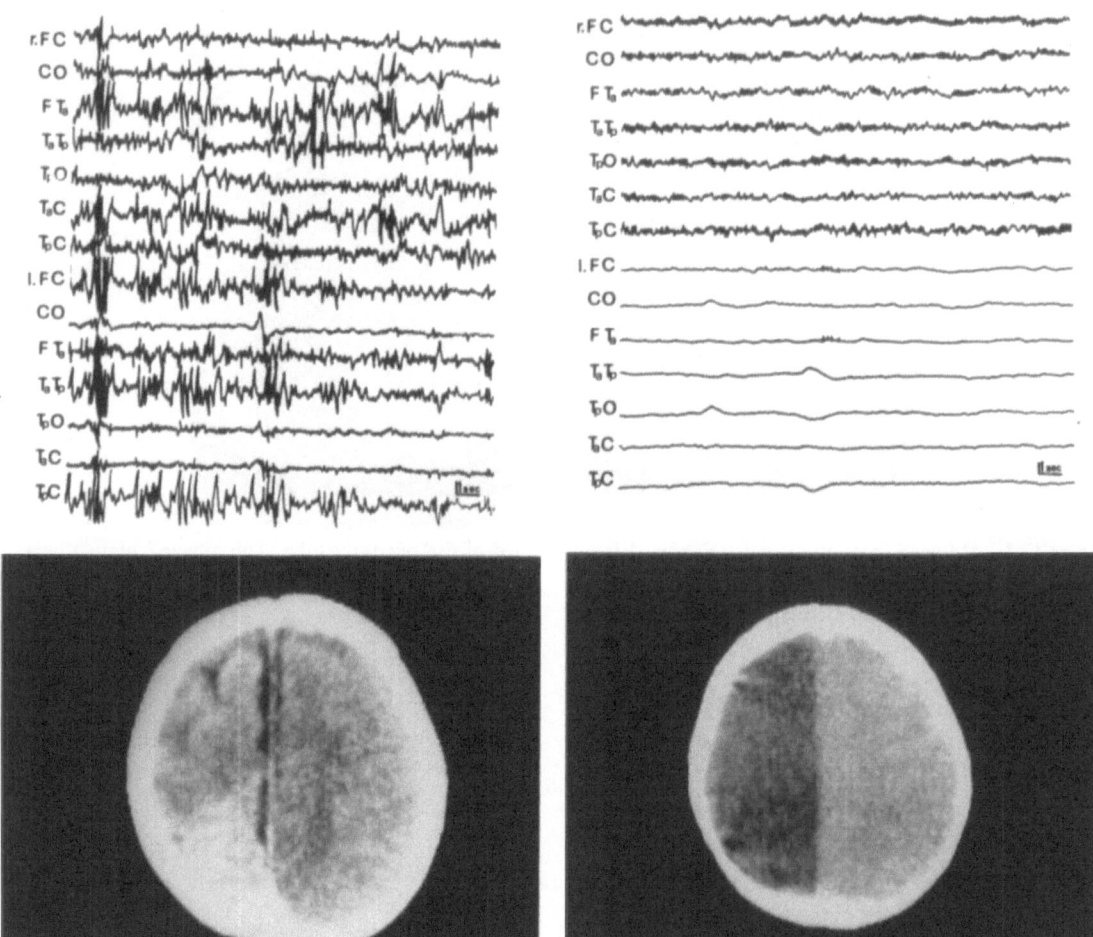

Figure 13.16. Preoperative (left) and postoperative (right) EEG and CT studies in a child with Sturge–Weber disease affecting the left cerebral hemisphere. The epileptic activity involving both cerebral hemispheres in the preoperative EEG study has completely disappeared after the removal of the affected left cerebral hemisphere.

Clinical Manifestations

With the exception of the very few cases in whom the Sturge–Weber disease is revealed by clinical manifestations such as subarachnoid hemorrhage[75] or gastrointestinal bleeding,[30] epilepsy is the presenting and most common clinical feature in nearly all the cases (Fig. 13.16).

Epilepsy, in fact, may occur in a very high proportion of patients (up to 85 to 89%).[21,25,30,76] In most instances focal seizures affecting the side of the body opposite the cerebral lesions, or generalized convulsions, begin in infancy.[21,30] The convulsive disorder begins less often in childhood or adolescence.[21]

The onset of epilepsy after the twentieth year of life is rare, even in patients showing the typical intracranial features of the condition.[25] The epilepsy seems to be less frequent (72%) when the cerebral calcifications are confined to the occipital lobe alone; on the other hand, epilepsy seems not to be significantly influenced by the extension (unilateral or bilateral) of the cutaneous nevus. In about half of the subjects, the initial epileptic paroxysm is a focal fit. Seizures are focal in about the same proportion of patients even in later clinical observations. Generalized nonfocal seizures represent about 21% of the cases while about 13% of the subjects present with both focal and nonfocal fits.[25]

Motor weakness, contralateral to the cerebral lesion, is the next most common symptom. Hemiplegia or hemiparesis may even be the first clinical manifestation of the disease, occurring in some patients as suddenly as in a vascular insult[77] or mimicking a status epilepticus.[25] When present since the first years of life, the motor deficit may determine a less than normal growth of the paretic limbs.

The disturbance of mentality, behavior, and speech varies widely from patient to patient. However, about one-third of the subjects at the initial evaluation, and half of them at later examinations, present with intellectual impairment.[21,29,74,78,79] In some cases the functional disturbances may be so severe as to prevent the subject from attending school, or to make him unaware of his surroundings. Epilepsy, the mental state, and loss of function (paresis, hemianopsia, sensory disturbances) are the most important clinical manifestations when considering the severity and the prognosis of the condition.

In a significant proportion of cases epilepsy correlates with signs of loss of function. In 1949, Lund,[25] by evaluating a total of 144 cases, 6 personal and 138 gathered from the literature, found that 60 of them presented with loss of function: 50 of these subjects had epilepsy (83%). Hypoplasia of the limb was noticed in 24 cases (22 of which had epilepsy). Paresis was present in a further 21 cases (18 of them with epilepsy). Epilepsy was also present in 10 of the remaining 15 patients, who presented with a varying but minor degree of loss of function.

Unfortunately, however, the occurrence of signs of loss of function and the time of onset of epilepsy are not so obvious as to establish their correlation. For example, in Lund's study paresis developed after the onset of epilepsy in 14 out of 40 patients with both paresis and epilepsy. However, in another nine cases paresis was present before the onset of epilepsy, even though in all of them the convulsions had begun within the first year of life. Also, the observation[25] of symptom-free intervals, often lasting years, during the clinical course of epilepsy in subjects with Sturge–Weber disease further limits the value of the seizures as a reliable indicator of the prognosis of the condition and,

eventually, of the necessity for alternative treatment.[77] However, it is a common experience that anticonvulsant medication may alleviate the milder cases, but fail to control seizures when they are numerous and severe. In such cases, the search for a therapeutic alternative—that is, the surgical excision of the epileptogenic cerebral lesion—is justified in order to avoid the progressive involvement of the "normal" brain and worsening of the clinical condition.

For several authors the disease tends to progress with age, thus limiting the effectiveness of medical treatment.[7,29,30,80] They have stressed that the evolution of the disease may be so severe as to require the patient to be confined to an institution or to determine his precocious death, usually before middle age.[18,81] The proliferation of the meningeal angioma with progressive displacement of brain matter, similar to that of a true neoplasm,[44] the continuous deposition of calcium,[18,29,42,77] the effect of chronic cortical vascular stasis and tissue hypoxia due to the changes in cerebral blood circulation (insufficient cortical venous drainage),[42,53,82] as well as acquired lesions such as Ammon's horn sclerosis, loss of ganglion cells in the hippocampal gyri, atrophy and sclerosis in Sommer's sector resulting from circulatory impairment, and tissue hypoxia associated with seizures,[76,79,83–85] have been proposed as possible causative factors accounting for the progression of the condition.

On the other hand, other authors have emphasized that almost half of the patients may lead a comfortable life, under anticonvulsant treatment, and with the help of ophthalmological treatment when required.[21] In these patients the mental symptoms are slight or entirely lacking, and the disease tends to have a rather benign course.[29] For example, in Peterman's series[21] of 31 patients, 25 of whom were followed for more than 5 years, 17 were found to have done well (2 patients without epilepsy, 15 with epilepsy but with episodes satisfactorily controlled by anticonvulsant medicaments; 3 of the patients in this group showed slight mental retardation, which, however, did not seem to interfere with school work), 10 to have done poorly (5 patients living at home in wretched health as the result of uncontrolled seizures, mental retardation, or progressive weakness, spasticity, movement disorders, or blindness; 5 subjects confined to institutions, all being unable to care for themselves because of severe seizures or mental retardation), and 4 to have died (3 patients after progressive deterioration in clinical condition, and 1 patient after craniotomy at 14 years).

Surgical Indications and Treatment

The treatment of Sturge–Weber syndrome consists primarily of attempts to control seizures medically. When the seizures cannot be controlled with anticonvulsant drugs, surgical treatment represents the only therapeutic alterative.[21,30,76–78, 82,86–92]

Obvious limits are experienced when evaluating the prognosis in each subject, owing to the variety of clinical expressions of the condition as well as its relatively unpredictable course. In fact, even though a progressive worsening of the epilepsy is observed in several cases, in others spontaneous improvement or even remission have been recorded. Furthermore, the rarity of the condition has prevented any one center from accumulating extensive experience; thus, the criteria for surgical indications remain largely based on the personal convictions of the neurosurgeon. For example, in 1972 Alexander[56] proposed operating on subjects with Sturge–Weber disease soon after 2 months of age, before the appearance of neurologic symptoms, in the assumption that early intervention represented the only measure apt to prevent irreversible damage of the brain not directly involved in the angiomatous lesion. Even at the present time, the main controversy concerns the advantage of early surgical operation versus later intervention. The matter here is obviously founded only on theoretical premises. Those authors who favor early surgical treatment consider that the operation not only stops the seizures but also improves learning capacity, thus avoiding progressive mental deterioration.[52,82,87,89,92–94] This opinion is based on the observation of good surgical outcomes, that is, control of epilepsy and relatively normal psychomotor development[82,92–94] in patients operated on in early life, compared to the ineffectiveness of operations on an already developed mental deficit in some cases treated in late childhood or adolescence,[82] in spite of an arrest of the epileptic attacks.

On the other hand, a more selective surgical approach, to be adopted only when an adequately prolonged clinical observation has excluded the possibility of controlling the seizures medically, has been advocated by other authors.[86,91] The lack of a reliable demonstration of the favorable effect of an early operation (insufficient number of treated cases) and the limited possibility of predicting the clinical evolution in the first months of life (risk of operating on children destined to have a normal mental development when the intervention is carried out in too early a phase) have been emphasized in order to justify such an attitude. A further element in favor of a selective approach might be furnished by the demonstration of the early occurrence of cerebral atrophic changes by CT or magnetic resonance imaging (MRI) investigations performed in the first days of life, a finding that challenges the real progressive nature of the disease. In other words, at least in some patients, the atrophic changes appear to result from prenatal damage rather than being produced by progressive postnatal pathologic processes. Serial neuroimaging examinations may also reveal the basically static nature of the lesions in many of these children. The possibility of cerebral hemorrhage, which was considered in the past positive justification for early surgical intervention,[8,84] is nowadays regarded to be so rare as to be of no practical value in making the decision. Severe mental retardation still represents a contraindication when considering whether to operate or not.[15,76,86,95]

A variety of surgical procedures has been utilized in the treatment of Sturge–Weber disease (Table 13.2).[8,15,76,82,88,91,96–99] With the exception of the few cases with bilateral lesions, where operations such as callosotomy may be indicated,[91] in nearly all the cases cortical excisions, lobectomy, or hemispherectomy represent possible therapeutic alterna-

Table 13.2. Surgical procedures in Sturge–Weber disease.

Procedures	Notes[a]
Ligation of the external carotid artery	First reported case: Cushing, 1906 (8)
Electrocoagulation	First reported case: Dimitri and Balado, 1933 (96)
Lobectomy	First reported case: Olivecrona, 1936 (15)
Hemispherectomy	First reported case: Cairns, 1951 (88): removal of the hemisphere in pieces as proposed by Krynauw, 1950 (99)
	Falconer and Rushworth, 1960 (82): removal of the hemisphere in one piece, as proposed by Obrador Alcade, 1950 and 1952 (97)
Callosotomy	First reported case: Lapras et al., 1971 (91) (bilateral forms)
Cortical excisions	First reported case: Rasmussen et al., 1972 (76)
Excision of the EEG focus	First reported case: Serfling and Parnitzke, 1954 (98)

[a] Numbers in parentheses are references.

tives owing to the unilateral and focal character of the condition.

Although cortical excisions, including the vascular malformation and the underlying calcified parenchymal tissue, or extended to areas where the EEG or the electrocorticographic examination have disclosed the presence of an EEG focus, have resulted in good control of epilepsy in some instances,[78] in most cases this type of operation has only allowed a reduction in epileptic activity and has been followed later on by recurrence of seizures.[30,77,80,82] Lobectomy and hemispherectomy, which associate the cortical excision and that of the underlying atrophic brain to the removal of the EEG focus, appear to be more effective than procedures limited to simple cortical excision, because of the multiple localization of the angiomatous and atrophic cerebral lesions that characterize Sturge–Weber disease (Fig. 13.4). Indeed, the most favorable results have been reported in patients who underwent removal of the affected cerebral hemisphere.[82,89,92–94,97] In fact, given proper indications, hemispherectomy in Sturge–Weber disease is well worthwhile, and its risk and

difficulties acceptable even when the operation is carried out in infancy. In infants, the procedure requires a particularly careful preoperative and postoperative replacement of blood loss. It should be remembered that in this age group, an otherwise unexplained and persisting hyperthermia may correspond to unexpectedly low levels of hemoglobin in the first postoperative days. In general, the reduced size of the affected cerebral hemisphere, because of the precociously occurring cerebral atrophy, makes the removal of the entire hemisphere en bloc relatively easy, limiting the need of piecemeal removal of the structure to only a very few cases.

As in older patients, the development of hydrocephalus following the operation represents the most common complication in infants, in spite of all the possible measures theoretically apt to decrease its incidence, such as, for example, preservation of the ependymal wall of the lateral cerebral ventricle, removal or coagulation of the choroid plexus, and reduction of the residual cavity by opportune closure of the dura mater. In infants, however, the disturbance of the intracranial fluid dynamics brought about by the operation may be diminished, at least to a certain extent, by the "compensative" growth of the intact cerebral hemisphere beyond the midline, and by the fact that the size of the hemicranium corresponding to the excised cerebral hemisphere is often significantly reduced.

Conclusions

Nowadays the diagnosis of Sturge–Weber disease offers less difficulty than in the past, owing to the contribution provided by modern neuroimaging techniques. However, the natural course and prognosis of the disease cannot be defined even at the present time. Although in some patients the clinical condition deteriorates in time, because of intractable seizures and progressive mental impairment, the state of other subjects remains rather stable, the epilepsy is controlled by medical treatment, and the mental symptoms are slight or entirely lacking. In cases where the epilepsy is intractable, surgical indications are relatively clear. Similarly, the decision to exclude patients with pronounced mental deterioration from surgical therapy is not a matter of discussion. On the other hand, surgical indication is still difficult when considering the intermediate forms, with a relatively unpredictable clinical course, where periods of remission alternate with phases of reexacerbation of the seizure disorder.

Among the surgical options, hemispherectomy, especially when performed in the first months of life, appears the most reliable therapeutic procedure in controlling epilepsy as well as in favoring psychomotor development.

References

1. Haberland C: The phakomatoses. In: Vinken PJ, Bruyn GW (eds.), Congenital Malformations of the Brain and Skull. Part II. Handbook of Clinical Neurology, Vol. 31. North-Holland, Amsterdam, 1977, pp. 1–34.
2. Hilal S, Solomon GE, Gold AP, Carter S: Primary cerebral arterial occlusive disease in children. Part II. neurocutaneous syndromes. Radiology 99:87–93, 1971.
3. Riccardi VM: Von Recklinghausen neurofibromatosis. N Engl J Med 305:1617–1627, 1981.
4. Yakolev PI, Guthrie RH: Congenital ectodermoses (neurocutaneous syndromes) in epileptic patients. Arch Neurol Psychiatr 26:1145–1197, 1931.
5. Schirmer R: Ein Fall von Teleangiektasie. Arch Ophthalmol 7:119–121, 1860.
6. Sturge WA: A case of partial epilepsy apparently due to a lesion of one of the vasomotor centres of the brain. Clin Soc Trans 12:162–167, 1879.
7. Kalischer S: Demonstration des Gehirns eines Kindes mit Teleangiektasie der linksseitigen Gesichts-Kopfhaut und Hirnoberfläche. Berl Kiln Wochenschr 34:1059–1067, 1897.
8. Cushing H: Cases of spontaneous intracranial hemorrhage associated with trigeminal nevi. JAMA 47:178–183, 1906.
9. Weber FP: Right-sided hemi-hypertrophy resulting from right-sided congenital spastic hemiplegia. J Neurol Psychopathol 3:134–139, 1922.
10. Krabbe KH: Facial and meningeal angiomatosis associated with calcification of the brain cortex: a clinical and anatomopathological contribution. Arch Neurol Psychiatr 32:737–755, 1934.
11. Krabbe KH, Wissing O: Calcifications de la pie-mère du cerveau (d'origine angiomateuse) demontrée par la radiographie. Acta Radiol (Stockholm) 10:523–532, 1929.
12. Dimitri V: Tumor cerebral congenito (angioma cavernosum). Rev Asoc Med Argent 36:1029–1037, 1923.
13. Marque A: Consideraciones sobre angiomas en la infancia. Rev Oto Neuro Oftel 1:202, 1927.
14. Brushfield T, Wyatt W: Hemiplegia associated with extensive naevus and mental defect. Br J Child Dis 24:98, 209, 1927.
15. Bergstrand H, Olivecrona H, Tönnis W: Gefässmissbildungen und Gefässgeschwülste des Gehirns. Thieme, Liepzig, 1936, p. 181.
16. Bergstrand H: Second International Neurological Congress (Abstracts), 1935, p. 124.
17. Roizin L, Gold G, Berman HH, Bonafede VI: Congenital vascular anomalies and their histopathology in Sturge–Weber–Dimitri syndrome. J Neuropathol Exp Neurol 18:75–97, 1959.
18. Alexander G, Norman RM: The Sturge–Weber Syndrome. J. Wright & Sons, Bristol, 1960.
19. Collignon J, Carlier G: Forme bilatéral de la maladie de Sturge–Weber avec anomalie rare du drainage veineux. Acta Neurol Belg 12:713–785, 1950.
20. Falkinburg LW, Silver ML, Kay MN, Stoll J: Sturge–Weber–Dimitri disease. Pediatrics 22:319–328, 1958.

21. Peterman AF, Hayles AB, Dockerty MB, Love JC: Encephalotrigeminal angiomatosis (Sturge–Weber disease). Clinical study of thirty-five cases. JAMA 167: 2169–2176, 1958.

22. Ambrosetto P, Ambrosetto G, Michelucci R, Bacci A: Sturge–Weber syndrome without port-wine facial nevus. Report of 2 cases studied by CT. Child's Brain 10:387–392, 1983.

23. Andriola M, Stolfi J: Sturge–Weber syndrome. Report of an atypical case. Am J Dis Child 123:507–510, 1972.

24. Lichtenstein BW: Sturge–Weber–Dimitri syndrome. Cephalic form of neurocutaneous hemangiomatosis. Arch Neurol Psychiatr 71:291–301, 1954.

25. Lund M: On epilepsy in Sturge–Weber disease. Acta Psychiatr Neurol 24:569–586, 1949.

26. Poser C, Taveras JM: Cerebral Angiography in encephalotrigeminal angiomatosis. Radiology 68:327–366, 1957.

27. Tönnis W, Friedmann G: Roentgenologic and clinical findings in 23 patients with Sturge–Weber disease. Zentalbl Neurochir 25:1–10, 1964.

28. Vouge M, Pasquini U, Salvolini U: CT findings of atypical forms of phakomatosis. Neuroradiology 20:99–101, 1980.

29. Myle G: Sémeiologie de l'angiomatose encéphlotrigéminée ou encéphalo-crânio-faciale. Acta Neurol Belg 12:713–785, 1950.

30. Chao DHC: Congenital neurocutaneous syndromes of childhood. III. Sturge–Weber disease. J Pediatr 55:635–648, 1959.

31. Kautzky R: Die Bedeutung der Hirnhaut-Innervation und ihrer Entwicklung für die Pathogenese der Sturge–Weber schen Frankheit. Dtsch Z Nervenh 161:505–510, 1949.

32. Cushing H, Bailey P: Tumors Arising from the Blood Vessels of the Brain. Charles C Thomas, Springfield, IL, 1928, pp. 17–22 and 49–59.

33. Streeter GL: The developmental alterations in the vascular system of the brain of the human embryo. Contrib Embryol (Carnegie Institution Washington) 8:5–38, 1918.

34. King G, Schwarz GA: Sturge–Weber syndrome (encephalotrigeminal angiomatosis). Arch Int Med Exp 94:743–757, 1954.

35. Di Trapani G, Di Rocco C, Abbamonti AL, Caldarelli M: Light microscopy and ultra-structural studies of Sturge–Weber disease. Child's Brain 9:23–36, 1982.

36. Miller SJH: Ophthalmic aspects of the Sturge–Weber syndrome. Proc Roy Soc Med 56:419–421, 1963.

37. Smith JL: Tomato-catsup in Sturge–Weber syndrome. Arch Ophthalmol 92:537, 1974.

38. Di Chiro G, Lindgren E: Radiographic findings in 14 cases of Sturge–Weber syndrome. Acta Radiol (Stockholm) 35:387–399, 1951.

39. Bonse G: Roentgenbefunde bei einer Phakomatose (Sturge–Weber kombiniert mit Klippel-Trénaunay). Fortschr Roentgenstr 74:727–729, 1951.

40. Guseo A: Ultrastructure of calcifications in Sturge–Weber disease. Virchows Arch Abt A Pathol Anat 366:352–356, 1975.

41. Haberland C, Perou M: Bone involvement in Sturge–Weber–Dimitri syndrome. Conf Neurol 28:413–422, 1966.

42. Nellhaus G, Haberland C, Hill BJ: Sturge–Weber disease with bilateral intracranial calcifications at birth and unusual pathologic findings. Acta Neurol Scand 43:314–347, 1967.

43. Van Bogaert L: Pathologie des angiomatoses. Acta Neurol Belg 50:525–610, 1950.

44. Wohlwill FJ, Yakolev PI: Histopathology of meningofacial angiomatosis (Sturge–Weber's disease). J Neuropathol Exp Neurol 16:341–364, 1957.

45. Hebold O: Haemangioma der weichen Hirnhaut bei Naevus vasculosus des Gesichts. Arch Psychiatr 51:445–456, 1913.

46. Volland O: Ueber zwei Fälle von zerebralem Angiome nebst Bemerkungen über Hirnangiome. Z Erforsch Behandl Junendl Schawachsinns 6:130–150, 1913.

47. Weber FP: A note on the association of extensive haemangiomatous naevus of the skin with cerebral (meningeal) haemangioma, especially cases of facial vascular naevus with controlateral hemiplegia. Proc Roy Soc Med 22:431–445, 1928/29.

48. Pagni CA, Wildi E: Pathogenetic hypothesis of intracortical calcifications in Sturge–Weber disease. Case report following lobectomy. Mod Prob Paediatr 18:250–257, 1977.

49. Peters G: Sturge–Weber'sche Krankheit. Handbuch der speziellen patologischen Anatomie und Histologie (Lubarsch-Henke-Rossle), Vol. 13. Springer-Verlag, Berlin, 1956, pp. 696–716.

50. Bentson JR, Wilson GH, Newton TH: Cerebral venous drainage pattern of Sturge–Weber syndrome. Radiology 101:1111–1118, 1971.

51. Norman MG, Schöne WC: The ultrastructure of Sturge–Weber disease. Acta Neuropathol 37:199–205, 1977.

52. Arseni C, Carp N: La maladie de Sturge–Weber. Ann Anat Pathol (Paris) 12:11–422, 1967.

53. Müller W: Zur Frage der Verkalkung bei der Sturge–Weber'sche Krankheit. Zentralbl Neurochem 21:67–74, 1961.

54. Shafer RN, Weiss DI: Congenital and Pediatric Glaucomas. C. V. Mosby, St. Louis, 1970, p. 60.

55. Stevenson RF, Thomson HG, Morin JD: Unrecognized ocular problems associated with port-wine stain of the face in children. Can Med Assoc J 111:953–954, 1974.

56. Alexander GL: Sturge–Weber disease. In: Vinken PJ, Bruyn GW (eds.), Handbook of Clinical Neurology. The Phakomatoses, Vol. 14. Elsevier, New York. 1972, pp. 223–240.

57. Chang C, Jackson GL, Baltz R: Isotopic cisternography in Sturge–Weber syndrome. J Nucl Med 11:551–553, 1970.

58. Chiron C, Raynaud C, Tzourio N, Diebler C, Dulac O, Zilbovicius M, Syrota A: Regional cerebral blood flow by SPECT imaging in Sturge–Weber disease: an aid for diagnosis. J Neurol Neurosurg Psychiatr 52:1402–1409, 1989.

59. Skoglund RR, Paa D, Lewis WJ: Elevated spinal-fluid protein in Sturge–Weber syndrome. Dev Med Child Neurol 20:99–102, 1978.

60. Huang YP, Wolf BS: Veins of the white matter of cerebral hemispheres (the medullary veins). Diagnostic importance in carotid angiography. Am J Roentgenol 92:739–755, 1964.

61. Coulam CM, Brow LR, Reese DF: Sturge–Weber syndrome. Semin Roentgenol 11:55–60, 1976.

62. Kuhl DE, Bevilacqua JE, Mishkin MM, Sanders TP: The brain scan in Sturge–Weber syndrome. Radiology 103:621–626, 1972.

63. Fanconi G: Sturge–Weber syndrom beim Neigeborenen: Ausgedehnte Naevi teleangiectatici, partieller Riesenwuchs und intrakranielle Verkalkung der rechten Hemisphäre, die im Lauf der ersten 1 1/2 Jahre eher zurückgehen. Helv Pediatr Acta 17:486–489, 1962.

64. Kitahara T, Maki Y: A case of Sturge–Weber disease with epilepsy and intracranial calcification at the neonatal period. Eur Neurol 17:8–12, 1978.

65. Gwinn JL, Lee FA: Radiological case of the month. Am J Dis Child 130:859–860, 1976.

66. Greenwald HM, Koota J: Associated facial and intracranial hemangiomas. Am J Dis Child 51:868–896, 1936.

67. Boltshauser E, Wilson J, Hoare RD: Sturge–Weber syndrome with bilateral intracranial calcifications. J Neurol Neurosurg Psychiatr 39:429–435, 1976.

68. Fiocchi A, Colombini A: Malattia di Sturge–Weber. Minerva Pediatr 30:579–584, 1978.

69. Gardeur D, Palmieri A, Mashaly R: Cranial computed tomography in the phakomatoses. Neuroradiology 25:293–304, 1983.

70. Maki Y, Semba A: Computed tomography of Sturge–Weber disease. Child's Brain 5:51–61, 1979.

71. New PJ, Scott W: Computed Tomography of the Brain and the Orbit. William & Wilkins, Baltimore, 1975, pp. 421–422.

72. Welch K, Naheedy MH, Abroms IF, Strand RD: Computed tomography of Sturge–Weber syndrome in infants. J Comput Assist Tomogr 4:33–36, 1980.

73. Enzman DR, Hayward RW, Norman D, Dunn RP: Cranial computed tomographic scan appearance of Sturge–Weber disease: unusual presentation. Radiology 172:721–724, 1977.

74. Chugani HT, Mazziotta JC, Phelps ME: Sturge–Weber syndrome: a study of cerebral glucose utilization with positron emission tomography. J Pediatr 114:244–253, 1989.

75. Anderson FH, Duncan GW: Sturge–Weber disease with subarachnoid hemorrhage. Stroke 5:509–511, 1974.

76. Rasmussen T, Mathieson G, Le Blanc P: Surgical therapy of typical and a form fruste variety of the Sturge–Weber syndrome. Suisse Neurol Neurochem Psychiatr 111:393–409, 1972.

77. Norlen G: The surgical treatment in Sturge–Weber's disease. Neurochirurgia 1:242–255, 1959.

78. Goscinski I, Kunicki A: On surgical treatment of Sturge–Weber syndrome. Acta Med Pol 13:229–236, 1972.

79. Masson M: La maladie de Sturge–Weber. Rev Prat 20:4455–4461, 1970.

80. Battin J, Got M, Vital Cl: Angiomatose de Sturge–Weber Évolution suivie pendant 7 ans, lobectomie occipitale et étude histologique des lésions cérébrales. Bordeaux Med 12:1767–1773, 1973.

81. Cohen HJ, Kay MN: Associated facial hemangioma and intracranial lesion (Weber–Dimitri disease). Am J Dis Child 62:606–612, 1941.

82. Falconer MA, Rushworth RG: Treatment of encephalotrigeminal angiomatosis (Sturge–Weber disease) by hemispherectomy. Arch Dis Child 35:433–447, 1960.

83. Courville BG: Morphology of small vascular malformations of the brain. J Neuropath Exp Neurol 2:274–284, 1963.

84. Livingston S, Eisner V, Brown WH, Boks LL: The Sturge–Weber syndrome. Postgrad Med 92:221–230, 1956.

85. Scholz W: Epilepsie. In: Bunke O (Ed.), Handbuch der Geisteskrankheiten. XI. Springer-Verlag, Berlin, 1930.

86. Achslogh J: Hémispherectomie dans un cas de maladie de Sturge–Weber. Acta Neurol Belgica 58:837–847, 1958.

87. Buttler G, Schulte FJ: Zur operativen Behandlung des Sturge–Weber syndroms. Neuropaediatrie 6:135–141, 1975.

88. Cairns H, Davidson MA: Hemispherectomy in the treatment of infantile hemiplegia. Lancet 2:411–415, 1951.

89. Caldarelli M, Di Rocco C, Rossi GF, Di Trapani G, Fileni A, Martino A, Moschini M: Indicazione chirurgica precoce nella sindrome di Sturge–Weber. Riv Ital Pediatr (IJP) 8:785–792, 1982.

90. Green JR, Foster J, Berens DL: Encephalotrigeminal angiomatosis (Sturge–Weber syndrome). Am J Roentgenal Radium Ther Nucl Med 64:391–398, 1950.

91. Lapras Cl, Dechaume J-P, Revol M, Nicolas A, Deruty R: A propos du traitement de la maladie de Sturge–Weber chez l'enfant. Pediatrie (Lyon) 26:789, 1971.

92. Venes JL, Linder S: Sturge–Weber–Dimitri syndrome. Encephalotrigeminal angiomatosis. In: Edwards MSB, Hoffman HJ (eds.), Cerebral Vascular Disease in Children and Adolescents. Williams & Wilkins, Baltimore, 1989, pp. 337–341.

93. Hendrick EB, Hoffman HJ, Hudson AR: Hemispherectomy in children. Clin Neurosurg 16:315–327, 1969.

94. Hoffman HJ, Hendrick EB, Dennis M, Armstrong D: Hemispherectomy for Sturge–Weber syndrome. Child's Brain 5:233–248, 1979.

95. Laine E, Gro Cl: L'Hémisphérectomie. Masson, Paris, 1956.

96. Dimitri V, Balado M: Angioma cerebral operado. Rev Asoc Med Argent 47:3045–3050, 1933.

97. Obrador Alcalde S: About surgical technique for hemispherectomy in cases of cerebral hemiatrophy. Acta Neurochir (Wien) 3:57–62, 1952.

98. Serfling HJ, Parnitzke H: Behandlungsmöglichkeiten bei der Sturge–Weberschen Erkrangung und die Problematik ihrer Anwendbarkeit. Wiss Z Univ Halle 3:989–995, 1954.

99. Krynau RA: Infantile hemiplegia treated by removing one cerebral hemisphere. J Neurol Neurosurg Psychiat 13:243–267, 1950.

CHAPTER 14

Coagulopathies and Vasculopathies

Piero A. Pellegrino, Luigi Zanesco, and Pier Antonio Battistella

These diseases, manifested by vascular occlusion, hemorrhage, or both, have a variety of causes. For didactic purposes, we are arbitrarily dividing this very heterogeneous group of lesions into three subgroups: (1) coagulopathies, (2) cerebrovascular disorders of cardiovascular origin, and (3) inflammatory and dysmetabolic vasculopathies.

Coagulopathies

It has now become customary before a neurosurgical intervention to assess accurately the patient's coagulation pattern by a screening that includes the platelet count and a certain number of key tests. An accurate history of any, even mild, hemorrhagic episodes is also very important as a warning of an abnormal coagulation status. A positive history in this sense must press for a more thorough investigation of the coagulation cascade by a specialist laboratory before starting the operation. By adopting these precautions, the risk for a neurosurgeon of being caught in unexpected coagulation deficit becomes really trivial. Bleedings during surgery, indeed, are usually related to mechanical factors. Hematologic and coagulation disorders that may give rise to cerebrovascular accidents in children are summarized in Table 14-1.

Congenital Diseases

Hemophiliac Syndromes

These disorders include hemophilia A (factor VIII deficiency) and hemophilia B or Christmas disease (factor IX deficiency), both transmitted with sex-linked recessive inheritance, and von Willebrand's disease or vascular hemophilia or pseudohemophilia (factor VIII and von Willebrand's factor deficiency), transmitted with an autosomal dominant pattern. The clinical expression of these syndromes is highly variable, so that mild cases may escape early identification, although an accurate history is often suggestive. In the general population about 50 out of 1 million persons suffer from the severe form of hemophilia, but approximately 1000 may present with the milder defect. Factor IX deficit is 7 to 10 times less frequent than classic hemophilia. von Willebrand's disease has an unknown incidence, probably higher than the

Table 14.1. Hematologic and coagulation disorders.

Congenital diseases
  Hemophiliac syndromes
    Hemophilia A
    Hemophilia B
    von Willebrand's disease
  Uncommon coagulation deficiencies
    Congenital afibrinogenemia
    Congenital factor XIII deficiency
    Protein C deficiency
    Antithrombin III deficiency
  Hemoglobinopathies
    Sickle cell disese
    Sickle cell trait
    Hemoglobin SC disease
    Thalassemia
Acquired disease
  Vitamin K deficiency
  Disseminated intravascular coagulation
  Idiopathic thrombocytopenic purpura
  Thrombocytosis
  Malignancies

other hemophiliac syndromes but the serious cases are definitely rarer. Cerebrovascular accidents exceptionally complicate this last coagulopathy and are usually limited to a variant known as severe von Willebrand's disease.

The diagnosis of hemophilia is based on laboratory evidence of decreased levels of factors VIII and/or IX. Severe hemophilia is defined by levels less than 1% of normal activity; it is moderately severe between 1 and 5%; and mild between 5 and 30%. Levels greater than or equal to 30% are generally safe. Intracranial hemorrhages, observed in 13% of affected patients,[1] still represent the most important cause of death. Only in 50% of cases is there a history of cranial trauma, usually mild and occurring 2 to 4 days before the onset of neurologic symptoms. Bleeding can be epidural, subdural, subarachnoid, intraventricular, parenchymal, and, less frequently, spinal, and the clinical picture depends on the site and quickness of the blood loss. The first diagnostic step is computerized tomography, while invasive procedures, such as spinal tap and angiography, may be performed after restoring the factor VIII level to over 60%.[2] In hemophiliac patients presenting with intracranial bleeding or undergoing a neurosurgical intervention, it is mandatory to correct immediately the coagulation deficit. The need for great amounts of factors VIII or IX in a very short time requires, in the case of intracranial hemorrhage, the use of cryoprecipitate or factor concentrate. Fresh frozen plasma, even if containing these factors, is contraindicated because of the excessive amounts necessary to reach safety levels in a matter of a few minutes. The replacement therapy in central nervous system (CNS) bleeding must be protracted for at least 2 weeks. The factor VIII level must reach about 100% of normality at the time of surgical treatment, remaining greater than 60% in the first four postoperative days, and greater than 20% in the following 10 days. When suspecting an intracranial hematoma, in the presence of headache and no laboratory confirmation, a 3-day "prophylactic" treatment with cryoprecipitate or factor concentrate is indicated.[3] In spite of the replacement therapy, many hemophiliac children continue to suffer from cerebrovascular hemorrhagic accidents and are left with some residual neurologic deficits.

Congenital Afibrinogenemia

This disorder, sustained by a practically complete absence of fibrinogen, and transmitted as an autosomal recessive characteristic, presents, also in the newborn, with severe bleedings in various organs, including the CNS. The hemorrhagic episodes are easily controlled by the use of fresh frozen plasma or fibrinogen concentrate (about 1 g/10 kg body weight). As the molecular half-life is 80 hr, treatment may be spaced every 4 to 5 days, also in the case of surgery. Once the bleeding problem has been solved, therapy must be stopped in order to avoid anti-fibrinogen antibodies or thromboembolic complications.[4]

Factor XIII Deficiency

The clinical manifestations consist of poor wound healing, and late wound bleeding due to a friable clot. Bleeding appears usually 1 to 2 days after trauma, and CNS hemorrhages are observed mainly in children. Coagulation screening tests are negative and the condition is diagnosed by finding an abnormal solubility of the clot in 5 M urea solution and a short euglobulin lysis time. Fresh frozen plasma (1 ml/kg body weight) once a week resolves the coagulation disturbance.

Protein C Deficiency

Protein C is a glycoprotein that inhibits factors V and VIII. Its deficiency, therefore, gives rise to thromboembolic phenomena accompanied by intravascular coagulation and cutaneous necrotic lesions.[5] Cerebrovascular complications, usually due to sinovenous thrombosis, are not rare and involve adolescents and young adults. The most severe deficit (homozygous?) is responsible for the neonatal marble fulminating purpura.

Antithrombin III Deficiency

This hereditary disorder, transmitted with an autosomal dominant pattern, is incompatible with life in its homozygous form. Heterozygous persons present from adolescence with a tendency to thrombotic events, which may appear in various organs, including the CNS, especially following trauma. Acquired varieties have also been reported, secondary to severe liver dysfunction, nephrosis, malnutrition, and heparin therapy. Treatment is based on the use of warfarin.

Sickle Cell Syndromes

The sickle cell syndromes constitute a most important group of hemoglobinopathies. The substitution of valine for glutamic acid in the number-6 position of the β-chain of hemoglobin represents the molecular basis of the disease (hemoglobin S, or HbS) and involves a change in the physical properties of hemoglobin: a tendency to aggregate and form watery crystals. These convert the erythrocytes into rigid, deformed cells unable to squeeze through the capillaries. Heterozygous persons are usually asymptomatic; however, occasionally, they can present with vascular accidents, such as splenic infarctions or vascular thrombosis, mainly in the youngster. The patient with true sickle cell anemia is homozygous for the gene for HbS. He has a severe hemolytic anemia and experiences repeated episodes of vascular occlusion in many organs. Frequent complications are pneumococcal or gram-negative bacterial infections. CNS involvement occurs in about 7% of children with sickle cell anemia and can result in a devastating, often fatal, accident. Hemiplegia, seizures, coma, speech defects, and visual disturbances are common signs and may resolve entirely, or improve, or remain constant. The treatment of CNS crises includes prompt and vigorous hydration, administration of oxygen, exchange transfusions to limit the extent of CNS sickling, and multiple transfusions of packed red cells. Computerized tomography (CT) scanning or cerebral arteriography are important to ruling out treatable disorders such as subdural hematoma, berry aneurysm, abscess, or tuberculoma, not so rare in sickle cell disease. Computerized tomography may show no abnormalities until 2 to 4 days after the initial crisis, when areas of edema and infarction are visible. Angiography should not be performed

until an exchange transfusion has been done, so that the hypertonic dye will not cause further intracerebral sickling. Strokes tend to be repetitive and progressive,[6] with the occurrence of secondary vascular anomalies (damage and proliferation of the intima, and stenosis at sites of bifurcation). Therefore, in a child who has experienced even just one cerebrovascular accident, it is justified to adopt maintenance transfusion therapy. This program, which has a profound influence on the morbidity of stroke, is designed to keep HbS at less than 30% and to lower the stroke recurrence rate to 10%, and should be carried out for at least 1 year or more.[7] In older children hemorrhages are more common than vascular occlusions.[8] These episodes, presenting with severe headache and meningismus, may progress rapidly and have a mortality rate of 50%. After stopping the blood loss by exchange transfusions, optimum hydration, oxygen, etc., the neurosurgeon will have to evaluate, together with the radiologist, the opportunity of evacuating the hematoma, even though in most cases surgery is not possible.

Acquired Diseases

Vitamin K Deficiency

Vitamin K is well represented in the human diet and its daily requirements are very small (about 1 μg/kg). In newborns and infants vitamin K synthesis by the intestinal bacterial flora represents the primary source. Vitamin K deficiency may be observed in several clinical contexts: hemorrhagic disease of the newborn, parenteral nutrition without vitamin K supplementation, protracted antibiotic therapy, biliary atresia or other malabsorption syndromes, and pharmacological antagonism (coumarin, salicylates, phenytoin). Hemorrhages due to vitamin K deficiency are nonspecific acute manifestations with a spectrum of extreme variability and CNS involvement, mainly in newborns and patients treated with antiblastic drugs.

This coagulopathy involves factors II, VII, IX, and X. Intravenous administration of 1 mg of vitamin K stops the hemorrhagic phenomena within 3 hr and corrects the coagulation deficits within 24 to 48 hr. Fresh plasma or prothrombin complex concentrate may be needed to arrest life-threatening bleeding or when surgery is contemplated.

Disseminated Intravascular Coagulation (DIC)

DIC or consumption coagulopathy, or defibrination syndrome, is an acquired disturbance usually associated with an underlying disease. An acute activation of physiologic coagulation and fibrinolysis with depletion of clotting factors result in both a hypocoagulability status and diffuse intravascular coagulation events. The pathogenic mechanism is related to the liberation of thromboplastin by the endothelial cells or of thromboplastin-like compounds by damaged tissues following trauma, burns, hemorrhagic shock, heat stress, or surgery. The primer may also be represented by infections, tumors (particularly promyelocytic leukemia), blood transfusions with hemolysis, and, finally, drugs or snake bite. The clinical spectrum is highly variable, depending on the underlying primary condition. Salient features of DIC, mainly in the acute form, are (1) presence of ecchymotic purpura, sometimes with surface bleeding, (2) anemia, and (3) variable circulatory failure with hypotension and shock. Laboratory data show thrombocytopenia, hypofibrinogenemia, prolongation of prothrombin time, and increase in the fibrin/fibrinogen degradation product. In the CNS the thromboplastin concentration is very high. Therefore DIC following head trauma, neurosurgical procedures, intracranial vascular accidents, etc., seems to be a frequent condition and cause of important injury to the brain.[9] In spite of controversies, heparin represents the only drug capable of stopping most of the activated coagulation factors, as long as adequate levels of antithrombin III are present. A continuous intravenous administration of heparin (300–600 U/kg/day) is preferred to the intermittent bolus that, sometimes, can make the hemorrhage worse. Frozen fresh plasma is added in order to provide antithrombin III. The use of ε-amino-caproic acid, a strong inhibitor of plasminogen activator, is still controversial. It does not seem to be effective in blocking the secondary fibrinolysis of DIC and, if used alone,

may produce thromboembolic complications.[3] The treatment of DIC must always include a serious attempt at eliminating the causal factors (infections, etc.) and at correcting the aggravating circumstances (hypotension, anemia, anoxia).

Idiopathic Thrombocytopenic Purpura (ITP)

ITP is an acute, usually autolimited, thrombocytopenia, characterized by a number of platelets less than $100,000/mm^3$, and sustained by autoantibodies linked to specific platelet antigens. Others hypothesize a different pathogenic mechanism based on IgG–viral immunocomplexes. In 80 to 90% of children a spontaneous cure occurs within 1 to 6 months. When lasting longer than 6 months, ITP is defined as chronic. One to 2% of patients, more often within the first month, suffer from an episode of intracranial hemorrhage. As demonstrated in a multicentric survey of more than 1,000 cases,[10] 22 patients had this complication and 8 of them died. Events favoring cerebrovascular accidents were a concomitant treatment with aspirin, a known inhibitor of platelet function, or a systemic hypertension, sometimes induced by protracted steroid therapy. Trauma, instead, was involved in only four cases. The intracranial hemorrhages may be more frequently intracerebral, subdural, or subarachnoid and, when suspected, a CT scan must be performed. The medical treatment of an acute and serious hemorrhagic episode consists of methylprednisolone (4 mg/kg i.v.) and infusion of IgG (400 mg/kg/day) for 5 days. Platelet concentrate is justified only if used very early and in adequate doses (at least 6 U/m²) or, even better, obtained by platelet pheresis. Platelets are usually administered only once in spite of their brief half-life. This is due to the very rapid activity of intravenous IgG. By this treatment platelets reach acceptable levels fairly rapidly. Subsequently, it is surgically possible to drain a hematoma when present. The emergency splenectomy has today been rejected since the same result may be obtained with the use of intravenous IgG (*medical splenectomy*). Management with steroids or IgG does not influence in any way the evolution of ITP, which cures spontaneously within a few weeks, other than in 10% of cases that become *chronically thrombocytopenic.*

Thrombocytosis

This disorder, which occurs when the platelet count exceeds 450,000/mm^3, often causes headache and occasionally thrombotic events in the brain.[11] Primary thrombocytosis, very rare in children, is related to myeloproliferative disorders, such as chronic leukemias, and polycythemia rubra vera. Secondary thrombocytosis is observed more frequently in the pediatric age group as a consequence of iron deficiency anemia, infectious or inflammatory conditions, or neoplasms. An increased number of circulating platelets is also common in asplenia syndrome and after surgical or functional splenectomy. Headache, vertigo, and mental slowness are the expression of global cerebral dysfunction, although the pathogenic mechanism is not yet completely understood. It has been suggested that an alteration of cerebral microcirculation similar to that occurring in polycythemia[12] may be involved, but definite proofs are still lacking. Less frequently, thrombocytosis is complicated by occlusion of cerebral vessels or sinovenous thrombosis with focal neurologic deficits. Usually no treatment is indicated. Secondary forms may be corrected by intervening on the underlying process. In symptomatic cases aspirin or dipyridamole, platelet pheresis, or chemotherapeutic agents are the keystones of management.[13]

Malignancies

Children with oncologic disorders are frequently at risk of cerebrovascular accidents.[14] In acute leukemia these complications may have different pathogenic mechanisms; (1) Hyperviscosity and leukostasis, especially with leucocyte counts greater than 100,000/mm^3. In this condition hemorrhage may be favored by other factors, such as lactic acidosis, vessel fragility due to leukemic infiltration of the vascular wall, thrombocytopenia, and hypoxia. (2) Disseminated intravascular coagulation, typical of the *promyelocytic* variant of acute myeloid leukemia and occurring in the first days of the disease,

sometimes as a prodromic sign: convulsions or a diffuse encephalopathy are the main clinical features. Not rarely, intracerebral DIC remains localized, and this may delay the diagnosis because laboratory evidence can be present only a few days later, or even never.[14] (3) Asparaginase treatment, which can produce, by an unclear mechanism, both thrombotic and hemorrhagic episodes: methotrexate is another drug potentially responsible for a similar clinical picture, and for focal vascular damage. Usually, clinical manifestations are reversible, and not linked to a vascular lesion. (4) Platelet-resistant thrombocytopenia, particularly in children undergoing a multitransfusional program: not rarely, children with leukemia in the terminal phase die of cerebrovascular accidents related to cerebral vascular damage, manifested by increased permeability, and a tendency to microhemorrhages with ensuing coma and respiratory insufficiency.

Sinovenous thrombosis, but also hemorrhage, has been observed also in young patients suffering from neuroblastoma with cranial and subdural metastases (exceptionally subarachnoid and intracerebral). In the terminal stage of solid tumors sepsis, DIC, and infections, together with the neoplastic progression, are frequent causes of cerebrovascular accidents. The management of these complications must always be addressed to the underlying disorder and contemplate strict cooperation between oncologists, hematologists, radiotherapists, and neurosurgeons.[15]

Cerebrovascular Disorders of Cardiovascular Origin

Cerebrovascular disorders of cardiovascular origin are relatively uncommon in children and adolescents, although in our institution (a large referral center as well as community hospital) they occur with some frequency. Since significant atherosclerosis is rare in the young, the etiological and predisposing factors are much different in the pediatric and adult populations and involve different diagnostic and therapeutic approaches. They occur mostly in four main etiopathogenetic contexts: (1) systemic hypertension, (2) polycythemia, (3) cerebral embolism, and (4) atherosclerosis.

Systemic Hypertension

It is well known that systemic hypertension may result in thrombosis, periventricular leukomalacia and/or bleeding, and intraventricular hemorrhage both in adults and children. Its incidence varies from 2.5% in the newborn to 1 to 2% in children to 10% in the adolescent group.[16] In younger children, most cases are secondary in nature while in adolescents 80 to 100% of hypertension is "essential."[16,17] We consider abnormal blood pressure values that are consistently above the ninety-fifth percentile for age.

In an analysis of 150 consecutive hypertensive children seen at our institution in the last 5 years, a little more than 75% of children with secondary hypertension had a renal abnormality. Of these, 50% have chronic glomerulonephritis or pyelonephritis, 25% a congenital renal malformation and 8% a renovascular disease. Hypertension due to endocrine disorders is quite uncommon.

Aortic Coarctation

Approximately 2% of secondary hypertension in childhood is due to aortic coarctation.[18] It is usually anatomically correctable by surgery but in 30% of operated patients hypertension persists or recurs. The incidence of berry-type intracranial aneurysms is increased in patients with aortic coarctation. The literature reports a 2.5 to 50% prevalence compared to 0.65 to 2% in the general population.[19] Some instances of sudden death in unoperated (and also operated) children with coarctation have been shown to be from rupture of the intracranial aneurysm.[19] In their recent work Roach and Riela advocate, in aortic coarctation patients after adolescence, the use of serial CT scans for preventing this potentially fatal complication.[20] Much rarer are cases of spontaneous paresis or paraplegia due to dilated intercostal arteries compressing the anterior spinal artery or to epidural hemorrhage.[21]

Clinical Manifestations

Whatever the cause, in general, clinical manifestations of hypertension in childhood will be directly related to the level and duration of high blood pressure. Because hypertensive children have fewer risk factors than adults, they develop complications like thrombosis or cerebral hemorrhage less frequently.

Even if cerebral hemorrhage has also been described in neonates with coarctation of the aorta,[22] it should be emphasized that this complication is infrequent in the pediatric age group. Instead, the occurrence of hypertensive encephalopathy presenting with headache, vomiting, ataxia, stupor, and coma is relatively frequent. Hypertensive encephalopathy is caused by cerebral hyperemia associated with damage to cerebral arterioles, increased permeability, and edema.[23,24] Seizures, both focal and generalized, are seen more frequently in infants and children than in adolescents. In malignant hypertension fundus examination will show papilledema, arterial spasm, hemorrhage, and exudates.

Polycythemia

Erythrocyte abnormalities, particularly changes in concentration (polycythemia, anemia) or structural changes in hemoglobin molecule, are known causes of cerebrovascular accidents. Polycythemia, which occurs when the erythrocyte count and the hemoglobin and hematocrit levels exceed the upper limits of normal, is usually associated with chronic arterial oxygen desaturation. This is the secondary form, which must be differentiated from the much rarer polycythemia rubra vera. This latter form affects almost exclusively adults and is characterized by polycythemia, leukocytosis, thrombocytosis, and bone marrow hyperplasia. The most frequent causes of secondary polycythemia are cyanotic congenital heart disease, like transposition of the great arteries, tetralogy of Fallot, tricuspid atresia, and chronic pulmonary conditions, like bronchiectasis and emphysema. In addition, there have been several observations in the literature that infratentorial neoplasms, especially cerebellar hemangioblastomas, kidney abnormalities such as cysts and hydronephrosis, hereditary hemorrhagic telangiectasia (Osler–Weber–Rendu disease), and hypoventilation of massive obesity (Pickwickian syndrome) may be associated with a polycythemic state.[25-27]

That the cerebral microcirculation is influenced by stasis in polycythemia (with or without thrombosis) is suggested by the elegant observations of Thomas et al.[12] of reduced cerebral blood flow and increased cerebrovascular resistance in the presence of high hematocrit. It is well known that when the hematocrit rises above 50% there is an exponential increase in the blood viscosity (Fig. 14.1). This, in turn, impedes perfusion in the cerebral microcirculation, resulting in symptoms such as headaches, dizziness, tinnitus, and mental slowness. While most neurological manifestations in polycythemia are expressions of global cerebral dysfunction, several studies in children with cyanotic congenital heart disease and chronic hypoxia have associated polycythemia to an increased stroke risk.[28-30] Occlusion of major arteries supplying the brain or thrombosis of venous channels, mainly the sagittal sinus, were the cause of massive infarctions, anemic and hemorrhagic, in infant and children.[28-31] Usually, cerebrovascular accidents in infants with cyanotic heart disease are favored by iron deficiency anemia and precipitated by severe dehydration, while in older children they are related to polycythemia and chronic hypoxia. Focal neurologic manifestations due to cerebrovascular accidents must be differentiated from cerebral abscess and cardiogenic emboli, which are also relatively frequent in this same group of patients.

Hyperviscosity may be treated by periodic erythropheresis, which results in increased cerebral blood flow and improvement in symptomatology.[12]

Cerebral Embolism

Arterial embolization to the brain in infants and children has been documented from thrombotic, neoplastic, infectious, lipoid, pneumatic, and foreign body sources.[28,30-39] Table 14.2 lists most of the known causes of cerebral embolism.

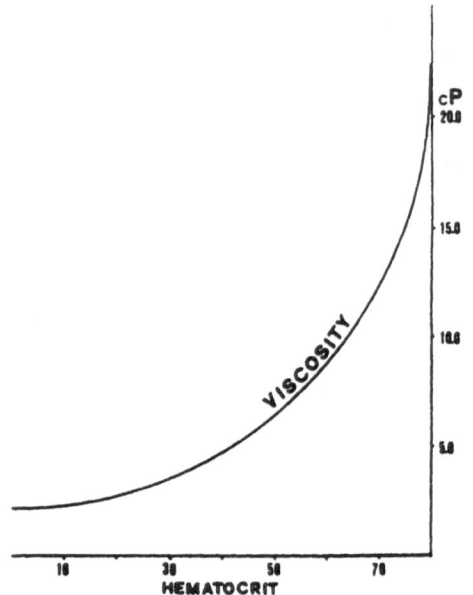

Figure 14.1. Relationship of hematocrit and viscosity. Marked increase in viscosity occurs at a hematocrit greater than 50%.

Cardiac Disease

No doubt that infants and children with congenital heart disease, especially a cyanotic type, are at particular risk of developing cerebral necrosis for a number of reasons. Right-to-left shunts, like those occurring in tetralogy of Fallot and transposition of great arteries, allow emboli

Table 14.2. Etiology of cerebral embolism.

Cardiac disease
   Rheumatic heart disease
   Congenital heart disease (mainly cyanotic)
   Paradoxical embolization
   Infective endocarditis
   Cardiac tumor (mainly myxoma)
   Cardiac arrhythmia
   Nonseptic endocarditis
   Myocardial infarction
   Cardiomyopathy
Pulmonary disease
   Pulmonary arteriovenous fistula
   Hereditary hemorrhagic telangiectasia
Trauma
   Arteriography
   Cardiac catheterization or surgery
   Air embolism (during neurosurgery or cardiac surgery)
   Fat embolism (fractures, cardiac surgery)
   Foreign body embolism (pellets, etc.)

from peripheral veins to bypass the lung filter and enter the systemic arterial circulation to the brain (paradoxical embolization). Any type of congenital heart disease, including ventricular septal defect, mitral stenosis, aortic stenosis, and others, and rheumatic valvular disease, such as mitral or aortic insufficiency, may be complicated by an infective endocarditis which, in turn, may give rise to major emboli to the brain or elsewhere in the body. Usually, *Staphylococcus aureus* endocarditis with more verrucous and friable vegetations is more prone to generate embolic events. In our experience of 35 cases of bacterial endocarditis in children, 7 were complicated by major emboli and 3 of these 7 showed cerebrovascular accidents.[40] Mitral valve prolapse, although rarely seen in children, may be responsible for embolic phenomena through different pathogenetic mechanisms: (1)

disruption of the endocardium of the myxomatous valve and thrombus formation,[41] (2) infective endocarditis, and (3) tachyarrhythmias. Cardiac catheterization, also in our experience, has been associated to small or large infarctions in the brain.[31] During surgery with cardiopulmonary bypass for congenital lesions, air emboli, thrombi, or foreign material may produce cerebral symptoms.

All cardiac tumors may be the source of peripheral embolism. This is a frequent manifestation of myxoma, the most common primary tumor of the heart occurring in 75% of cases in the left atrium.[36] Embolism is observed in about 45% of cases of left atrial myxoma[36] and the brain is affected in about 50%.

We have recently had the opportunity to care for a 6-year-old child who presented with sudden onset of right hemiparesis and aphasia. A CT scan showed a left parietal hypodense area with indirect signs of perifocal edema. A prompt and complete cardiac work-up led us to a diagnosis of left atrial myxoma, which was successfully removed 5 weeks after diagnosis[42] (Figs. 14.2 and 14.3). A CT scan 3 years later disclosed a clear-cut left parietal infarction area (Fig. 14.4).

Pulmonary Disease

Pulmonary arteriovenous fistula, isolated or in the context of hereditary hemorrhagic telangiectasia, has been associated with neurologic deficits as a result of paradoxical emboli.[43] Chronic hypoxemia, polycythemia, and brain abscesses are other possible causes of cerebral dysfunction in both situations.[43,44]

Trauma

Air embolism during cerebral arteriography has recently been described by Voorhies and Fraser and diagnosed by computerized tomography.[38] Because of the evanescent nature of air bubbles in the vasculature a precise documentation of cerebral air embolism is difficult. In our institution most cases of air embolism to the brain in children have been observed following open heart surgery with cardiac bypass. In these cases, if postoperative neurologic abnormalities, like alteration of consciousness, seizure, and

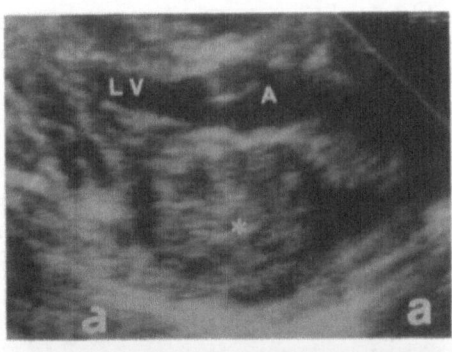
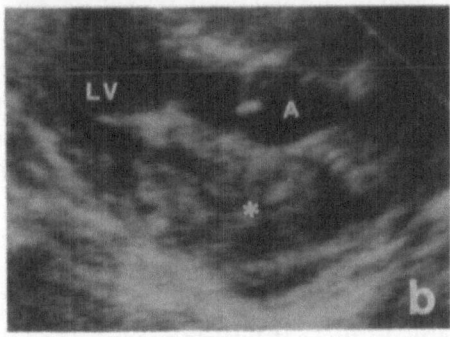

Figure 14.2. Two-dimensional echocardiogram. Long-axial view in a case of left atrial myxoma showing a large mass (asterisk) adherent to the atrial wall and occupying most of the left atrial cavity in systole (**a**) and protruding through the mitral valve toward the left ventricle in diastole (**b**). A, Aortic root; LV, left ventricle.

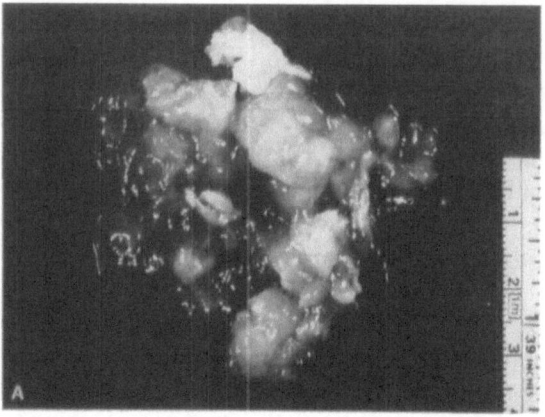

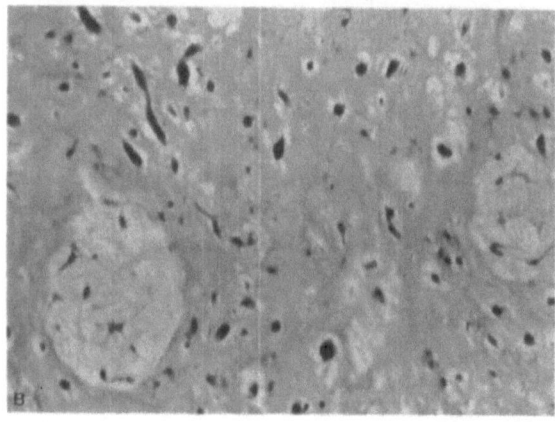

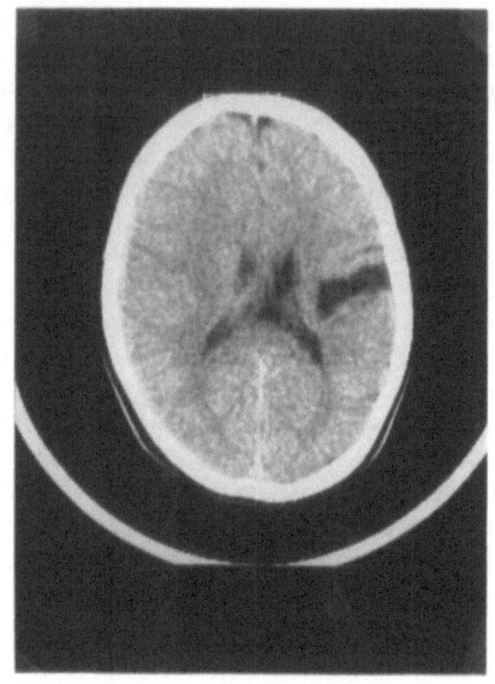

Figure 14.4. Unenhanced CT scan (same case as in Figs. 14.2, 14.3) shows a sharply demarcated hypodense area of left parietal infarction.

Figure 14.3. (A) Macroscopic appearance of the surgically removed left atrial myxoma (same case as in Fig. 14.2). Irregularly lobulated, papillary gelatinous mass presenting with hemorrhagic areas. (B) Microscopic appearance. Spindle-shaped and stellate cells embedded in acid mucopolysaccharide ground substance. (Hematoxylin-eosin; × 180.)

focal neurological deficits, are present, embolism should be considered, as well as brain damage due to hypoxia or hypotension.

There are good published accounts of posttraumatic fat embolism in children,[45] following cardiac surgery and, most interestingly, after intravenous fat infusions in infants.[37] Paresis, coma, and electroencephalographic changes are the most frequent neurologic disturbances. Diagnosis of fat embolism can only be made with certainty in vivo by detection of retinal fat embolism or from biopsy. Whatever the cause, brain necrosis consequent to arterial thromboembolism is, usually, ischemic but in

the case of embolus fragmentation or of mycotic emboli the lesion may become hemorrhagic owing to reperfusion and hemorrhage into the necrotic area.

The diagnosis of cerebral embolism must be entertained in any child with (1) sudden onset of clinical symptoms and presence of maximal brain dysfunction at the time of onset, (2) a certain or probable source of emboli, like cyanotic congenital heart disease, infective endocarditis, etc., and (3) signs of major emboli in other districts of the body.[46] In fact, the prompt recognition and treatment of any underlying medical condition, although it probably will not improve the neurologic deficit, will serve to prevent further progression of the embolic phenomena or new complication.

Atherosclerosis

Unlike in adults, atherosclerosis plays a definitely minor pathogenetic role in strokes in children. The vascular changes are very much similar to those found in adults and consist mainly of changes in the intima of arteries, with lipid, fibrin, platelets, calcium, and fibrous tissue deposition, and in the media. Also, angiographically the arteriopathy observed is usually nonspecific,[47] being characterized by vascular occlusion, irregularities of the arterial lumen, tortuosity, and evidence of collateralization, and should be differentiated from other lesions responsible of ischemic strokes in children, such as hemoglobinopathies, polycythemia, cerebral embolism secondary to cardiac disorders, arteritis, and fibromuscular dysplasia. Even if early atherosclerotic changes are an occasional finding in autopsies of children and adolescents,[48,49] they are rarely a cause of cerebrovascular accidents. These have been described mainly in patients with progeria, juvenile diabetes, and children with familial lipid disorders.[47,48,50,51] Glueck et al. have recently

reported on eight children who had familial lipoprotein disorders and evidence of thromboembolic cerebrovascular disease. Most of them presented with low levels of plasma high-density lipoprotein cholesterol.[51] The authors postulate the possible pathogenic relationship between lipoprotein abnormalities and endothelial damage and thrombosis of cerebral arteries, supporting their assumption also with the in vitro studies by Tauber et al.[52] of a protective effect of high-density lipoprotein on bovine vascular endothelial cells.

Inflammatory and Dysmetabolic Vasculopathies

This group of disorders is responsible for arterial thromboembolism, sinovenous occlusions, or parenchymal or subarachnoid hemorrhages.[53] The classification is difficult because of the multiple etiology, the markedly different clinical manifestations, and the heterogeneity in the pathological substrate (Table 14.3).

Inflammatory Vasculopathies

Infectious Vasculitis

The CNS infections represent the most frequent cause of vasculitis. Radiologic findings compatible with cerebral infarction have been observed in about one-third of patients with bacterial meningitis.[54] The risk of cerebrovascular complications, in addition, is inversely related to age.[55]

Systemic Lupus Erythematosus (SLE)

This autoimmune disease is observed in the first decade of life in less than 5% of cases. Clinical symptomatology is due to arterial and venous thrombotic events, hemorrhage, but also metabolic derangements, or pharmacologic side effects.[56] Neurologic complications, which are very frequent in SLE (13 to 30% of cases[57]), consist mainly of seizures, psychiatric disturbances, headache and chorea, and more

Table 14.3. Inflammatory and dysmetabolic vasculopathies.

Inflammatory
  Infectious vasculitis
  Collagen disease
    Lupus erythematosus
    Lupus anticoagulants
    Polyarteritis nodosa
    Rheumatoid arthritis
    Rheumatic fever
  Giant cell arteritis
    Takayasu's arteritis
    Temporal arteritis
  Granulomatous arteritis
  Hypersensitivity vasculitis
  Other arteritis
    Transient embologenic aortoarteritis
    Kawasaki disease
    Behçet's disease
Dysmetabolic
  Homocystinuria
  Fabry's disease
  Kinky-hair syndrome (Menkes' disease)
  Hemolitic–uremic syndrome
  MELAS syndrome
Other vasculopathies
  Malignant atrophic papulosis (Degos' disease)
  Pseudoxanthoma elasticum
  Fibromuscular dysplasia

rarely myelopathy, ataxia, polyradiculoneuritis, and pseudotumor cerebri. Laboratory data show increases in the sedimentation rate and C-reactive protein, anemia, leukopenia, presence of anti-nuclear antibodies, positivity of the LE cells test, and hypocomplementemia. The cerebrospinal fluid (CSF) may demonstrate a mild increase in the protein level and pleiocytosis in about one-third of cases.[58] Nonspecific anomalies are often discovered in electroencephalograms (EEGs); this is useful for monitoring the course of the disease. Neuroradiologic abnormalities are recognized in 50% of cases, mainly in the active phase.[59]

Lupus Anticoagulants

This syndrome, characterized in adults by recurrent thrombosis, repeated abortions, and thrombocytopenia, has been recently described also in childhood.[60] It may be observed in association with SLE and other collagenopathies, malignancies, and treatment with phenothiazines, but also with no apparent causes.[61] Lupus anticoagulants are acquired IgG or IgM immunoglobulins that, by interference with the phospholipid portion of the prothrombin activator complex, increase the partial thromboplastin time and inhibit coagulation. Paradoxically, the clinical manifestations are thrombotic in nature, consisting mainly of focal neurologic deficit, headache, myelopathy, and polyradiculoneuritis, as reported in a recent paper.[62] DIC must enter in the differential diagnosis.

Polyarteritis Nodosa

About one-third of pediatric patients present with neurologic manifestations, such as convulsions, headache, and focal deficit.[53] Less frequently, this disorder is complicated by peripheral neuropathy because of involvement of the vasa nervorum. A vasculitic process of the small and medium-sized arteries, more evident at the bifurcation level, is the main pathologic feature. Arteriography may show segmentary restriction of the vessel caliber and, occasionally, microaneurysmatic dilations, responsible for infarctions and hemorrhages, respectively. Laboratory evidence is based on leukocytosis,

anemia, increased sedimentation rate, and proteinuria. The complement is normal, and anti-nuclear antibodies and rheumatoid factor are absent. In infancy this disorder displays clinical[63] and pathologic[64] characteristics similar to Kawasaki disease.

Juvenile Rheumatoid Arthritis

Neurologic symptomatology, observed in a minority (6 to 10%) of patients, occurs either acutely, as convulsive encephalopathy,[65] or chronically, as meningitis.[66] In this disorder more than 50% of patients show EGG abnormalities related to ischemic lesions secondary to the vasculitic process.

The neurologic manifestation of rheumatic fever is chorea minor or Sydenham's chorea, an extrapyramidal disturbance that in about 25% of cases represents the only expression of the disease. The differential diagnosis becomes more difficult in those patients (30%) in whom there is no laboratory evidence of previous streptococcal infection. In all cases it is important to determine the level of ceruloplasmin and to search for the presence of anti-nuclear antibodies in order to rule out Wilson's disease and SLE, respectively. Long-term penicillin prophylaxis prevents cardiac complications and possible recurrences of the disease.[67]

Other Autoimmune Arteritis

Very rarely CNS arteritic manifestations have been reported, mainly in adults, during the course of other multisystemic diseases such as scleroderma. This disorder in its focal expression may also involve the CNS, giving rise to seizures, focal deficits, and recurring headaches. Neurologic symptoms, also severe, have been observed in the mixed connective tissue disease.[68]

In both Sjögren's syndrome and isolated CNS angiitis neurologic disturbances have been described only in adult series, in 25 to 60%[69] and 80% of cases,[53] respectively. The pathologic picture in the latter disorder discloses abnormalities of the small cerebral arteries responsible for focal disturbances.

Takayasu's Disease

This arteritic process of the great arteries presents mainly in patients of the second and third decades, but recent pediatric reports are not lacking.[70] While in the youngster the abdominal aorta and its major branches are affected, in young adults the stenotic process is more often localized in the aortic arch and carotid subclavian arteries ($> 50\%$), or vertebral arteries (20%). The clinical picture, nonspecific at the beginning of the disease, may then be complicated by transient ischemic attacks or, more rarely ($< 10\%$), strokes due to thromboembolism.[70] Decreased amplitude in the peripheral pulses (*pulseless disease*), and bruits and murmurs at the neck and in the supraclavicular region, can be appreciated.

The etiology is still unknown but the hypergammaglobulinemia and good response to immunosuppressive treatment suggest an autoimmune mechanism.[71] The pathologic characteristic of this disorder is a granulomatous inflammation of the media and adventitia of the large vessels with cellular infiltrates and fibrosis.[71] At angiography, segmentary restrictions and aneurysmal dilatations are seen.

Temporal Arteritis

Very rare in the young, this panarteritis spares the intracranial district. Recurrent headaches, ischemic optic neuropathy, and masseter claudication are the prominent clinical features. The biopsy of the superficial temporal artery, which appears tortuous and firm on physical examination,[72] supports the diagnosis by demonstrating mononuclear and giant cell infiltrates, inner elastic fragmentation, and intimal proliferation.

Granulomatous Arteritis

Of rare occurrence in children, this entity includes Wegener's granulomatosis, a necrotizing vasculitis of the small arteries with occasional involvement of the peripheral nervous system,[73] and Churg–Strauss allergic granulomatosis.[74] Another rare necrotizing vasculitis is the granulomatous angiitis that may give rise to neurologic manifestations, also in the young.[75] Brain disturbances, in addition, have been observed in sarcoidosis.[76]

Hypersensitivity Vasculitis

Acute necrotizing inflammation of the capillaries and small arteries with rare CNS involvement characterize these disease entities. They are mostly related to the assumption of drugs, such as sulfonamides, penicillin, salicylates, thiazides, amphetamines, and diet pills,[77] and to viral[54] or mycoplasma[78] infections. The cat-scratch disease may be accompanied by a diffuse encephalopathy and, less frequently, focal neurologic dysfunction without permanent sequelae.[79] The role of pericarotid inflammation in the vascular occlusive pathology is still controversial.[80]

Transient Embologenic Aortoarteritis

This inflammatory disorder of the aorta and cervical vessels of adolescents and young adults[81] must be differentiated from Takayasu's disease.[82] Clinically, this entity presents with repetitive embolic occlusion of intra- and extracranial vessels of the brain. Focal fragmentation of elastic lamellae in the media, edema of the intima, and mural thrombosis are seen in pathologic specimens.

Kawasaki Disease

The mucocutaneous lymph node syndrome, characterized by erythematous papular rash, hyperpyrexia, cervical adenopathy, conjunctivitis, desquamation of hands and feet, and anemia, exhibits the highest incidence in the first 2 years of life. While cardiac complications occur in more than 50%[63,64,83] of cases, neurologic disturbances are rarer[63,64,83] and related to arteritis of small and medium-sized vessels. Unlike coronary aneurysms, cerebral aneurysms have never been documented.[63] Encouraging results have been obtained by the use of high doses of intravenous gammaglobulin.[84,85]

Behçet's Disease

Very rare in children, this disorder may determine neurologic symptomatology in 10 to 30% of cases, with different pictures of meningoencephalitis or intracranial hypertension secondary to sinovenous dural thrombosis.[86,87]

Dysmetabolic Vasculopathies

Homocystinuria

This rare inborn error of methionine metabolism, recessively transmitted and due to a cystathionine synthase deficiency, causes an increase of homocystine in the blood and urine.[88] The damage, induced by homocystine on the vascular endothelium with secondary platelet activation, is accompanied by thrombotic phenomena mainly at the level of large and medium-sized vessels. Very recent papers, instead, have emphasized the role of clotting abnormalities.[89] Clinical expression is multisystemic, namely skeletal, cutaneous, and ocular. At the CNS level thromboembolic arterial and venous events determine hemiparesis, mental retardation (50%), convulsions (10 to 15%), and frequent psychiatric manifestations.[90,91] Heterozygous adults are at increased risk for premature atherosclerosis, a fact not yet demonstrated in children.[88] Treatment with pyridoxine results in reduced incidence of thromboembolic complications in about 50% of patients.[88]

Fabry's Disease

Fabry's disease, or angiokeratoma corporis diffusum, is an X-linked lysosomal disorder due to α-galactosidase A deficiency. Symptomatology begins in the first decade with burning or shooting pains due to sensory neuropathy, and typical cutaneous lesions, that is, punctate reddish-black skin eruptions localized about the hips and genitalia. Glycolipid accumulation in the endothelium and myofibers of the vessel wall results in thrombotic phenomena, while hemorrhage may occur secondary to renal dysfunction and systemic hypertension. Focal neurologic signs, convulsions, and psychosis are sustained by multifocal thrombosis of small cerebral vessels. Plasmapheresis, by decreasing the plasma levels of ceramide-triexoside, has recently been proposed in the treatment of this disease.[92]

Kinky-Hair Syndrome

This rare disorder of copper metabolism has an X-linked recessive pattern of inheritance. The metabolic defect is probably localized in the copper transport across cellular compartments.[93] Pili torti (steely or kinky hair), hypopigmentation of skin, hypothermia, major motor seizures, developmental delay, and osteoporosis are part of the multisystemic expression. Fragmentation of elastic lamina and marked intimal thickening are evident in pathologic specimens. Arterial thrombosis or aneurysmal dilatations and rupture cause cerebral degeneration or subdural effusions.[94] Angiography shows tortuosity of the vessels and precocious degenerative changes.

Hemolytic–Uremic Syndrome

In this entity, presenting with sudden onset of hemolytic anemia, thrombocytopenia, and uremia, the cardinal feature is endothelial damage with secondary hemolysis and platelet destruction. Neurologic complications occur in more than 30% of patients[95] and consist of alteration of consciousness, seizures, hemiparesis, coma, and dysregulation of breathing. Recent papers suggest that marked improvement is possible also in cases with CNS disturbances.[95,96] The pathogenesis of CNS symptoms is not clear. Three mechanisms have been postulated: (1) metabolic derangement (hyponatremia, hypocalcemia, hypoglycemia), (2) systemic hypertension, and (3) cerebral microangiopathy with thrombi.[97]

Recently we treated an 8-year-old girl affected by hemolytic-uremic syndrome presenting with abdominal pain of several weeks' duration and followed by severe status epilepticus, anuria, and cortical blindness. A CT scan performed a few weeks after coma revealed cerebral atrophy and bilateral occipital infarction (Fig. 14.5).

Treatment includes management of dyselectrolytemia and high blood pressure, and dialysis when necessary. The use of antiplatelet agents is controversial because of the possibility of a hemorrhagic infarction.[98]

MELAS Syndrome

Mitochondrial encephalopathy, lactic acidosis, and strokes (MELAS) compose a rare multisystem entity characterized also by short stature, weakness, sensory-neural hearing loss, recurrent

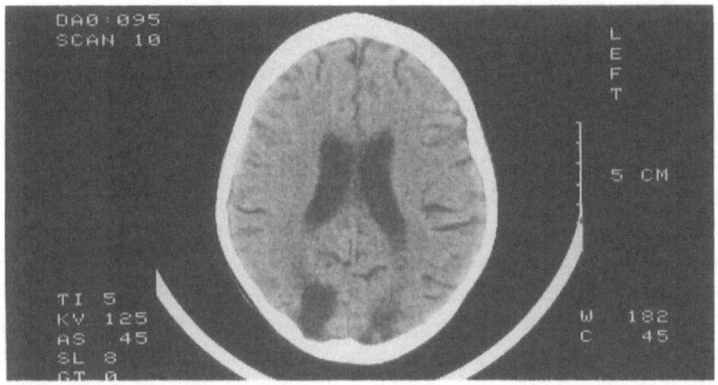

Figure 14.5. Unenhanced CT scan demonstrates cortical atrophy and ventricular enlargement associated with hypodense areas of infarction in both occipital regions (right more than left).

migraine-like attacks, seizures, and focal neurologic dysfunction.[99] Pathologically the vessels are unaffected but the clinical course may be confused with that of a vasculitis. Neuroradiologic investigations reveal focal, mainly parietooccipital, infarct-like areas and calcifications, or hypodensity in the basal ganglia.[100]

Other Vasculopathies

Malignant Atrophic Papulosis

This unusual multisystem progressive vasculopathy has recently been reported also in the pediatric age group.[101] Pathognomonic skin lesions are the early sign of this occlusive arteriopathy, which is limited to the small arteries. The pathologic substrate differs from that of collagen diseases for the very mild perivascular inflammatory component. Alternating areas of narrowing and ectasia in distal intracranial branches (*beaded appearance*) are demonstrable at angiography. The evolution is often fatal and insensitive to any treatment.

Pseudoxanthoma Elasticum

This systemic hereditary disorder is sustained by pathology of the connective tissue. Usually recognized from the skin manifestations, it rarely presents also with neurologic symptomatology due to progressive occlusion or rupture of the cerebral vessels.[102]

Fibromusculr Dysplasia

This nonatheromatous angiopathy of unknown etiology involves the small and medium-sized vessels. The renal district and the extracranial portion of the internal carotid artery are affected more frequently than the posterior cerebral arteries.[103] An intracranial vessel involvement, never observed in adult cases, has recently been documented in children.[104–106] Pathologic features consist of alternating areas of thickening (hypertrophy and fibrosis of the media and hyperplasia of the intima) and thinning of the media of the arterial wall, resulting in the typical angiographic pattern of a string of beads. Aneurysmal dilatation may be found only in adult series. Focal deficits or seizures constitute the neurologic manifestations.[107] Antiplatelet agents are the treatment of choice in children.[108]

References

1. Eyster ME, Gill FM, Blatt PM, Hilgartner MW, Ballard JO, Kinney TR: Central nervous system bleeding in hemophiliacs. Blood 51:1179–1188, 1978.

2. Humphreys RP: Computed tomography and the early diagnostic lumbar puncture,. Can Med Assoc J 121:150–151, 1979.

3. Hilgartner MW, McMillan CW: Common inherited coagulation deficiencies. In: Miller DR, Baenher RL (eds.), Blood Disease of Infancy and Childhood. C. V. Mosby, St. Louis, 1984, pp. 867–890.

4. MacKinnon HH, Fekete JF: Congenital afibrinogenemia: vascular changes and multiple thrombosis induced by fibrinogen infusions. Can Med Assoc J 140:547–551, 1971.

5. Griffin JN: Clinical studies of protein C. Semin Thromb Hemost 10:162–167, 1984.

6. Sarnaik S, Soorya D, Kim J, Ravindranath Y, Lusher J: Periodic transfusions for sickle cell anemia and CNS infarction. Am J Dis Child 133:1254–1261, 1979.

7. Russell MO, Goldberg HL: Effect of transfusion therapy on arteriographic abnormalities and on recurrence of stroke in sickle cell disease. Blood 63:162–166, 1984.

8. Powars D, Wilson B: The natural history of stroke in sickle cell disease. Am J Med 65:461–471, 1978.

9. Clark, JA, Finelli RE, Netsky MG: Disseminated intravascular coagulation following cranial trauma—case report. J Neurosurg 52:266–269, 1980.

10. Stuart MJ, Kelton JG: The platelet. In: Nathan DG, Oski F (eds.), Hematology of Infancy and Childhood. W. B. Saunders, Philadelphia, 1987, pp. 1351–1373.

11. Jabaily J, Iland HJ, Laszlo J, Massey EW, Faguet GB, Briere J, Landaw SA, Pisciotta AV: Neurologic manifestations of essential thrombocythemia. Ann Intern Med 99:513–517, 1983.

12. Thomas DJ, Du Boulay GH, Marshall J, Russell RRW, Wetherley-Mein G, Pearson TC, Symon L, Zilkha E: Cerebral blood flow in polycythemia. Lancet 2:161–163, 1977.

13. Panlilio AL, Reiss RF: Therapeutic plateletpheresis in thrombocythemia. Transfusion 19:147–152, 1979.

14. Packer RJ, Rorke LB, Lange BL, Siegel KR, Evans AE: Cerebrovascular accidents in children with cancer. Pediatrics 76:194–201, 1985.

15. Lange B, d'Angio G, Ross AJ, O'Neill JA, Packer RJ: Oncologic emergencies. In: Pizzo P, Poplack D (eds.), Pediatric Oncology. Lippincott, Philadelphia, 1989, pp. 799–812.

16. Londe S: Causes of hypertension in the young. Pediatr Clin North Am 25:55–65, 1978.

17. Loggie J, New MI, Robson A: Hypertension in the pediatric patient: a reappraisal. J Pediatr 94:685–699, 1979.

18. Harlan JL, Doty DB, Brandt B III, Ehrenhaft JL: Coarctation of the aorta in infants. J Thorac Cardiovasc Surg 88:1012–1019, 1984.

19. Shearer WT, Rutman JY, Weinberg WA, Goldring D: Coarctation of the aorta and cerebrovascular accident: a proposal for early corrective surgery. J Pediatr 77:1004–1009, 1979.

20. Roach ES, Riela AR: Intracranial aneurysm. In: Roach ES, Riela AR (eds.), Pediatric Cerebrovascular Disorders. Futura, Mount Kisko, NY, 1988, pp. 143–160.

21. Kirklin JW, Barrat-Boyes BG: Cardiac Surgery. Churchill Livingstone, Edinburgh, 1986, p. 1044.

22. Young RSK, Liberthson RR, Lalneraitis EL: Cerebral hemorrhage in neonates with coarctation of the aorta. Stroke 13:491–494, 1982.

23. Johannson B, Strandgaard S, Lassen NA: On the pathogenesis of hypertensive encephalopathy: the hypertension breakthrough of autoregulation of cerebral blood flow with forced vasodilatation, flow increase, and blood–brain-barrier damage. Circ Res 34 (Suppl 1):167–174, 1974.

24. Trompeter RS, Smith RL, Hoare RD, Neville BGR, Chantler C: Neurological complications of arterial hypertension. Arch Dis Child 57:913–917, 1982.

25. Silverstein A, Gilbert H, Wasserman RL: Neurologic complications of polycythemia. Ann Int Med 57:909–916, 1962.

26. Berlin NI: Diagnosis and classification of the polycythemias. Semin Hematol 12:339–351, 1975.

27. Grotta JC, Manner C, Pettigrew LC, Yatsu FM: Red blood cell disorders and stroke. Stroke 17:811–817, 1986.

28. Tyler RH, Clark DB: Cerebrovascular accidents in patients with congenital heart disease. Arch Neurol Psychiatry 77:483–489, 1957.

29. Pellegrino PA, Fassetta G, Scalambrin A: Neurologic complications of cyanotic congenital heart disease in children. Acta Paediatr Lat 28:204–218, 1975.

30. Phornputkul C, Rosenthal A, Nadas AS, Berenberg W: Cerebrovascular accidents in infants and children with cyanotic congenital heart disease. Am J Cardiol 32:329–334, 1973.

31. Terplan KL: Patterns of brain damage in infants and children with congenital heart disease. Am J Dis Child 125:175–185, 1973.

32. Golden GS: Strokes in children and adolescents. Stroke 9:169–171, 1978.
33. Cottrill CM, Kaplan S: Cerebral vascular accidents in cyanotic congenital heart disease. Am J Dis Child 125:484–487, 1973.
34. Tharakan J, Ahuja GK, Manchanda SC, Khanna A: Mitral valve prolapse and cerebrovascular accidents in the young. Acta Neurol Scand 66:295–302, 1982.
35. Marks MI: Pediatric Infectious Diseases for the Practitioner. Springer-Verlag, New York, 1985, pp. 632–635.
36. Tipton BK, Robertson JT, Robertson JH: Embolism to the central nervous system from cardiac myxoma. J Neurosurg 47:937–940, 1977.
37. Barson AJ, Chiswick ML, Doig CM: Fat embolism in infancy after intravenous fat infusions. Arch Dis Child 53:218–223, 1978.
38. Voorhies RM, Fraser RAR: Cerebral air embolism occurring at angiography and diagnosed by computerized tomography. J Neurosurg 60:177–178, 1984.
39. Vascik JM, Tew JM: Foreign body embolization of the middle cerebral artery: review of the literature and guidelines for management. Neurosurgery 11:532–536, 1982.
40. Pellegrino PA: Infective endocarditis in children (abstract). 6th Annual Meeting of the European Society for Paediatric Infectious Diseases. Padua, 27–29 April, 1988, p. 4.
41. Braunwald E: Valvular heart disease. In: Braunwald E (ed.), Heart Disease. A Textbook of Cardiovascular Medicine, Vol. 2. W. B. Saunders, Philadelphia, 1984, pp. 1089–1095.
42. Del Torso S, De Martin PG, Marcadella M, Milanesi O, Pellegrino PA, Battistella PA: Ischemic cerebral stroke: clinical assessment and echocardiographic diagnosis in a case of atrial myxoma. Ital J Pediatr 13:93–96, 1987.
43. Sisel RJ, Parker BM, Bahl OP: Cerebral symptoms in pulmonary arteriovenous fistula. A result of paradoxical emboli? Circulation 41:123–128, 1970.
44. Reilly PJ, Nostrant TT: Clinical manifestations of hereditary hemorrhagic telangiectasia. Am J Gastroenterol 79:363–367, 1984.
45. Weisz GM, Schramek A, Abrahanson J, Barzilai A: Fat embolism in children: tests for its early detection. J Pediatr Surg 9:163–167, 1974.
46. Yamaguchi T, Minematsu K, Choki J-I, Ikeda M: Clinical and neuroradiological analysis of thrombotic and embolic cerebral infarction. Jap Circ J 48:50–58, 1984.
47. Daniels SR, Bates S, Lukin RR, Benton C, Third J, Glueck CJ: Cerebrovascular arteriopathy (arteriosclerosis) and ischemic childhood stroke. Stroke 13:360–365, 1982.
48. Rosenthal IM, Bronstein IP, Dallenbach FD, Pruzansky S, Rosenwald AK: Progeria. Pediatr 18:565–577, 1956.
49. Velican C, Velican D: Atherosclerosis involvement of human intracranial arteries with special reference to intimal necrosis. Atherosclerosis 43:59–69, 1982.
50. Janaki S, Baruah JK, Jayaram SR, Saxena VK, Sharma SR, Gulati MS: Stroke in the young: a four-year study. Stroke 6:318–320, 1975.
51. Glueck CJ, Daniels SR, Bates S, Benton C, Tracy T, Third JLHC: Pediatric victims of unexplained stroke and their families: familial lipid and lipoprotein abnormalities. Pediatrics 69:308–316, 1982.
52. Tauber JP, Cheng J, Gospodarowicz D: Effect of high and low density lipoproteins on proliferation of cultured bovine vascular endothelial cells. J Clin Invest 66:696–708, 1980.
53. Moore PM, Cupps TR: Neurological complications of vasculitis. Ann Neurol 14:155–167, 1983.
54. Taft TA, Chusid MJ, Sty JR: Cerebral infarction in *Hemophilus influenzae* type B meningitis. Clin Pediatr 25:177–180, 1986.
55. Ment LR, Ehrenkranz RA, Duncan CC: Bacterial meningitis as an etiology of perinatal cerebral infarction. Pediatr Neurol 2:276–280, 1986.
56. Kaell AT, Shetty M, Lee BCP, Lockshin MD: The diversity of neurologic events in systemic lupus erythematosus. Prospective clinical and computed tomographic classification of 82 events in 71 patients. Arch Neurol 43:273–276, 1986.
57. Yancey CL, Doughty RA, Athreya BH: Central nervous system involvement in childhood SLE. Arth Rheum 24:1389–1395, 1981.
58. Silber TJ, Chatoor I, White PH: Psychiatric manifestations of systemic lupus erythematosus in children and adolescents. Clin Pediatr 23:331–335, 1984.
59. Aisen AM, Gabrielsen TO, McCune WJ: MR imaging of systemic lupus erythematosus involving the brain. AJR 144:1027–1031, 1985.
60. Kelley RE, Berger JR: Ischemic stroke in a girl with lupus anticoagulant. Pediatr Neurol 3:58–61, 1987.
61. Huges GRV, Harris NN, Ghavari AE: The anticardiolipin syndrome. J Rheumatol 13:486–489, 1986.

62. Levine SR, Welch KMA: The spectrum of neurological diseases associated with antiphospholipid antibodies. Arch Neurol 44:876–883, 1987.

63. Laxer RM, Dunn HG, Flodmark O: Acute hemiplegia in Kawasaki disease and infantile poliarteritis nodosa. Dev Med Child Neurol 26:814–821, 1984.

64. Lapointe JS, Nugent RA, Graeb DA, Robertson WD: Cerebral infarction and regression of widespread aneurysms in Kawasaki's disease: case report. Pediatr Radiol 14:1–5, 1984.

65. Hadchouel M, Prieur A, Griscelli C: Acute hemorrhagic, hepatic and neurologic manifestations in juvenile rheumatoid arthritis. Possible relationship to drugs or infection. J Pediatr 106:561–566, 1985.

66. Yarom A, Rennebohm RM, Levinson JE: Infantile multisystem inflammatory disease. A specific syndrome? J Pediatr 106:390–396, 1985.

67. Berrios X, Quensney F, Morales A, Blazquez J, Bisno AL: Are all recurrences of "pure" Sydenham chorea true recurrences of acute rheumatic fever? J Pediatr 107:867–872, 1985.

68. Oetgen WJ, Boice JA, Lawless OJ: Mixed connective tissue disease in children and adolescents. Pediatrics 67:333–337, 1981.

69. Molina R, Provost TT, Alexander EL: Peripheral inflammatory vascular disease in Sjogren's syndrome, association with nervous system complications. Arth Rheum 28:1341–1347, 1985.

70. Kohrman MH, Huttenlocher PR: Takayasu arteritis: a treatable cause of stroke in infancy. Pediatr Neurol 2:154–159, 1986.

71. Hall S, Barr W, Lie JT, Stanson AW, Kazmier FJ, Hunder GG: Takayasu arteritis. A study of 32 North American patients. Medicine 64:89–99, 1985.

72. Small P: Giant cell arteritis presenting as a bilateral stroke. Arth Rheum 27:819–821, 1984.

73. Orlowski JP, Clough JD, Dyment PG: Wegener's granulomatosis in the pediatric age group. Pediatrics 61:83–90, 1978.

74. Hanson V: Systemic lupus erythematosus, dermatomyositis, scleroderma and vasculitides in childhood. In: Kelley WN, Harris ED Jr, Ruddy S, Sledge CB (eds.), Textbook of Rheumatology. W. B. Saunders, Philadelphia, 1985, pp. 1327–1348.

75. Sabharwal UK, Keogh LH, Weisman MH, Svaifler NJ: Granulomatous angiitis of the nervous system: case report and review of the literature. Arth Rheum 25:342–345, 1982.

76. Pattishall EN, Strope GL, Spinola SM, Denny FW: Childhood sarcoidosis. J Pediatr 108:169–177, 1986.

77. Forman HP, Levin S, Stewart B, Patel M, Feinstein S: Cerebral vasculitis and hemorrhage in an adolescent taking diet pills containing phenylpropanolamine: case report and review of literature. Pediatrics 83:737–741, 1989.

78. Maytal J, Resnick TJ: A TIA-like syndrome associated with *Mycoplasma pneumoniae* infection. Pediatr Neurol 1:308–311, 1985.

79. Lewis DW, Tucker SH: Central nervous system involvement in cat-scratch disease. Pediatrics 77:714–721, 1986.

80. Isler W: Stroke in childhood and adolescence. Eur Neurol 23:421–424, 1984.

81. Guerra RR, Hernandez-Batres F: Transient embolic aorto-arteritis: presentation of a patient. Stroke 12:869–873, 1981.

82. Wickremasinghe HR, Peiris JB, Thenabadu PN, Sheriffdeen AH: Transient emboligenic aortoarteritis. Noteworthy new entity in young stroke patients. Arch Neurol 35:416–422, 1978.

83. Terasawa K, Ichinose E, Matsuishi T, Kato H: Neurologic complications in Kawasaki disease. Brain Dev 5:371–374, 1983.

84. Newburger JW, Takahashi M, Burns JC, Beiser AS, Chung KJ, Duffy CE, Glode MP, Mason WH, Reddy V, Sanders SP: The treatment of Kawasaki syndrome with intravenous gamma globulin. N Engl J Med 315:341–347, 1986.

85. American Academy of Pediatrics. Committee on Infectious Diseases. Intravenous γ-globulin use in children with Kawasaki disease. Pediatrics 82:122, 1988.

86. Davis LE, Hodgin UG, Kornfeld M: Recurrent meningoencephalitis recovery from Behcet's disease. Western J Med 145:238–239, 1986.

87. Rakover Y, Adar H, Tal I, Lang Y, Kedar A: Behcet disease: long-term follow up of three children and review of the literature. Pediatrics 83:986–992, 1989.

88. Mudd SH, Skovby F, Levy HL, Pettigrew KD, Wilcken B, Pyeritz RE, Andria G, Boers GH, Bromberg IL, Cerone R: The natural history of homocystinuria due to cystationine beta-synthase deficiency. Am J Hum Genet 37:1–31, 1985.

89. Palareti G, Salardi S, Piazzi S, Legnani C, Poggi M, Grauso F, Caniato A, Coccheri S, Cacciari E: Blood coagulation changes in homocystinuria: effects of pyridoxine and other specific therapy. J Pediatr 109:1001–1006, 1986.

90. Abbott MH, Folstein SE, Abbey H, Pyeritz RE:

Psychiatric manifestations of homocystinuria due to cystathionine beta-synthase deficiency: prevalence, natural history and relationship to neurologic impairment and vitamin B_6-responsiveness. Am J Med Genet 26:959–969, 1987.

91. Schwab FJ, Peyster RG, Brill CB: CT of cerebral venous sinus thrombosis in a child with homocystinuria. Pediatr Radiol 17:244–245, 1987.

92. Dau PC: Plasmapheresis—therapeutic or experimental procedure. Arch Neurol 41:647–653, 1984.

93. Menkes JH: Kinky hair disease: twenty-five years later. Brain Dev 10:77–79, 1988.

94. Danks DM: Hereditary disorders of copper metabolism in Wilson's disease and Menkes' disease. In: Stanbury JB, Wyncaarden JB, Frederickson DS, Goldstein JL, Brown MS (eds.), The Metabolic Basis of Inherited Disease. McGraw-Hill, New York, 1983, pp. 1261–1268.

95. Sheth KJ, Swick HM, Haworth N: Neurological involvement in hemolytic-uremic syndrome. Ann Neurol 19:90–93, 1986.

96. Steele BT, Murphy N, Chuang SH, McGreal D, Arbus GS: Recovery from prolonged coma in hemolytic uremic syndrome. J Pediatr 102:402–404, 1983.

97. Steinberg A, Ish-Horowitcz M, El Peleg O, Mor J, Branski D: Stroke in a patient with hemolytic-uremic syndrome with a good outcome. Brain Dev 8:70–72, 1986.

98. Crisp DE, Siegler RI, Bale JF, Thompson JA: Hemorrhagic cerebral infarction in the hemolytic-uremic syndrome. J Pediatr 99:273–276, 1981.

99. Pavlakis SG, Philips PC, Di Mauro S, De Vivo DC, Rowland LP: Mitochondrial myopathy, encephalopathy, lactic acidosis and stroke like episodes (MELAS): a distinctive clinical syndrome. Ann Neurol 16:481–488, 1984.

100. Allard JC, Tilak S, Carter AP: CT and MR of MELAS syndrome. AJNR 9:1234–1238, 1988.

101. Sotrel A, Lacson AG, Huff KR: Childhood Kohlmei-Degos' disease with typical skin lesions. Neurology 33:1146–1151, 1983.

102. Iqbal A, Alter M, Lee SH: *Pseudoxanthoma elasticum*: a review of neurological complications. Ann Neurol 4:18–20, 1978.

103. Frens DB, Petajan JH, Anderson R, Deblanc HJ: Fibromuscular dysplasia of the posterior cerebral artery: report of a case and review of the literature. Stroke 5:161–166, 1974.

104. Sheilds WD, Ziter FA, Osborn AG, Allen J: Fibromuscular dysplasia as cause of stroke in infancy and childhood. Pediatrics 59:899–901, 1977.

105. Lemathieu SF, Marchau MM: Intracranial fibromuscular dysplasia and stroke in children. Neuroradiology 18:99–102, 1979.

106. Emparanza JI, Aldamiz-Echevarria L, Perez-Yarza E: Ischemic stroke due to fibromuscular dysplasia. Neuropediatrics 20:181–182, 1989.

107. Abdul-Rahman AM, Abu-Salih HS, Brun A, Kin H, Ljunggren B, Mizukami M, Moquist-Olsson I, Sahlin CH, Svendgaard NA, Thulin CA: Fibromuscular dysplasia of the cervicocephalic arteries. Surg Neurol 9:217–222, 1978.

108. Wesen CA, Elliott BM: Fibromuscular dysplasia of the carotid arteries. Am J Surg 151:448–451, 1986.

CHAPTER 15

Ischemic and Hemorrhagic Lesions of the Newborn

Alan Hill and Joseph J. Volpe

Hypoxic–ischemic and hemorrhagic cerebral injury in the newborn are a major cause of morbidity and mortality in the neonatal period as well as major determinants of neurological handicap observed in older infants and children, for example, cerebral palsy, mental retardation, and seizures. The overall extent and distribution of hypoxic–ischemic and hemorrhagic cerebral injury are determined by the severity and duration of the insult, and by the degree of maturation of the newborn brain at the time of the insult. Thus, the patterns of cerebral injury observed in the premature newborn often differ significantly from those observed in the term newborn.

In this chapter, we will discuss the major pathogenic mechanisms and patterns of hypoxic–ischemic and hemorrhagic cerebral injury in the newborn. Although hypoxic–ischemic and hemorrhagic injury will be discussed separately, they frequently occur together and the close relationship between the two cannot be overemphasized.

Hypoxic–Ischemic Cerebral Injury

Pathogenesis

Hypoxic–ischemic cerebral injury occurs as a consequence of inadequate delivery of oxygen to cerebral tissue, secondary usually to a combination of hypoxemia and ischemia. Although the two forms of insult invariably occur together with one or the other predominating, it is convenient to discuss them separately.

In the newborn infant, disturbances of respiratory function, cardiac function, and sepsis often play a major role in the pathogenesis of cerebral hypoxic–ischemic injury (Tables 15.1 and 15.2). The effects of these disturbances of respiratory and cardiac function on overall cardiopulmonary function and on systemic blood pressure are particularly detrimental because of the dysfunctional cerebrovascular autoregulation in the sick newborn (especially the premature newborn). The cerebral metabolic derangements that result from the combination of hypoxemia and ischemia lead to disturbed cell function and, if the insult is severe enough, to irreversible cellular injury.

Nature and Timing of Cerebral Insult

Approximately 90% of hypoxic–ischemic cerebral injury manifested in the neonatal period is sustained during the antepartum and intrapartum periods.[1] However, recent studies suggest that the importance of intrapartum asphyxia as a sole direct cause of cerebral palsy may have been overemphasized in the past. In fact, a significant proportion of asphyxiated infants have evidence of developmental anomalies, which raises the possibility that a prior insult, sustained much earlier in gestation, may have predisposed to further hypoxic–ischemic injury at the time of delivery.[2,3] However, there exists a substantial group of term newborns who sustain significant antepartum/intrapartum hypoxic–ischemic cerebral injury that is manifested by an acute clinical encephalopathy during the first few days of life.[1] Moreover, there is experimental evidence in primates that intrapartum asphyxia alone can injure the brain and that the nature of the insult may influence

Table 15.1. Major causes of cerebral hypoxemia.

Major mechanism	Example	Principal age group affected
Intrauterine asphyxia	Placental insufficiency	Premature and term
Postnatal respiratory insufficiency	Meconium aspiration	Term
	Recurrent apnea	Premature and term
	Hyaline membrane disease	Premature
Severe right-to-left shunts	Persistent fetal circulation	Term
	Patent ductus arteriosus	Premature

Table 15.2. Major causes of cerebral ischemia.

Major mechanism	Example	Principal age group affected
Intrauterine asphyxia	Placental insufficiency	Premature and term
Postnatal cardiac insufficiency	Congenital heart disease	Term
	Acquired cardiac problems, transient myocardial ischemia	Term
	Patent ductus arteriosus	Premature
Postnatal hypotension	Sepsis	Premature and term

the topography of injury, for example, acute, total asphyxia will affect principally brainstem structures, whereas prolonged, partial asphyxia results in diffuse cortical injury.[4]

Arterial Blood Supply

The circulatory response to significant perinatal asphyxia involves redistribution of cardiac output such that there is an initial increase in blood flow to vital organs, including the brain.[1] However, subsequently, systemic hypotension may supervene and result in decreased cerebral perfusion.

The stage of maturation of the cerebral arterial architecture at the time of the insult is an important determinant of the topography of injury. Thus, in the term newborn, diminished cerebral blood flow affects predominantly cerebral cortex, either diffusely, in instances of severe cerebral hypoperfusion, or in the parasagittal watershed zones between anterior, middle, and posterior cerebral arteries in instances where there is less severe cerebral hypoperfusion. In contrast, in the premature newborn, the parasagittal cerebral cortex is relatively resistant to hypoxic–ischemic insult, due to persistence of anastomoses between

meningeal arteries.[1,5] The principal watershed zone in the premature infant is located in the periventricular white matter, between subependymal vessels and penetrating branches of anterior, middle, and posterior cerebral arteries. Consequently, with mild ischemic insult, the major injury occurs in the periventricular white matter, although with increasing severity of insult, cortex may be included also.

Occlusion of individual cerebral vessels results in focal cerebral infarction within the territory of perfusion of the involved vessel. In the term newborn, the middle cerebral artery is involved in more than 50% of cases.[1] Focal injury occurs much less commonly in the premature newborn and is often multifocal as a result of occlusion of numerous small vessels.[1]

Significance of Impaired Cerebrovascular Autoregulation

Cerebrovascular autoregulation is the mechanism of arteriolar vasoconstriction and vasodilation that maintains relatively constant cerebral perfusion over a wide range of systemic arterial blood pressures. There is increasing experimental evidence to suggest that even mild degrees of hypoxic–ischemic insult may impair this mechanism and result in a "pressure-passive" relationship between systemic blood pressure and cerebral blood flow.[6] Clearly, this occurrence has major implications concerning hypoxic–ischemic cerebral injury in the sick newborn infant in whom systemic hypotension occurs commonly.

Significance of Increased Intracranial Pressure

In contrast to the brain of older children and adults, the newborn brain is relatively resistant to cerebral edema following hypoxic–ischemic insult. In fact, increased intracranial pressure (ICP) appears to occur only *following* severe hypoxic–ischemic cerebral insult in term newborns and has not been documented convincingly at any time in the preterm infant, that is, in the absence of severe periventricular–intraventricular hemorrhage (PVH–IVH) and/or hydrocephalus. Furthermore, following severe hypoxic–ischemic insult, increased ICP most probably is a consequence of extensive prior tissue necrosis.[7,8] Thus, in a recent study of 32 asphyxiated term newborns, increased ICP (> 10 mmHg) occurred in only 7 severely asphyxiated infants, 3 of whom died and 4 of whom developed severe neurological sequelae (e.g., microcephaly and spastic quadriplegia). The ICP was maximum between 2 and 3 days of age, which corresponds to the time when decreased tissue attenuation on computed tomography (CT) scans of the head was maximal. Autopsy studies of the three infants who died demonstrated extensive cerebral necrosis. Similar observations have been reported in asphyxiated newborns studied by direct ICP measurements with a subarachnoid bolt.[9] Consideration of autopsy data and the temporal profile of elevated ICP suggest that prior cerebral necrosis is the most probable cause of brain swelling, and that the use of antiedema medications in this context, for example, mannitol and dexamethasone, may reduce ICP but is unlikely to improve outcome.

Diagnosis

The diagnosis of hypoxic–ischemic encephalopathy is based on an accurate obstetric and neonatal history and on detailed serial neuro-

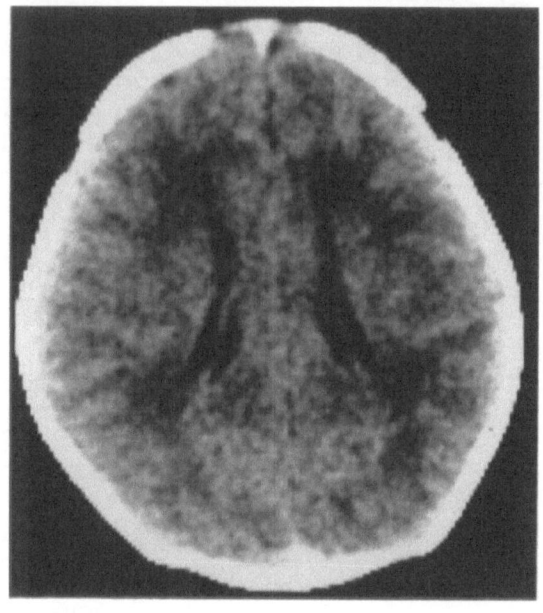

A

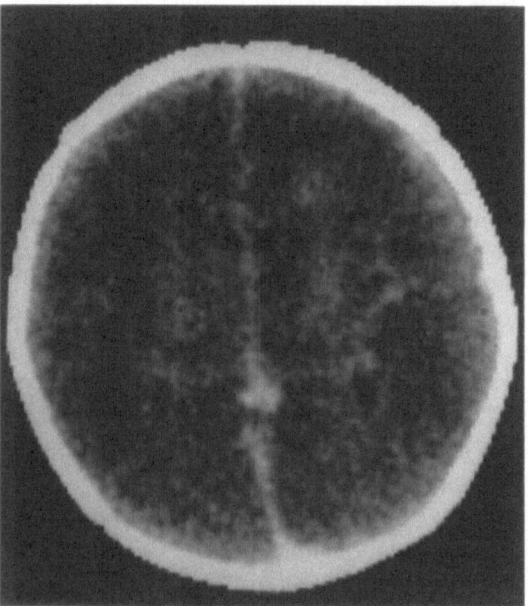

B

Figure 15.1. (A) CT scan in axial plane of normal term newborn. Note relative attenuations of gray and white matter. **(B)** CT scan of term newborn with severe hypoxic–ischemic encephalopathy. Note diffuse decrease in attenuation with almost complete loss of differentiation between gray and white matter.

logical examinations in the newborn period. In addition, diagnosis may be supported by a variety of investigations, for example, fetal blood sampling, electroencephalography (EEG), and CT and ultrasound scanning of the head. The severity of hypoxic–ischemic encephalopathy, classified usually as mild, moderate, or severe,[1,10] correlates well with neurological outcome.

The choice of adjunctive investigations varies according to the gestational age of the infant. Thus, cranial ultrasonography is the technique of choice in the premature newborn for diagnosis of intraventricular hemorrhage (IVH) and in periventricular parenchymal injury, for example, periventricular leukomalacia (PVL). In the latter instance, ultrasonography may demonstrate increased periventricular echoes during the first few days of life, followed by cyst formation in these regions during subsequent weeks.[1,11,12] The cysts may disappear over the ensuing months when only ventricular enlargement remains to mark the site of white matter loss. Limitations of this technique relate to difficulties in its ability to identify mild injury and to distinguish between hemorrhagic and ischemic injury.[12,13] CT is the technique of choice for assessment of hypoxic–ischemic injury in the term newborn. Thus, diffusely decreased attenuation of cerebral tissue observed on CT scans performed 2 to 4 days following insult correlates closely with poor outcome[8] (Fig. 15.1). Computed tomography is of less value for assessment of the premature newborn, due to the normally high water content of the premature brain and poor differentiation between white and gray matter.[14] Magnetic resonance imaging (MRI) is associated with practical difficulties during the stage of acute encephalopathy in the newborn, for example, prolonged scanning time, inability to use ferromagnetic life-support equipment. However, MRI is of value for the diagnosis of PVL in older children with spastic diplegia.[15,16]

In addition to the aforementioned radiologic techniques, the evolution of cerebral injury may be assessed with EEG[10,17] and measurement of brainstem auditory-evoked responses (BAER).[18]

Neuropathology and Clinicopathological Correlations

The clinical features of hypoxic–ischemic encephalopathy in the newborn are determined principally by the severity and extent of the cerebral injury. Recent use of cerebral imaging techniques, for example, ultrasound, CT, and MRI, allows definition of the topography of the lesions. Although the clinical presentations in the newborn period of the various patterns of cerebral injury may be similar, accurate localization of the topography of the injury permits better prediction of specific long-term neurological sequelae. Because the specific neuropathological patterns are determined to such a large extent by the stage of maturation of the immature brain at the time of insult, we will summarize separately clinicopathological correlations in term and premature newborns (Tables 15.3 and 15.4).

Table 15.3. Major neuropathological patterns of hypoxic–ischemic cerebral injury in the premature newborn.

Pattern of injury	Anatomic location	Long-term outcome
Selective neuronal necrosis	Diencephalon, brainstem, cerebral cortex	Spastic quadriplegia, cranial nerve dysfunction, ?attention deficit
Periventricular leukomalacia	Periventricular white matter (usually bilateral)	Spastic diplegia/quadriplegia, visual impairment (intellectual deficits)
Focal/multifocal cerebral necrosis	Cerebral cortex and subcortical white matter in a vascular distribution	Hemiparesis, focal seizures
Periventricular hemorrhagic lesions	Periventircular white matter (unilateral)	Hemiplegia, quadriplegia, intellectual deficits

Table 15.4. Major neuropathological patterns of hypoxic–ischemic cerebral injury in the term newborn .

Pattern of injury	Anatomic location	Long-term outcome
Diffuse/selective neuronal necrosis	Cerebral cortex, thalamus, cerebellum, brainstem, spinal cord	Intellectual deficits, seizures, spastic quadriplegia, brainstem dysfunction
Parasagittal cerebral injury	Parasagittal cortex and subcortical white matter	Spastic quadriplegia, intellectual deficits
Status marmoratus of basal ganglia	Basal ganglia, thalamus	Choreoathetosis, mental retardation
Focal/multifocal cerebral necrosis	Cerebral cortex/subcortical white matter in a vascular distribution	Hemiparesis, focal seizures

Diffuse Hypoxic-Ischemic Cerebral Injury

Diffuse hypoxic–ischemic cerebral injury occurs as a consequence of diminished cerebral perfusion. Clearly the severity of the neonatal clinical signs relates to the severity of insult. There is depression in the level of consciousness, which relates presumably to dysfunction of cerebral hemispheres and/or brainstem. Seizures may result from cortical injury. Disturbances of muscle tone and power may be a consequence of injury at many levels of the neural axis, for example, cerebral cortex, brainstem, spinal cord. Disturbed sucking or swallowing, poor facial movement, and tongue fasciculations may reflect injury to neurons of lower cranial nerves in the brainstem.

In instances where hypoxic–ischemic injury has been especially severe, there may be clinically recognizable brain swelling (e.g., bulging anterior fontanelle or suture separation). These clinical observations imply a bad prognosis, because they reflect cerebral edema, most probably secondary to tissue necrosis. The long-term outcome of such infants is poor. A CT scan of such an infant is illustrated in Figure 15.2. In the premature infant, injury to cerebral cortex is more difficult to recognize, perhaps because of the relative immaturity of the developing cortex.

Parasagittal Cerebral Injury

In the term newborn, the parasagittal region of the cerebral cortex and subcortical white matter is located at a watershed of arterial supply of the anterior, middle, and posterior cerebral arteries. This situation renders this region especially vulnerable to decreases in cerebral perfusion. Consequently, cerebral hypoperfusion that is insufficient to cause diffuse neuronal necrosis may produce more localized injury to the parasagittal region.

In the newborn period, such injury may manifest as weakness and hypotonia of the proximal extremities, with greater involvement

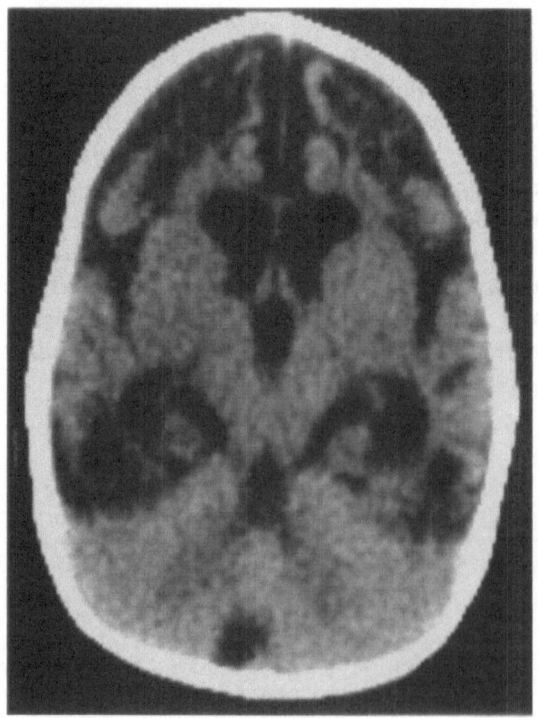

Figure 15.2. CT scan in axial plane at 10 months of age of an infant who was born at term with severe hypoxic–ischemic encephalopathy. Note marked atrophy.

of upper than lower limbs. The long-term clinical correlate of parasagittal injury is spastic quadriplegia. Intellectual deficits in this group of children may relate to injury to visual and auditory association areas in the watershed zones. The extent and location of this lesion has been demonstrated by technetium and occasionally CT scans in the newborn period.[19,20] More recently, positron emission tomography has demonstrated decreased cerebral blood flow to the affected parasagittal regions.[21]

Status Marmoratus of the Basal Ganglia and Thalamus

This uncommon type of neonatal brain injury occurs in the term newborn and is characterized by necrosis of the neurons of basal ganglia and thalamus. Histologically, there is hypermyelination in the injured structures and this does not become apparent until one or more years following the injury. The characteristic neuropathological appearance, that of marbled basal ganglia, gives the entity its name.

The clinical correlate in the newborn period is not known. However, the long-term clinical correlates include, particularly, movement disorders (e.g., tremor, dystonia, choreoathetosis) and, less commonly, intellectual impairment secondary to concomitant injury to thalamus and/or cerebral cortex.

Periventricular Leukomalacia

Periventricular leukomalacia occurs most commonly in infants born prematurely and involves necrosis of cerebral white matter, dorsal and lateral to the external angles of the lateral ventricles. The most common sites are the region of the optic radiations at the trigone of the lateral ventricles and the frontal white matter near the foramen of Monro. The vulnerability of these regions relates to their location in the watershed zones between major cerebral arteries in periventricular white matter. The prevalence of PVL in autopsies of infants born prematurely increases as a function of the duration of postnatal survival and the frequency and severity of cardiorespiratory disturbances. Secondary hemorrhage may occur in areas of PVL. This form of hemorrhage may coexist with IVH,

another common cerebral lesion of the premature newborn (see later discussion).

The clinical correlate of PVL in the newborn period has not been defined in detail because of difficulties in the identification of more subtle abnormalities of tone and power in very sick premature infants. However, there are infants in whom decreased power in the lower extremities may be recognized. Diagnosis of PVL in the newborn period is possible with ultrasonography, which, on coronal projections, may demonstrate increased echodensities adjacent to the external angles of the lateral ventricles and, on parasagittal projections, in the region of the trigone. Subsequent serial ultrasound scans, after approximately 2 or 3 weeks, may reveal small cystic lesions in the areas occupied previously by the increased echodensities. Subsequently these small cysts may not be visualized on ultrasound scans. Imaging with CT and MRI permits recognition of PVL in later infancy and childhood. Thus, CT scans at several months of age reveal a characteristic pattern of diminished periventricular white matter, an irregular outline of the lateral ventricles, and deep and prominent sulci reaching the ventricular surface (Fig. 15.3). Similar lesions are observed on MRI.

The long-term correlate of PVL is spastic diplegia, a form of quadriplegia in which lower extremities are affected more than upper extremities. In severe cases, cortical visual impairment is often associated. It should be realized that following severe hypoxic–ischemic cerebral insult in the premature newborn, PVL may represent only part of more diffuse hypoxic–ischemic brain injury.[1] The long-term clinical correlate therefore may also include cognitive abnormalities and seizures.

Focal or Multifocal Ischemic Cerebral Injury

Focal or multifocal ischemic cerebral injury may result from venous or arterial occlusion. Large infarcts tend to occur more commonly in the term newborn, whereas multiple small infarcts tend to occur in the premature newborn. Large lesions have a propensity to become cystic and, on occasion, communicate with the lateral ventricles. The most common cause of focal

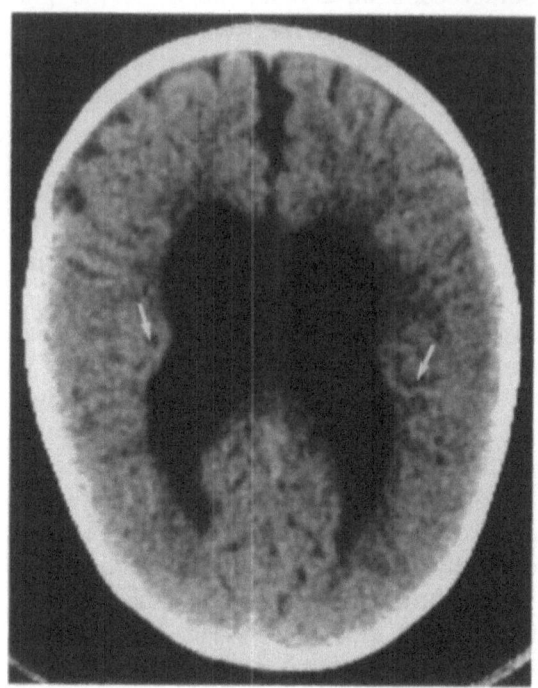

Figure 15.3. CT scan in axial plan demonstrates decreased periventricular white matter, prominent deep sulci (arrows), and irregular contour of lateral ventricles.

cerebral injury in the newborn is considered to be thromboembolism, secondary to disseminated intravascular coagulation, placental infarction, polycythemia, involuting fetal vessels, or punctured or catheterized vessels. In addition, focal lesions may occur often inexplicably, as part of a diffuse cerebral insult. In a large number of term infants with focal cerebral infarction there is no history of trauma, asphyxia, or other adverse occurrence. During the neonatal period, the clinical correlates consist of decreased tone or weakness (recognized often as decreased movement and power) of one side of the body and/or focal seizures. The long-term prognosis often includes hemiparesis. The focal ischemic lesions may be recognized occasionally with ultrasound scanning but are diagnosed more accurately by CT.

Management of Hypoxic–Ischemic Lesions

The management of hypoxic–ischemic encephalopathy has been discussed in detail

elsewhere.[1] Because of the propensity for uncontrolled seizures and the possibility that such seizures may cause additional brain injury, either through compromise of cardiorespiratory function, depletion of the high-energy stores of the brain, or accumulation of excitotoxic amino acids, vigorous treatment with anticonvulsant medications is essential. In term infants who have clinically recognizable brain swelling, there is controversy regarding management. At the present time, there are no controlled studies that demonstrate a beneficial effect of the use of drugs to reduce brain swelling.

Hemorrhagic Cerebral Injury

The types of intracranial hemorrhage that occur in the newborn are similar to those that occur in older patients. Most of the major varieties of hemorrhagic cerebral injury can occur in relation to craniocerebral trauma, for example, epidural, subdural, subarachnoid, intracerebellar, and intracerebral hemorrhage. With improvements in obstetric management, these types of hemorrhage are observed only uncommonly and are discussed in detail elsewhere.[1] Because of the recent improved survival of very premature newborns, periventricular–intraventricular hemorrhage (PVH–IVH) is the most common type of intracranial hemorrhage encountered in the newborn and will be discussed in greater detail below.

Periventricular–Intraventricular Hemorrhage

Pathogenesis

PVH–IVH originates most commonly during the first 3 days of life from rupture of fragile capillaries within the subependymal germinal matrix.[1,22,23] This structure, which serves as the major source of neuronal glial precursors, is located, in the third trimester, in the subventricular zone, primarily in the region of the head of the caudate nucleus, and usually gradually resolves by term. Hence, PVH–IVH occurs uncommonly in the term newborn in whom the causes are more diverse, for example, residual germinal matrix, choroid plexus, vascular malformation, or tumor.[1] In more than 80% of cases, hemorrhage spreads subsequently throughout the ventricular and subarachnoid spaces. Hemorrhagic infarction of periventricular cerebral parenchyma and subsequent formation of a porencephalic cyst may accompany severe IVH[13]

Numerous intravascular, vascular, and extravascular factors have been identified in the pathogenesis of PVH–IVH.[1,19,20] Because of the immaturity of cerebrovascular autoregulation in the premature brain (discussed previously), exposure of the fragile capillaries of the germinal matrix to fluctuations of cerebral arterial and/or venous pressures may result in rupture of these vessels and consequent hemorrhage. The propensity to rupture may be enhanced by prior hypoxic–ischemic injury to the endothelial lining of vessels. Approximately 15% of infants with PVH–IVH exhibit unilateral hemorrhagic necrosis in the periventricular white matter. Recent studies have demonstrated that such parenchymal hemorrhage represents venous infarction, rather than "extension" of IVH, and that this lesion appears to be distinct neuropathologically from hemorrhagic PVL (discussed earlier).[22,23]

Clinical Features

There is a wide spectrum of clinical presentation of PVH–IVH, ranging from absence of detectable abnormalities to a catastrophic neurological deterioration with major systemic abnormalities, including rapid fall in hematocrit, hypotension, bulging fontanelle, and acidosis, as well as such neurological abnormalities as coma, decerebrate posturing, and cranial nerve deficits. Clearly, the severity of clinical abnormalities relates to the extent of hemorrhage and to concomitant hypoxic–ischemic cerebral injury. Not more than approximately 50% of premature newborns with PVH–IVH may be identified on the basis of clinical abnormalities alone.[1,23]

Diagnosis

Accurate diagnosis depends particularly on the use of imaging techniques, principally cranial

ultrasonography[1,23,24] (Fig. 15.4). Although CT and MRI are similarly effective for demonstration of PVH–IVH, their clinical application is limited by practical problems, for example, exposure to ionizing radiation, lack of portability of equipment, and long scanning times.[23] Several schemes for classification of severity of PVH–IVH have been developed based on the quantity of blood in the ventricles and the presence of parenchymal involvement. The optimal timing of scanning is around 3 days of age when 90% of PVH–IVH can be detected. Repeat scanning at the end of the first week of life is necessary to detect maximal extent of lesions.[1,23] Subsequently, further scans may be performed periodically to detect complications, such as periventricular hemorrhagic infarction and posthemorrhagic hydrocephalus.

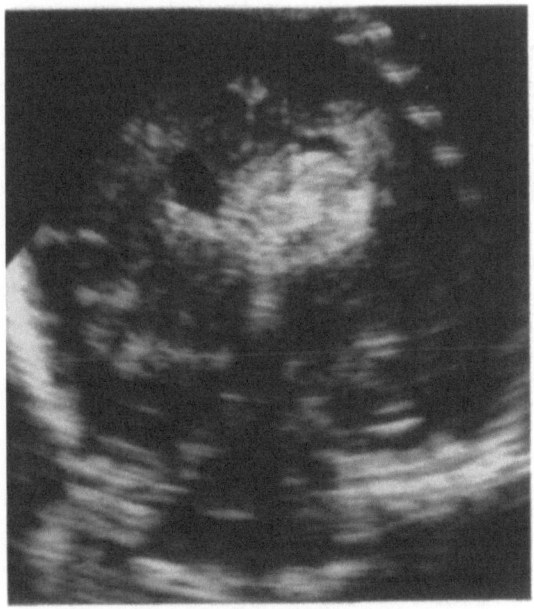

Figure 15.4. Ultrasound scan of head in coronal plane of infant born at 28 weeks of gestation. Note large intraventricular hemorrhage on left and subependymal germina matrix hemorrhage on right. Note also increased echoes in periventricular white matter at angle of anterior horn of left lateral ventricle. These increased echoes in periventricular region most probably represent hemorrhagic infarction.

Prevention and Management of Periventricular–Intraventricular Hemorrhage

Rational management strategies for PVH–IVH must be based on pathogenic factors.[23,24] Clearly, the best method for prevention of IVH would be to prevent premature delivery. If premature delivery is inevitable, optimal management of labor and delivery should be ensured by transportation of the infant in utero to a high-risk perinatal center. Several prenatal pharmacologic interventions, for example, phenobarbital and vitamin K, are currently under investigation for prevention of PVH–IVH. Antenatal steroids to reduce the severity of respiratory distress syndrome may indirectly influence the likelihood of PVH–IVH. Several postnatal interventions have been studied, for example, prevention of fluctuating cerebral blood flow velocity by muscle paralysis of the ventilated preterm infant, prevention of other hemodynamic disturbances, correction of coagulation abnormalities, and the use of medications, including phenobarbital, indomethacin, ethamsylate, and vitamin E.[23,24] At the present time, no single interventional strategy is of sufficiently proven benefit to warrant recommendation for routine clinical use, except for muscle paralysis of the subset of infants with fluctuating cerebral blood flow velocity. Once PVH–IVH has occurred, major effort must be directed toward supportive care of the infant and surveillance for complications, for example, periventricular infarction and posthemorrhagic ventricular dilation.

Major Complications of Periventricular–Intraventricular Hemorrhage

Periventricular Hemorrhagic Infarction

Approximately 15% of infants with IVH (usually severe) develop unilateral or strikingly asymmetric hemorrhagic necrosis in the periventricular white matter. Careful neuropathological studies indicate that this lesion represents venous infarction, which is distinguishable neuropathologically from hemorrhagic PVL, although the two lesions may coexist.[13,23,25]

Posthemorrhagic Ventricular Dilation

Posthemorrhagic ventricular dilation, related to disturbed cerebrospinal fluid (CSF) dynamics, develops commonly following severe PVH–IVH.[1,20] In the majority of cases, ventriculomegaly develops gradually over several weeks, secondary to an obliterative arachnoiditis in the posterior fossa that obstructs the flow of CSF.[26] At the present time, the optimal management of posthemorrhagic ventriculomegaly has not been defined unequivocally. Serial ultrasound scans are required to detect increasing ventricular size, because increases in head circumference measurements may be a relatively late manifestation of progressive ventriculomegaly. In approximately 50% of cases, ventricular dilation arrests or resolves spontaneously.[1] In the remainder, a variety of interventional strategies have been used, including serial lumbar punctures,[1,27] administration of drugs to decrease cerebrospinal fluid production,[1,28] external ventriculostomy,[1,29] or placement of a ventriculoperitoneal shunt.[1,30] Before embarking on treatment, it is important to be certain that the ventricular dilation relates to disturbed CSF dynamics rather than loss of cerebral tissue, that is, atrophy, which is not accompanied by increased ICP.

Outcome

It has been established that the major determinant of outcome of infants with PVH–IVH is the presence of periventricular parenchymal injury, which is usually considered to be principally hypoxic–ischemic in origin.[1,13] If extensive parenchymal involvement is present, patients die or develop significant neurological sequelae. With more localized parenchymal lesions, outcome tends to be more favorable if involvement is limited to frontal, parietal, or occipital regions.[13,23]

The relationship between posthemorrhagic ventricular dilation and subsequent neurological impairment is less clear, although there is increasing experimental and clinical evidence that progressive ventriculomegaly accompanied by rising ICP may be detrimental.[1,23]

References

1. Volpe JJ: Neurology of the Newborn. W. B. Saunders, Philadelphia, 1987.
2. Nelson KB, Ellenberg JH: Antecedents of cerebral palsy: multivariate analysis of risk. N Engl J Med 315:81–86, 1986.
3. Freeman JM, Nelson KB: Intrapartum asphyxia and cerebral palsy. Pediatrics 82:240–249, 1988.
4. Myers RE: Four patterns of perinatal brain damage and the conditions of occurrence in primates. Adv Neurol 10:232–234, 1975.
5. DeReuck JL: Cerebral angioarchitecture and perinatal brain lesions in premature and fullterm infants. Acta Neurol Scand 70:391–395, 1984.
6. Lou HC: The "lost autoregulation hypothesis" and brain lesions in the newborn—an update. Brain Dev 10:143–146, 1988.
7. Mujsce DJ, Boyer MA, Vannucci RC: CBF and brain edema in perinatal cerebral hypoxia–ischemia. Pediatr Res 21:494A, 1987.
8. Lupton BA, Hill A, Roland EH, Whitfield MF, Flodmark O: Brain swelling in the asphyxiated term newborn: pathogenesis and outcome. Pediatrics 82:139–146, 1988.
9. Clancy R, Legido A, Newel R, et al.: Continuous intracranial pressure monitoring and serial electroencephalographic recordings in severely asphyxiated term newborns. Am J Dis Child 142:740–747, 1988.
10. Sarnat HB, Sarnat MS: Neonatal encephalopathy following fetal distress: a clinical and electroencephalographic study. Arch Neurol 33:696–705, 1976.
11. Dubowitz LMS, Bydder GM, Mushin J: Developmental sequence of periventricular leukomalacia. Arch Dis Child 60:349–355, 1985.
12. Grant EG: Sonography of the premature brain: intracranial hemorrhage and periventricular leukomalacia. Neuroradiology 28:476–490, 1986.
13. Guzzetta F, Shackelford GD, Volpe S, Perlman JM, Volpe JJ: Periventricular intraparenchymal echodensities in the premature newborn: critical determinant of neurologic outcome. Pediatrics 78:995–1006, 1986.
14. Flodmark O, Becker LE, Harwood-Nash D, Fitzhardinge PM, Fitz CR, Chuang SH: Correlation between computed tomography and autopsy in premature and full-term neonates that have suffered perinatal asphyxia. Radiology 137:93–103, 1980.
15. Flodmark O, Lupton BA, Li D, Stimac GK, Roland EH, Hill A, Whitfield MF, Norman MG: MR imaging of periventricular leukomalacia in childhood. AJNR 10:111–118, 1989.
16. Baker LL, Stevenson KD, Enzmann DR: End-stage periventricular leukomalacia: MR evaluation. Radiology 168:809–815, 1988.
17. Holmes G, Rowe J, Hafford J, Schmidt R, Testa M, Zimmerman A: Prognostic value of the electroencephalogram in neonatal asphyxia. Electroencephalogr Clin Neurophysiol 53:60–72, 1982.
18. Hakamada S, Watanabe K, Hara K, Miyazaki S: The evolution of visual and auditory evoked potentials in infants with perinatal disorder. Brain Dev 3:339–344, 1981.
19. O'Brien MJ, Ash JM, Gilday DL: Radionuclide brain scanning in perinatal hypoxia/ischemia. Dev Med Child Neurol 21:161–173, 1979.
20. Pasternak JF: Parasagittal infarction in neonatal asphyxia. Ann Neurol 21:202–204, 1987.
21. Volpe JJ, Herscovitch P, Perlman JM, Kreusser KL, Raichle ME: Positron emission tomography in the asphyxiated term newborn: parasagittal impairment of cerebral blood flow. Ann Neurol 17:287–296, 1985.
22. Volpe JJ: Intraventricular hemorrhage in the premature infant—current concepts. Part I. Ann Neurol 25:3–11, 1989.
23. Volpe JJ: Intraventricular hemorrhage and brain injury in the premature infant: diagnosis, prognosis and prevention. Clin Perinatol 16:387–411, 1989.
24. Volpe JJ: Intraventricular hemorrhage in the premature infant—current concepts. Part II. Ann Neurol 25:109–116, 1989.
25. Takashima S, Mito T, Ando Y: Pathogenesis of periventricular white matter hemorrhages in preterm infants. Brain Dev 8:25–30, 1986.
26. Hill A, Volpe JJ: Normal pressure hydrocephalus in the newborn. Pediatrics 68:623–629, 1981.
27. Kreusser KL, Tarby TJ, Hill A, Kovnar E, Volpe JJ: Serial lumbar punctures at least temporary amelioration of neonatal posthemorrhagic hydrocephalus. Pediatrics 75:719–724, 1985.
28. Taylor DA, Hill A, Fishman MA, Volpe JJ: Treatment of posthemorrhagic hydrocephalus with glycerol. Ann Neurol 10:297, 1981.
29. Kreusser KL, Tarby DJ, Taylor D, Kovnar E, Hill A, Conray JA, Volpe JJ: Rapidly progressive posthemorrhagic hydrocephalus. Am J Dis Child 138:633–637, 1984.
30. Bada HS, Salmon JH, Pearson DH: Early surgical intervention in posthemorrhagic hydrocephalus. Child's Brain 5:109–115, 1979.

CHAPTER 16

Inflammatory Conditions

Massimo Caldarelli

Cerebral vessels can be affected by inflammatory pathologies either as part of a systemic disease or as a primary vasculitis involving only the central nervous system (CNS).[1–3]

These conditions are very rare, particularly in the pediatric population. Among the various forms, those related to CNS infections are by far the most common, while others are often so exceptional in children as to justify only isolated case reports. For this reason, this chapter will mainly describe the cerebral vasculitides associated with leptomeningeal infections (arteritis, thrombophlebitis, bacterial aneurysms), as well as the other rarer forms of vasculitis.

Cerebral Vasculitis Complicating Leptomeningitis

Leptomeningitis is still a major concern in the pediatric population, particularly in the early stages of life.[4–6] Despite the advent of efficacious antibiotic therapy, the mortality and morbidity for this disease remain elevated (up to 0.4% of all live births).[4,7–9]. The newborn (and the preterm babies in particular) seem specifically prone to leptomeningitis caused by gram-negative bacteria (like *Escherichia coli*, *Proteus*, *Klebsiella*, *Pseudomonas*), or group B strepto-coccus.[4,6,10] Infants and children may be affected as well, even though to a lesser extent. In this group other infectious agents are involved, like *Meningococcus*, *Hemophilus influenzae*, and *Pneumococcus*.[6,10] Also, *Mycobacterium tuberculosis* may be responsible for leptomeningitis, and its frequency is continuously increasing in the pediatric population, even in developed countries.[11]

Whatever the causative factor may be, the pathological appearance of the affected brain is quite similar. The hallmark of bacterial meningitis is an infiltration of the pia–arachnoid layers by inflammatory cells (firstly polymorphonuclear cells, and mononuclear in a later phase) which fill the subarachnoid space, either locally or diffusely. Generally, the purulent exudate is particularly thick and abundant at the cranial base, and within the basal cisterns, but it may also spread along the cerebrospinal fluid (CSF) pathways of the convexity, within the cerebral sulci, and extend into the cerebral parenchyma, along the Virchow–Robin spaces.[12–16]

The anatomical location of the cerebral arteries and veins, which run through the subarachnoid spaces and are bathed by the CSF, explains their actual involvement during the course of a leptomeningeal infection.[2,17] Microscopically, the acute phase is characterized by polymorphonuclear leukocyte infiltration of the arterial wall (particularly the adventitia and the subintimal layer), leading to a narrowing, and occasionally, to the obstruction of the vascular lumen.[12,13,14,18,19] On the other hand, the subacute and chronic phases are characterized by the prevalence of proliferative processes, with partial or total destruction of the internal elastic lamina and reduction (until total closure) of the arterial lumen.[13,18,20–22]

Obviously, an arterial occlusion should lead to cerebral infarction, but this actually is not as frequent as one might expect. The relatively long duration of the processes that lead to vascular obstruction may justify the development of a valid collateral circulation that reduces the adverse effect of cerebral ischemia. On the contrary, vasculitis associated with tuberculous or granulomatous meningitis, which is characterized by the prevalence of proliferative phenomena, also in the acute phase, is more likely to become complicated by arterial obstruction and, consequently, by infarction.[3,23,24]

Some particular aspects have been referred to as typical of a definite infectious agent; for instance, group B streptococcal meningitis is often associated with a necrotizing arteritis, which is complicated by hemorrhagic parenchymal necrosis, while ischemic necrosis is more likely to occur with *H. influenzae* or *Pseudomonas* meningitis.[2,22]

Even more rarely, cerebral vasculitis may be caused by a spirochetal, fungal, viral, or rickettsial infection.[2,5,6,16,21,25] The pathological findings in mycotic and spirochetal arteritis (meningovascular lues) look like those of tuberculous vasculitis, and are characterized by the striking predominance of chronic proliferative endoarteritis, which may lead to vascular obstruction. Also, fungal infections may be complicated by CNS vasculitis. These fungal vasculitides are becoming more widespread in immunodepressed people; in particular, children affected by leukemia or those undergoing bone marrow transplantation, are prone to harboring such opportunistic infections as candidiasis or aspergillosis, and consequently may present cerebrovascular complications related to vascular compromise by these biological agents.[22] Rickettsial and viral infection of the CNS are both characterized by a necrotizing vasculitis.[26–30] That, complicating the nowadays almost extinct congenital rubella syndrome, is responsible for focal obstruction of the vessel walls accompanied by proliferative phenomena that might lead to an ischemic infarction (in 65% of cases).[31,32] Another rare variety of viral arteritis has been described in recent years in association with herpes zoster ophthalmicus (granulomatous angiitis of the CNS).[33] This rare complication, observed also in children,[34] has been attributed to the spread of the zoster infection to the homolateral carotid or vertebral arteries (and their main branches), mediated by the ophthalmic branch of the trigeminal nerve.[35]

Together with the arteries, cerebral veins are also affected by leptomeningeal infections. Their walls are likewise infiltrated by inflammatory cells; moreover, due to the increased deformability of the venous wall by the dense inflammatory exudate, phlebitis is often already complicated by thrombus formation in the acute phase of the disease.[4,5,36–39] Occlusion of multiple veins is required to produce cerebral infarction, which is characteristically hemorrhagic and is more frequently seen in the brain cortex and subcortical white matter[8] as well as the subependymal areas.[13,16] Brain edema acts as a favoring factor in the process of thrombus formation.[4,38,39] The incidence of infarcts has been estimated to be as high as 30% in autoptic cases,[8,16] but this value is probably overestimated when one considers all the cases of leptomeningeal infections, not only the fatal ones.

Such vascular accidents may be suspected on a clinical basis, when the course of a leptomeningitis is complicated by the acute onset of neurological signs, such as seizure disorders, alteration of consciousness, focal deficits, and cranial nerve palsies.[4–6] In these cases an arterial or venous obstruction may be hypothesized and neuroradiology can confirm the clinical suspicion.

In the pre-CT era, cerebral angiography was the main instrument for a correct diagnosis. Its widespread utilization during the course of a leptomeningeal infection was sustained by many authors, especially when considering the low rate of complications related to this procedure[40,41] (Fig. 16.1). Angiographic alterations include (1) segmental constrictions of the cerebral arteries, associated with dilatations of variable lengths[42–46] (these dilatations may be either primary or secondary,[24] the result of a local failure in autoregulation or a focal increase in metabolism),[24,47] (2) narrowing (until complete occlusion) of the main arterial trunks of the cranial base and, to a lesser extent, of the convexity branches,[42–46] and (3) luminal alterations, mostly segmental, along the subarachnoidal course of the internal carotid artery and its branches.[42–46] Although such narrowings and luminal alterations are more frequently associated with tuberculous meningitis (Fig. 16.2), they are also common to the other forms

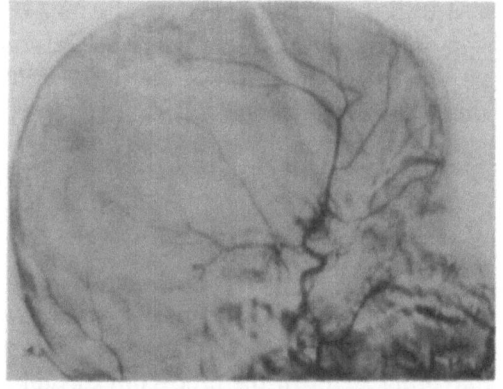

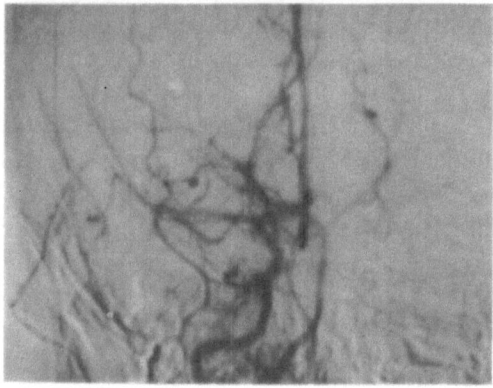

Figure 16.1. Right retrograde cerebral angiography performed in a child with neonatal bacterial meningitis (*Hemophilus influenzae*); lateral (top) and anteroposterior (AP) views. The middle cerebral artery is not visualized because of severe spasm and/or obstruction, due to arteritis. Note also the bowing of the anterior cerebral artery, corresponding to acute hypertensive hydrocephalus.

of meningitis and may be explained as the constriction exerted by the inflammatory exudate[24,48–51] or also, at least in part, as the localized effect of brain edema; however, they seem more likely attributable to the cellular infiltration of the vessel wall (adventitia and media) together with endothelial alterations.[7,12–15] These segments of narrowing may be short or long, with smooth or irregular ("shaggy") margins.[22] The latter aspect has been considered as almost pathognomonic of vasculitis related to leptomeningeal infections.[24] It is worth noting that anatomopathological investigations performed on fatal cases usually failed to demonstrate thrombosis of the lumen,[12,13,52,53] which had, however, been

detected by cerebral angiography in the same patients. This observation would suggest that the actual occurrence of ischemic accidents must require the concomitant occurrence of functional events such as, for instance, transitory vessel wall edema or cerebral spasm.[19,24]

Actually, the CT scan (and echoencephalography in infants with open anterior fontanel) has almost substituted for cerebral angiography in diagnosing CNS complications related to leptomeningitis.[9,54,55] In particular, cerebral infarcts secondary to arteritis or phlebitis (in the acute phase of the disease) appear as hypodense areas localized, respectively, either in the territory of a cerebral artery or in the cerebral cortex and adjacent subcortical white matter with scant or no contrast enhancement. In a later phase, from the second week on, contrast enhancement becomes apparent.[9,56] These lesions are generally so typical as not to require any additional angiographic examination in order to assess their occlusive nature (arteritic or phlebitic). At follow-up CT, they evolve into circumscribed areas of cerebral atrophy or, if the infarct is large enough, into porencephaly, usually within 2 to 3 weeks[9] (Fig. 16.2).

Quite recently, echoencephalography has been suggested as a means to detect cerebral vasculitis at an earlier stage than can be detected by the CT scan.[57] Neonates harboring different infections of the CNS, like congenital rubella, cytomegalovirus, human immunodeficiency virus (HIV) infections, or who may also be affected by connatal neurosyphilis (conditions all characterized by the occurrence of a necrotizing vasculitis) demonstrate on cranial sonography a "bright" aspect of the perforating arteries of the basal ganglia (which are normally not conspicuous), while the CT scan fails to demonstrate any abnormality in the same area. This particular aspect has been correlated with the vasculitic inflammation, characterized by perivascular infiltrates of mononuclear cells or also by the deposition of hyalinized material, both of which are processes leading to thickening and eventually to mineralization of the arterial walls.

Treatment of vasculitis associated with a leptomeningeal infection is essentially medical and the same as that of leptomeningitis.[3–6]

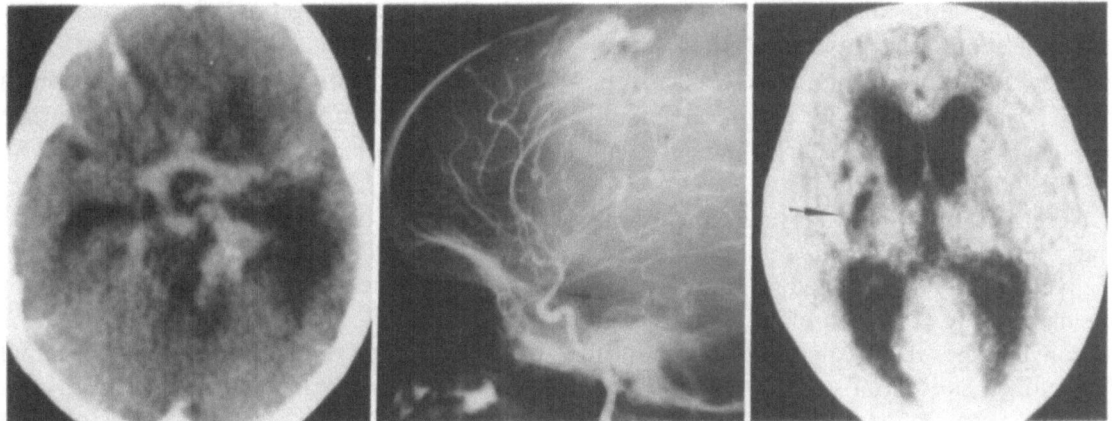

Figure 16.2. Five-year-old boy affected by tuberculous meningitis. Axial contrast-enhanced CT scan taken in the acute phase of the disease (left) shows the hyperdense exudate filling the basal cisterns and a hypodense inflammatory/ischemic lesion of the right temporal lobe. Note also the dilatation of the left temporal horn in acute hydrocephalus. Cerebral angiography (center) demonstrates a focal narrowing of the supraclinoid portion of the internal carotid artery (arrow), together with signs of ventricular dilatation under tension. Follow-up noncontrast CT scan (right), taken 3 months later, reveals a lacunar infarct (arrow) in the left basal ganglia.

Generally, antibiotic therapy, together with resolution of the meningeal infection, leads to a resolution of the vasculitic process, although neurological deficits secondary to the ischemic (or hemorrhagic) insult may remain unchanged.

Bacterial (Mycotic) Aneurysms

In 1885 Osler[58] first utilized the term *mycotic* aneurysm to describe an aneurysm developing from an inflammatory process of the arterial wall, leading to its weakening and, eventually, its rupture. Although decreasing in recent years due to antibiotic therapy, such pathology still deserves the attention of neurosurgeons for the potentially life-threatening complications. The incidence of bacterial aneurysms is estimated to be as high as 2 to 5% of all intracranial aneurysms,[59,60] and those observed in the pediatric age group represent 27 to 55%.[60-63] This latter observation accounts for the interest of pediatric neurosurgeons in this pathology.

The etiology is bacterial, although fungi may be responsible on rare occasions.[64-67] The most important and well-documented source of infection is represented by septic emboli detached from the cardiac vegetation of a septic endocarditis, which may remain stationary within the lumen of a small artery (more commonly the distal branches of the middle cerebral artery), or invade the arterial wall via the vasa vasorum. Mycotic aneurysms complicate the course of endocarditis in 3 to 15% of cases.[59-61,68] While the classical endocarditis that develops in congenital heart defects or artificial cardiac valves, or which complicates rheumatic heart disease, is at present declining in developed countries, that related to acquired nonrheumatic heart disease or intravenous drug abuse is becoming a major concern.[63]

Another possible pathogenesis of this condition is the extension into the vessel wall of a neighboring infection, like purulent or tuberculous meningitis,[69-71] sinus infection,[66] or cavernous thrombophlebitis[62,72-74] (the latter, prevalent among children, involves specifically the intracavernous tract of the internal carotid artery).

Whichever the portal entry may be, the infective process produces localized arteritis that involves progressively the adventitia, the muscularis, and the elastic lamina. The main pathological findings in the acute phase are represented by endothelial cell swelling and proliferation, fibrinoid necrosis of the media, and infiltration of the adventitia. These processes lead to the segmental weakening of the arterial wall, responsible for aneurysmal dilatation (which is typically fusiform) and eventually rupture and hemorrhage.[75]

The classical picture of a mycotic aneurysm is that of a subarachnoid (and/or intraparenchymal) hemorrhage. Before rupture, these aneurysms may cause neurological deficit signs or convulsions, which complicate the indolent course of an endocarditis or a meningitis.[63]

In the case of an associated cavernous thrombophlebitis, clinical signs related to the structures running within the cavernous sinus may be the presenting picture. When a mycotic aneurysm is suspected, potential sources for septic emboli should be sought, by means of multiple blood cultures, ENT evaluation, heart auscultation, echocardiography, and lumbar puncture for CSF examination.

Besides the information provided by the CT scan (subarachnoid clots, intraparenchymal hemorrhage, and occasionally direct visualization of the aneurysm), demonstration of a mycotic aneurysm relies on four-vessel cerebral angiography.[40,41,61,68,76] The malformation is usually fusiform, rather than saccular; it is located peripherally, rather than in the circle of Willis (typically in the terminal branches of the middle cerebral artery), generally not at bifurcations. Often the malformations are multiple and small and may change in size and shape on successive angiograms.[41,69,77] In this regard many authors have suggested repeated examinations (up to one every 7 to 10 days) to rule out the development of new aneurysms or to assess their evolution, during the course of antibiotic therapy.[64,70,71,76,77] There is no agreement as to whether the asymptomatic child affected by endocarditis should undergo routine cerebral angiography to rule out silent mycotic aneurysms; on the contrary, this procedure is reserved for all those presenting abnormal CT scans or CSF examination.[66]

Treatment of mycotic aneurysms is basically medical and consists of prolonged antibiotic therapy, continued for 4 to 6 weeks.[60–62,68,69] Surgical management is controversial. In fact, there are reports demonstrating the efficacy and safety of antibiotic therapy alone in managing bacterial aneurysms[70,74,78] while others consider the high mortality rates associated with rupture and claim surgical excision at the time of diagnosis to be the optimal treatment for all single, peripheral mycotic aneurysms, whether their location be proximal or peripheral.[67–69] Although no agreement exists on this matter, surgery is generally considered advisable for peripheral single aneurysms (especially in those requiring craniotomy for intraparenchymal bleeding), while proximal or multiple aneurysms are treated with antibiotics and closely followed angiographically, with their increase in size being the criterion for surgery.[63] Preoperative antibiotic therapy is always advisable in order to favor fibrosis of the friable aneurysm wall, which makes surgical maneuvers less dangerous.[76] In consideration of their nature and shape, the excision of mycotic aneurysms should be accompanied by excision of a segment of the parent artery, and by removal of the neighboring infected tissues.[60,63,68,78] Intracavernous carotid aneurysms, like those of the circle of Willis, should be treated medically whenever possible, and followed angiographically. Surgery, consisting of carotid artery ligation, should be reserved for those aneurysms that continue to enlarge regardless of antibiotic therapy, or if ophthalmoplegia worsens.[62,63,74]

In the case of urgent cardiac surgery performed on a child harboring a mycotic aneurysm, many authors claim that definitive treatment (medical and/or surgical) of the aneurysm should precede cardiac surgery, owing to the increased risk of its rupture after cardiac valve replacement,[63,80] while others prefer cardiac surgery first, in order to remove the source of infection and possible emboli.[76]

Other Vasculitides

Besides the other more common vasculitides associated with leptomeningeal infections, there is a particular variety of infectious arteritis that affects specifically the carotid artery.[81–83] Pathological findings consist of perivascular infiltration of polymorphonuclear cells and of fibrinoid necrosis of the media, alterations that affect mainly the supraclinoid portion of the internal carotid artery and its major branches.[81] Clinically, carotid arteritis is manifested by the acute onset of hemiplegia, generally without seizures. Angiography demonstrates severe narrowing or obstruction of the supraclinoid portion of the internal carotid artery, beginning above the ophthalmic artery and extending to the carotid bifurcation, and a less severe narrowing of the adjacent portions, in particular the beginning of the lenticulostriate arteries.[41,81,82] A severe infection of the upper respiratory tract, reported in as many as 60% of cases, suggests the possible role of an extracranial inflammatory disease (nasopharyngeal or tonsillar), which might secondarily involve the arterial wall through the lymphatic drainage.[84,85]

Immune-related diseases [rheumatic fever, juvenile rheumatoid arthritis (RA), systemic lupus erythematosus (SLE), thrombotic thrombocytopenic purpura (TTP), and polyarteritis nodosa (PAN)], which are quite rare in the pediatric age, may all be complicated by CNS vasculitis, with an incidence varying from 6% (rheumatoid arthritis) to 80% (thrombotic thrombocytopenic purpura) of cases.[86,87] From a pathological point of view, these vasculitides are characterized by lymphoid and histiocytic infiltration of the arterial wall, causing a granulomatous angiitis,[88,89] and by fibrinoid necrosis. These pathological findings suggest a hypersensitivity pathogenesis. Angiography may demonstrate segmental arteritis (RA, SLE), arterial beadings (PAN), or even thrombotic vascular occlusion (TTP).[89]

From a clinical point of view, acute psychosis with convulsions, confusion, and increased intracranial pressure are the main signs, while ocular signs (like internuclear ophthalmoplegia) are less frequent.[86] An isolated angiitis of the CNS (also referred to as granulomatous angiitis) was described in adults for the first time in 1959[90] and thereafter also in children and adolescents.[91] This vasculitis is characterized, from a pathological point of view, by a mononuclear infiltration of the walls of small arteries and veins of the CNS, with a predilection for the medial and adventitial layers. Fibrinoid necrosis may also be present.

These alterations have been attributed[91] both to a direct toxic (or infectious) insult to the vessel wall, or to an immune mechanism. Although "primary" (or idiopathic) in nature, this vasculitis probably has an infectious etiology, due to the possible association with zoster or HIV infections.[34,35,91] Likewise, the described association with lymphoma or leukemia raises the possibility of widespread dissemination of a viral infection in profoundly immunodepressed patients.[92] Focal neurologic deficits or higher cortical dysfunction are generally the clinical signs that focus the attention of the clinician on the possible CNS involvement during the course of a disease characterized by vague symptomatology (fever, myalgias, arthralgia, weight loss).[86] Angiography, which is the diagnostic procedure of choice, reveals a typical pattern characterized by the alternation of areas of stenosis and ectasia ("sausage" pattern). Vague luminal irregularities or narrowings are less common.[93]

Acquired immunodeficiency syndrome (AIDS) is complicated by a CNS pathology in approximately 80 to 100% of cases. Apart from vasculitides stemming from opportunistic infections (toxoplasmosis, cytomegalovirus, tuberculosis, etc.) there are specific vascular alterations typical of AIDS.[94,95] These include (1) a mild to moderate fibrous thickening of the wall of small arterioles; (2) calcification of small vessel walls, with calcium deposits in the perivascular area and surrounding brain parenchyma (particularly evident in pediatric patients)[96]; and (3) granulomatous angiitis with intimal proliferative lesions. All these lesions may be responsible for cerebral infarcts, which are generally mild, and, occasionally, for hemorrhage. Finally, a necrotizing arteritis characterized by fibrinoid necrosis may be observed in the final stages of such systemic disorders as disseminated intravascular coagulation or hemolytic uremic syndrome,[22] as well as after radiation therapy.[97-99]

A necrotizing vasculitis (both arteritis and thrombophlebitis) has been reported in association with drug abuse,[22,100-102] particularly with intravenous and also oral assumption of metamphetamines. This form of drug addiction is also becoming a major problem in adolescents. The vascular abnormalities described in this condition are represented by alternating areas of narrowing and dilation of the anterior and middle cerebral arteries.[102-104]

Fibromuscular Dysplasia

Fibromuscular dysplasia (or hyperplasia) is a rare nonatherosclerotic, noninflammatory vascular disease of unknown etiology, which primarily involves medium-sized splanchnic arteries, particularly the renal, and to a lesser extent the carotid arteries.[105,106]

This rare disorder is characterized, from a pathological point of view by prevalent involvement of the intimal, medial, or adventitial layers of the arterial wall, although the most common variety is that affecting the media (medial fibroplasia). The pathological findings are a marked hyperplasia of the media, with fibrosis of the adventitia, associated with areas of thinning and disruption of the elastic lamina[105,106]; these alterations are responsible for segmental stenosis (focal, multifocal, or tubular), alternating or not with segments of dilatation.[104,106,107] The cephalic arterial involvement is fundamentally a disease in old women (more than 50 years old), although a few cases have been described in children and adolescents.[22,106,108-110]

The carotid arteries are characteristically affected along their extracranial course, with a predilection for the C1–C2 level. Angiographically the disease is characterized by single or multiple stenoses,[40,41,107] either smooth or irregular, alternating with segmental dilatations and giving the affected artery a characteristic "beaded" appearance. In about 20% of cases aneurysms of the intracranial arteries have been reported, sometimes multiple,[41,105,106] although a more elevated incidence (up to 50%) has been described by others.[106]

Carotid fibromuscular dysplasia may be an incidental finding, but it is more commonly observed in association with "major" neurological disturbances (such as transient ischemic attacks, cerebral infarcts, syncope, or subarachnoid hemorrhage) or "minor" abnormalities (headache, tinnitus, vertigo, etc.). The actual incidence of symptomatic cases is difficult to assess, as angiography is essential for diagnosis and patients undergoing cerebral angiography are a selected group. Besides the association with intracranial aneurysms, adult cases of cerebrovascular fibromuscular dysplasia may be complicated by spontaneous dissection of the internal carotid artery, presenting with a sudden onset of headache or neck pain, blurred vision, and/or Horner's syndrome, and signs of transient or permanent cerebral ischemia.[105,106]

Among the various surgical techniques suggested (resection of the pathologic segment, patch angioplasty, intraluminal dilatation, extra-intracranial bypass) graduated intraluminal dilatation is considered by most surgeons the method of choice.[106]

Percutaneous transluminal angioplasty has recently been performed successfully.[106]

References

1. Bickerstaff ER: Cerebrovascular disease in infancy and childhood. In: Vinken PJ, Bruyn GW (eds.), Handbook of Clinical Neurology. Vascular Disease of the Nervous System. Elsevier, New York, 1972, pp. 340–351.

2. Stehbens WE: Pathology of the Cerebral Blood Vessels. C. V. Mosby, St. Louis, 1972, pp. 604–622.

3. Golden GS: Vascular diseases of the brain. Curr Probl Pediatr 8:1–28, 1978.

4. Bell, WE, McCormick WF: Neurologic Infections in Children. W. B. Saunders, Philadelphia, 1981.

5. Weil ML: Infections of the nervous system. In: Menkes JH (ed.), Textbook of Child Neurology. Lea & Febiger, Philadelphia, 1985, pp. 316–431.

6. Volpe JJ: Neurology of the Newborn. W. B. Saunders, Philadelphia, 1987, pp. 548–635.

7. Dodge PR, Swarzz MN: Bacterial meningitis: a review of selected aspects. II. Special neurologic problems, postmeningitic complications and clinicopathological correlations. N Engl J Med 272:1003–1009, 1965.

8. Berman PH, Banker BQ: Neonatal meningitis. A clinical and pathological study of 29 cases. Pediatrics 38:6–24, 1966.

9. Diebler C, Dulac O: Pediatric Neurology and Neuroradiology. Springer-Verlag, Berlin, 1987. pp. 139–183.

10. Smith ES: Purulent meningitis in infants and children. A review of 409 cases. J Pediatr 45:425–436, 1954.

11. Wilkinson HA, Ferris EJ, Muggia AL, Cantù RC: Central nervous system tuberculosis: a persistent disease. J Neurosurg 34:15–22, 1971.

12. Adams RD, Kubik CS, Bonner FJ: Clinical and pathological aspects of influenzal meningitis. Arch Pediatr 65:354–376, 1948.

13. Cairns H, Russell DS: Cerebral arteritis and phlebitis in pneumococcal meningitis. J Pathol Bact 58:649–665, 1946.

14. Rorke LB, Pitts FW: Purulent meningitis. The pathologic basis of clinical manifestations. Clin Pediatr 2:64–71, 1963.

15. Harriman DGF: Bacterial infections of the central nervous system. In: Adams JH, Corsellis JAN, Duchen LW (eds.), Greenfield's Neuropathology. 4th Ed. Wiley, New York, 1984, pp. 236–259.

16. Friede RL: Developmental Neuropathology, 2nd Ed. Springer-Verlag, New York, 1989, pp. 169–197.

17. Feigin RD, Dodge PR: Bacterial meningitis: new concepts of pathophysiology and neurological sequelae. Pediatr Clin North Am 23:541–556, 1976.

18. Friede RL: Cerebral infarcts complicating neonatal meningitis. Acute and residual lesions. Acta Neuropathol (Berlin) 23:245–253, 1973.

19. Yamashima T, Kashihara K, Ikeda K, Kubata T, Yamamoto S: Three phases of cerebral arteriopathy in meningitis: vasospasm and vasodilatation followed by organic stenosis. Neurosurgery 16:546–553, 1985.

20. Smith JF, Landing BH: Mechanisms of brain damage in H. influenzae meningitis. J Neuropathol Exp Neurol 19:248–265, 1960.

21. Rorke LB: Pathology of cerebral vascular disease in children and adolescents. In: Edwards SB, Hoffman HJ (eds.), Cerebral Vascular Disease in Children and Adolescents. Williams & Wilkins, Baltimore, 1989, pp. 95–138.

22. Lyons EL, Leeds NE: The angiographic demonstration of arterial vascular disease in purulent meningitis. Radiology 88:935–938, 1967.

23. Dastur DK, Udani PM: The pathology and pathogenesis of tuberculous encephalopathy. Acta Neuropathol (Berlin) 6:311–326, 1966.

24. Leeds NE, Goldberg HI: Angiographic manifestations in cerebral inflammatory disease. Radiology 98:595–604, 1971.

25. Ferris EJ, Levine HL: Cerebral arteritis: classification. Radiology 109:327–341, 1973.

26. Brownell B, Tomlinson AH: Virus diseases of the central nervous system. In: Adams JH, Corsellis JAN, Duchen LW (eds.), Greenfield's Neuropathology, 4th Ed. Wiley, New York, 1984, pp. 260–303.

27. Desmonts G, Couvreur J: Congenital toxoplasmosis. N Engl J Med, 290:1110–1112, 1974.

28. Koeppen AH, Lansing LS, Peng SK, Smith RS: Central nervous system vasculitis in cytomegalovirus infection. J Neurol Sci 51:395–410, 1981.

29. Marques Dias MJ, Harmant-van Rijckevorsel G, Landrieu P, Lyon G: Prenatal cytomegalovirus disease and microgyria: evidence for perfusion failure, not disturbance of histogenesis, as the major cause of fetal cytomegalovirus encephalopathy. Neuropediatrics 15:18–24, 1984.

30. Diebler C, Dusser A, Dulac O: Congenital toxoplasmosis: clinical and neuroradiological evaluation of the cerebral lesions. Neuroradiology, 27:125–130, 1985.

31. Rorke LB: Nervous system lesions in the congenital rubella syndrome. Arch Otolaryngol 98:249–251, 1973.

32. Townsend JJ, Stroop WG, Baringer JR, Wolinsky JS, McKerrow JH, Berg BO: Neuropathology of progressive rubella panencephalitis after childhood rubella. Neurology 32:185–190, 1982.

33. McKenzie RA, Forbes GS, Karnes WE: Angiographic findings in herpes zoster arteritis. Ann Neurol 10:458–464, 1981.

34. Walker RJ, Gammal TE, Allen MB: Cranial arteritis associated with herpes zoster: case report with angiographic findings. Radiology 107:109–110, 1973.

35. Hilt DC, Buchholz D, Krumholz A, Weiss H, Wolinsky JS: Herpes Zoster ophthalmicus and delayed contralateral hemiparesis caused by cerebral angiitis: diagnosis and management approaches. Ann Neurol 14:543–553, 1983.

36. Krayenbühl H: Cerebral venous and sinus thrombosis. Clin Neurosurg 14:1–24, 1966.

37. Kalbag RM: Cerebral venous thrombosis. Oxford University Press, London, 1967.

38. Chiras J, Dubs M, Bories J: Venous infarctions. Neuroradiology 27:593–600, 1985.

39. Dunn DW, Daum RS, Weisberg L, Vargas R: Ischemic cerebrovascular complications of Hemophilus influenzae meningitis. Arch Neurol 39:650–652, 1982.

40. Raimondi AJ: Pediatric Neuroradiology. W. B. Saunders, Philadelphia, 1972, pp. 662–679.

41. Harwood Nash DC, Fitz CR: Neuroradiology in Infants and Children. C. V. Mosby, St. Louis, 1972, pp. 855–871, 960.

42. Davis DO, Taveras JM: Radiological aspects of inflammatory conditions affecting the central nervous system. Clin Neurosurg 14:192–210, 1966.

43. James AE, Hodges FJ III, Jordan CE, Mathews EH, Heller R: Angiography and cisternography in acute meningitis due to *Hemophilus influenzae*. Radiology 103:601–606, 1972.

44. Segall HD, Rumbaugh CL, Bergeron RT, Teal JS: Neuroradiology in infections of the brain and meninges. Surg Neurol 1:178–186, 1973.

45. Raimondi AJ, Di Rocco C: Cerebral angiography in meningocerebral inflammatory diseases in infancy and childhood: a study of thirty-five cases. Neurosurgery 3:37–44, 1978.

46. Raimondi AJ, Di Rocco C: The physiopathogenetic basis for the angiographic diagnosis of bacterial infections of the brain and its coverings in children. I. Leptomeningitis. Child's Brain 5:1–13, 1979.

47. Davis DO, Dilenge D, Schlaepfer W: Arterial dilatation in purulent meningitis. Case report. J Neurosurg 32:112–115, 1970.

48. Greitz T: Angiography in tuberculous meningitis. Acta Radiol Diagn 2:369–378, 1964.

49. Lehrer H: The angiographic triad in tuberculous meningitis. A radiographic and clinicopathological correlation. Radiology 87:829–835, 1966.

50. Frech RS: Tuberculous meningitis. Radiology 91:1129–1134, 1968.

51. Mathew NT, Abraham J, Chandy J: Cerebral angiographic features in tuberculous meningitis. Neurology (Minneapolis) 20:1015–1023, 1970.

52. Heading DL, Glasgow LA: Occlusion of internal carotid artery complicating *Hemophilus influenzae* meningitis. Am J Dis Child 131:854–856, 1977.

53. Snyder RD, Storving J, Cushing AH, Davis LE, Hardy TL: Cerebral infarction in childhood bacterial meningitis. J Neurol Neurosurg Psychiatr 44:581–585, 1981.

54. Cockrill HH, Dreisbach J, Lowe B, Yamauchi T: Computed tomography in leptomeningeal infections. Am J Roentgenol 130:511–515, 1978.

55. Zimmerman RA, Patel S, Bilaniuk LT: Demonstration of purulent bacterial intracranial infections by computed tomography. Am J Roentgenol 127:155–165, 1976.

56. Rao KCVG, Knipp HC, Wagner EJ: CT findings in cerebral sinus and venous thrombosis. Radiology 140:391–398, 1981.

57. Littlewood Teele R, Hernanz-Schulman M, Sotrel A: Echogenic vasculature in the basal ganglia of neonates: a sonographic sign of vasculopathy. Radiology 169:423–427, 1988.

58. Osler W: The Gulsonian lectures on malignant endocarditis. Br Med J 1:467–470, 1885.

59. Cantù RC, Le May M, Wilkinson HA: The importance of repeated angiography in the treatment of mycotic-embolic intracranial aneurysms. J Neurosurg 25:189–193, 1966.

60. Roach MR, Drake CG: Ruptured cerebral aneurysms caused by micro-organisms. N Engl J Med 273:240–244, 1965.

61. Bohmfalk GL, Story JL, Wissinger IP, Brown WE Jr: Bacterial intracranial aneurysm. J Neurosurg 48:369–382, 1978.

62. Rout D, Sharma A, Mohan PK, Rao VRK: Bacterial aneurysms of the intracavernous carotid artery. J Neurosurg 60:1236–1242, 1984.

63. Andrews BT, Hudgins RJ, Edwards MSB: Mycotic aneurysms in children. In: Edwards MSB, Hoffman HJ (eds.), Cerebral Vascular Disease in Children and Adolescents. Williams & Wilkins, Baltimore, 1989, pp. 275–282.

64. Goldman JA, Fleischer AS, Leifer W, Parent A, Schwarzman SW, Raggio J: *Candida albicans* mycotic aneurysm associated with systemic lupus erythematosus. Neurosurgery 4:325–328, 1979.

65. Mielke B, Weir B, Oldring D, von Vestarp C: Fungal aneurysm. Case report and review of the literature. Neurosurgery 9:578–582, 1981.

66. Morriss FH Jr, Spock A: Intracranial aneurysm secondary to mycotic orbital and sinus infection. Report of a case implicating *Penicillium* as an opportunistic fungus. Am J Dis Child 119:357–362, 1970.

67. Hadley MN, Martin NA, Spetzler RF, Johnson PC: Multiple intracranial aneurysms due to *Coccidioides immitis* infection. J Neurosurg 66:453–456, 1987.

68. Frazee JG, Cahan LD, Winter J: Bacterial intracranial aneurysms. J Neurosurg 53:633–641, 1980.

69. Heidelberger KP, Layton WM Jr, Fisher RG: Multiple cerebral mycotic aneurysms complicating posttraumatic *Pseudomonas* meningitis. J Neurosurg 29:631–635, 1968.

70. Suwanwela C, Suwanwela N, Chruchinda S, Hongsaprabhas C: Intracranial mycotic aneurysms of extravascular origin. J Neurosurg 36:552–559, 1972.

71. Ojemann RG, Crowell RM: Infectious intracranial aneurysms. In: Ojemann RG, Crowell

RM (eds.), Surgical Management of Cerebrovascular Disease. Williams & Wilkins, Baltimore, 1983, pp. 255–263.

72. Devadiga KV, Mathai KV, Chandy J: Spontaneous cure of intracavernous aneurysm of the internal carotid artery in a 14-month-old child. Case report J Neurosurg 30:165–168, 1969.

73. Eguchi T, Nakagomi T, Teraoka A: Treatment of bilateral mycotic intracavernous carotid aneurysms. J Neurosurg 56:443–447, 1982.

74. Tomita T, McLone DG, Naidich TP: Mycotic aneurysm of the intracavernous portion of the carotid artery in childhood. J Neurosurg 54:681–684, 1981.

75. Molinary GF, Smith L, Goldstein MN, Satran R: Pathogenesis of cerebral mycotic aneurysms. Neurology (Minneapolis) 23:325–332, 1973.

76. Morawetz RB, Karp RB: Evolution and resolution of intracranial bacterial (mycotic) aneurysms. Neurosurgery 15:43–49, 1984.

77. Pootrakul A, Carter LP: Bacterial intracranial aneurysm: importance of sequential angiography. Surg Neurol 17:429–431, 1982.

78. Bingham WF: Treatment of mycotic intracranial aneurysms. J Neurosurg 46:428–437, 1977.

79. Venger BH, Aldama AE: Mycotic vasculitis with repeated intracranial aneurysmal hemorrhage. Case report. J Neurosurg 69:775–779, 1988.

80. Bullock R, van Dellen JR: Rupture of bacterial intracranial aneurysms following replacement of cardiac valves. Surg Neurol 17:9–11, 1982.

81. Shillito J Jr: Carotid arteritis: a cause of hemiplegia in childhood. J Neurosurg 21:540–551, 1964.

82. Harwood-Nash DC, McDonald P, Argent W: Cerebral arterial disease in children. An angiographic study of 40 cases. Am J Roentgenol 111:672–686, 1971.

83. Isler W: Acute hemiplegias and hemisyndromes in childhood. Clin Dev Med 41/42, 1971.

84. Bickerstaff ER: Aetiology of acute hemiplegia in childhood. Br Med J 2(July 11):82–87, 1964.

85. Hilal SK, Solomon GE, Gold AP, Carter S: Primary cerebral arterial occlusive disease in children. I. Acute acquired hemiplegia. Radiology 99:71–86, 1971.

86. Swaiman KF, Wright FS: The Practice of Pediatric Neurology. C. V. Mosby, St. Louis, 1982, pp. 799–811.

87. Devinsky O, Petito CK, Alonso DR: Clinical and neuropathological findings in systemic lupus erythematosus: the role of vasculitis, heart emboli, and thrombotic thrombocytopenic purpura. Ann Neurol 23:380–384, 1988.

88. Younger DS, Hays AP, Brust JCM, Rowland LP: Granulomatous angiitis of the brain. An inflammatory reaction of diverse etiology. Arch Neurol 45:514–518, 1988.

89. Mumenthaler M: Inflammatory angiopathy. In: Toole JF (ed.), Cerebrovascular Disorders. Raven, New York, 1984, pp. 299–311.

90. Cravioto H, Feigin I: Noninfectious granulomatous angiitis with a predilection for the nervous system. Neurology 9:599–609, 1959.

91. Calabrese LH, Mallek JA: Primary angiitis of the central nervous system. Report of 8 cases, review of the literature, and proposal for diagnostic criteria. Medicine 67:20–39, 1988.

92. Borenstein D, Costa M, Jannotta F, Rizzoli H: Localized isolated angiitis of the central nervous system associated with primary intracerebral lymphoma. Cancer 62:375–380, 1988.

93. Cupps T, Moore P, Fauci A: Isolated angiitis of the central nervous system. Prospective diagnostic and therapeutic experience. Am J Med 74:97–105, 1983.

94. Mizuawa H, Hirano A, Llena JF, Shintaku M: Cerebrovascular lesions in acquired immune deficiency syndrome (AIDS). Acta Neuropathol (Berlin) 76:451–457, 1988.

95. Vinters HV, Guerra WF, Eppoliti L, Keith PE III: Necrotizing vasculitis of the central nervous system in a patient with AIDS-related complex. Neuropathol Appl Neurobiol 14:417–424, 1988.

96. Belman AL, Lantos G, Horoupian D, Novick BE, Ultman MH, Dickson DW, Rubinstein A: AIDS: calcification of the basal ganglia in infants and children. Neurology 36:1192–1199, 1986.

97. Kagan AR, Bruce DW, Di Chiro G: Fatal foam cell arteritis of the brain after irradiation for Hodgkin's disease: angiography and pathology. Stroke 2:232–238, 1971.

98. Painter MJ, Chutorian AM, Hilal SK: Cerebrovasculopathy following irradiation in childhood. Neurology 25:189–194, 1975.

99. Price RA, Birdwell DA: The central nervous system in childhood leukemia. III. Mineralizing microangiopathy and dystrophic calcification. Cancer 42:717–728, 1978.

100. Rumbaugh CL, Bergeron RT, Scanlon RL, Teal JS, Segall H, Zanz H, McCormick R: Cerebral vascular changes secondary to amphetamine abuse in the experimental animal. Radiology 101:345–351, 1971.

101. Brust JCM: Stroke and substance abuse. In: Barnett HJM, Mohr JP, Stein BM, Yatsu FM (eds.), Stroke: Pathophysiology, Diagnosis and

Management. Churchill Livingstone, Edinburgh, 1986, pp. 903–917.

102. Kaye BR, Fainstat M: Cerebral vasculitis associated with cocaine abuse. JAMA 258:2104–2106, 1987.

103. Margolis MT, Newton TH: Methamphetamine ("speed") arteritis. Neuroradiology 2:179–182, 1971.

104. Leeds NE, Malhotra V, Zimmerman RD: The radiology of drug addiction affecting the brain. Semin Roentgenol 18:227–233, 1983.

105. Mettinger KL, Ericson K: Fibromuscular dysplasia and the brain: observations on angiographic, clinical and genetic characteristics. Stroke 13:46–52, 1982.

106. Lüscher TF, Lie JT, Stanson AW, Houser OW, Hollier LH, Sheps SG: Arterial fibromuscular dysplasia. Mayo Clin Proc 62:931–952, 1987.

107. Houser OW, Baker HL Jr, Sandok BA, Holley KE: Cephalic arterial fibromuscular dysplasia. Arch Neurol 38:616–618, 1971.

108. Anderson PE: Fibromuscular hyperplasia in children. Acta Radiol (Diagn) 10:205–210, 1970.

109. Lemahieu SF, Marchau MM: Intracranial fibromuscular dysplasia and stroke in children. Neuroradiology 18:99–102, 1979.

110. Shields WD, Ziter FA, Osborn AG: Fibromuscular dysplasia as a cause of stroke in infancy and childhood. Pediatrics 59:899–901, 1977.

CHAPTER 17

Moyamoya Disease

Kiyoshi Sato and Takeyoshi Shimoji

Introduction

At the fourteenth meeting of the Japanese Neurosurgical Society in 1955, Shimizu and Takeuchi reported a new disease entity designated as dysplasia of both internal carotid arteries[1]. This appears to be the first report of what we now refer to as moyamoya disease[2]. A succession of reports by a number of Japanese neurosurgeons[3–6] of a similar disease followed, and the pathology of the disease was found to be characterized by the bilateral formation of abnormal netlike vessels at the base of the brain, associated with bilateral stenosis and/or occlusion of the arteries composing the circle of Willis.

Although considerable investigations have been conducted, the etiology of moyamoya disease is still unknown. Accordingly, the fact that the etiology is unknown is included as a criterion in diagnosis of moyamoya disease. The name *moyamoya disease* was coined by Suzuki and Kakaku[2] in 1969: the Japanese word indicated the hazy, puff-of-smoke angiographic appearance of the abnormal netlike vessels developed in the base of the brain. Initially thought to be a disease affecting only Japanese,[7] cases of similar moyamoya disease began to be reported from 1965 on in North America and Europe by Weidner[8], Krayenbuhl[9], and Taveras.[10] At present, cases are being reported throughout the world regardless of race, although not to the extent as in Japan. The clinical features of moyamoya disease are quite specific in some cases involving children, but a diagnosis of the disease can only be made angiographically, demonstrating the aforementioned abnormality of the cerebral vessels.

In the present chapter, the general features of moyamoya disease are described by illustrating some of the cases we have experienced at Juntendo University (Tokyo, Japan) during the past 10 years.

Clinical Presentation

Although moyamoya disease may occur at any age, there are two peaks in the age distribution: under 10 years and in the 30s.[12] This appears to be more frequent in females. The youngest child in our series was 12 months old. On the basis of the clinical presentation moyamoya disease may be classified in four types: (1) transient ischemic attack (TIA), (2) infarction, (3) epilepsy, and (4) hemorrhage. Symptoms of the first three types appear almost exclusively in children, resulting from brain ischemia. Conversely, the hemorrhagic type occurs mainly in adults[11].

In children, the most typical symptoms of cerebral ischemia are recurrent (sometimes alternating) episodes of such focal neurological deficits as monoparesis, hemiparesis, paraparesis, or speech disturbances. Motor paresis may occur, without constancy, on either side. Hyperventilation, induced on specific occasions as when playing the flute or harmonica or blowing on hot noodle soup to cool it, often causes onset of neurological deficits, followed by their complete remission. TIAs most often occur during the first 4 years, decreasing in incidence thereafter. Intellectual deterioration and neurological deficits increase with the lapse of time. TIA-type cases in which there is no remission of recurring neurological deficits, or cases in which such deficits appearing at the time of the initial attack become permanent, are designated as infarction-type cases.

Numerous cases of the epileptic type characterized by the occurrence of seizures, as evidence by abnormal epileptic discharges recorded on an electroencephalogram, also have been reported. In addition, cases also have been observed in which headaches are the only symptom and no other neurological deficits are detected.

Intracranial hemorrhage as an initial presentation of moyamoya disease is common in adults but quite rare in children[12]. This is either (1) intracerebral hemorrhage in the vicinity of the lateral ventricle due to bleeding from the moyamoya vessels, which may be accompanied by intraventricular hemorrhage, (2) subarachnoid hemorrhage resulting from the rupture of a pseudoaneurysm, formed in the abnormal network of vessels at the base of the brain, or (3) the result of rupture of a saccular aneurysm that has developed in the vertebrobasilar system.[13-15] The occurrence of a saccular aneurysm may probably be attributed to hemodynamic factors of increased blood flow in the posterior circulation compensating for a reduction in anterior circulation blood flow resulting from occlusion of the carotid[13]. The severity of moyamoya disease varies with the age of onset. It is most severe in infants and young children under 5 years of age, a timespan during which progressive motor deficit and intellectual deterioration are produced[16].

Concerning family history in the case of moyamoya disease, filioparental cases and cases affecting twins and siblings have been reported, representing a familial incidence of more than 7% of about 600 cases reported in Japan. Such being the circumstances, moyamoya disease may be considered a disease with a congenital or hereditary background.[17-19] Suzuki and Kodama[12], however, speculated that such chronic infections as respiratory infections, including tonsillitis, bronchitis, and pneumonia, or paranasal sinusitis may be causes of moyamoya disease because such chronic infections in and above the upper cervical area have been found in the past history of patients with the disease.

Angiographic Features

Cerebral angiographic features commonly observed in moyamoya disease include stenotic or occlusive changes, abnormal netlike neovascularization, and progressive changes. Stenosis and/or occlusion of the supraclinoid portion of the internal carotid artery on both sides results frequently in extension of the stenotic or occlusive processes into the proximal portions of the anterior and middle cerebral arteries. Abnormal netlike vessel formations arise at the base of the brain bilaterally and are contributed to by lenticulostriate, choroidal, thalamoperforating, premammillary, thalamostriate, and other newly formed circle of Willis vessels. In addition to the aforementioned features, progression of the disease may result in (1) an abnormal netlike formation of vessels at the frontal base, with blood supply coming through the anterior and posterior branches of the ophthalmic artery (ethmoidal moyamoya[12]) (Fig. 17.1), (2) dilatation of the basilar artery and development of "moyamoya" vessel formation by perforating branches of the posterior cerebral artery (posterior basal moyamoya,[20] (3) a well-developed posterior pericallosal artery (Fig. 17.2), and (4) development of extra- and intracranial transdural leptomeningeal collaterals between the pial vessels and those arising from the external carotid artery, which include meningeal branches of the internal maxillary, superficial temporal, and occipital arteries (vault moyamoya[12]) (Fig. 17.3).

According to Suzuki and Takaku[2], these angiographic features may be divided into six stages in terms of the progression of the carotid fork occlusion, as illustrated in Table 17.1. Although their staging was not obtained by serial angiography, there are considerable reports and observations that support these angiographically identifiable classifications (Fig. 17.4). In the early stages, stenosis of the supraclinoid portion of the internal carotid artery occurs (stage 1). With progression of the disease, compensatory dilatation of the main intracerebral arteries and the abnormal netlike formation of basal perforating vessels takes place (stage 2) (Fig. 17.5A). When carotid stenosis progresses to occlusion, there is

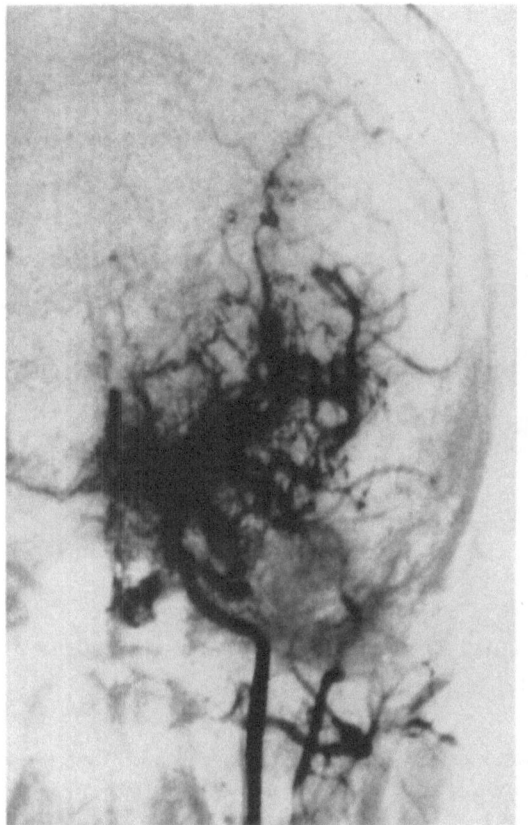 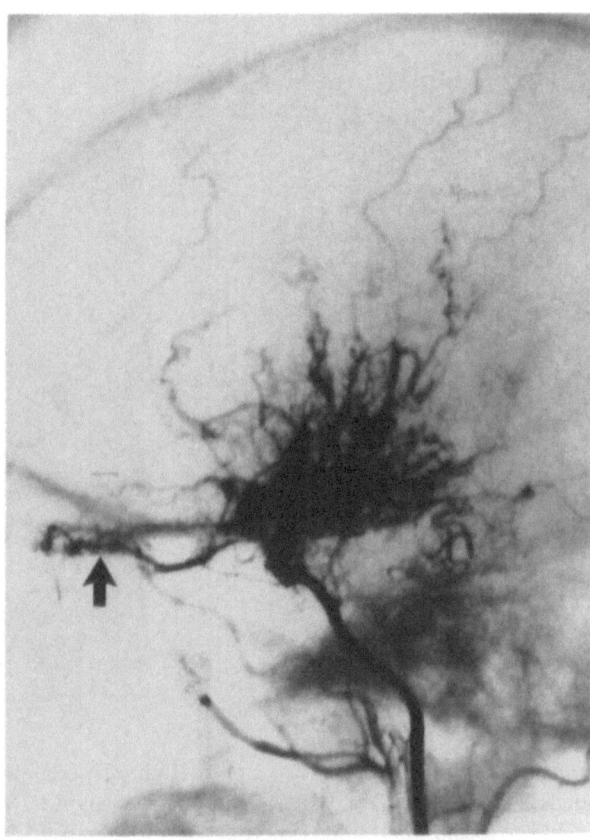

Figure 17.1. Typical left carotid angiograms [anteroposterior (AP; top) and lateral (bottom) views] of moyamoya disease (stage 3). Note occlusion of carotid bifurcation and abnormal vascular network at the base of the brain (basal moyamoya). The arrow indicates ethmoidal moyamoya.

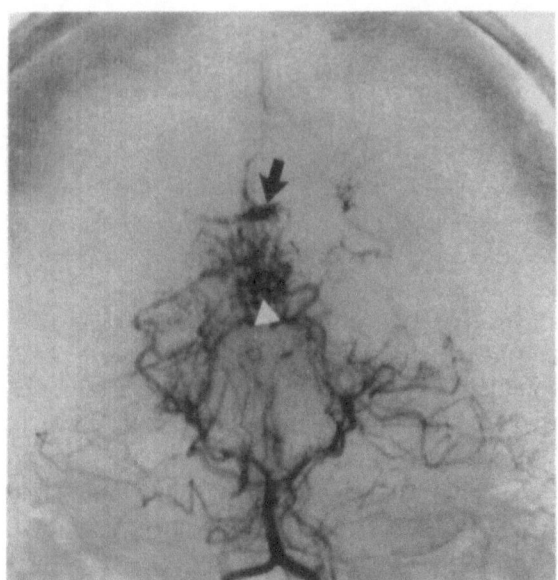 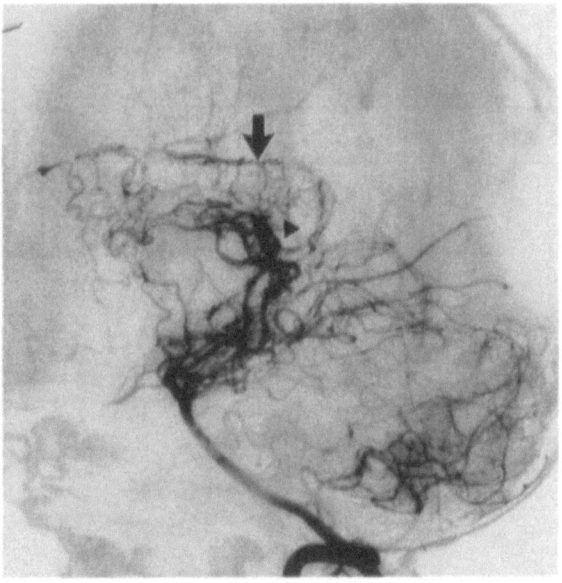

Figure 17.2. The left vertebral angiograms [AP (top) and lateral (bottom) views] show posterior basal moyamoya (arrowhead) and prominent posterior pericallosal artery (arrow).

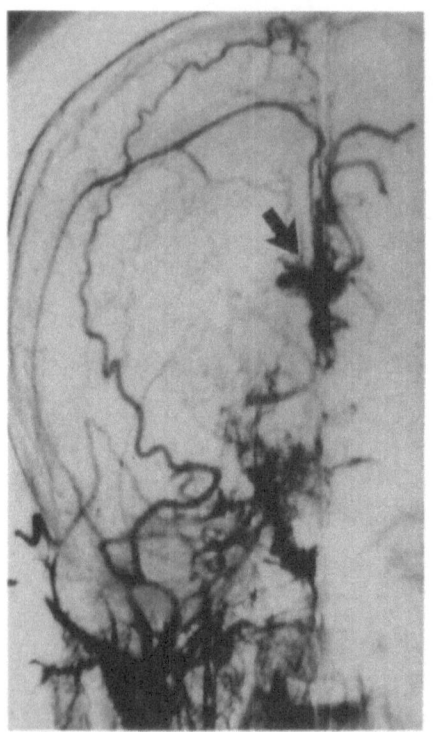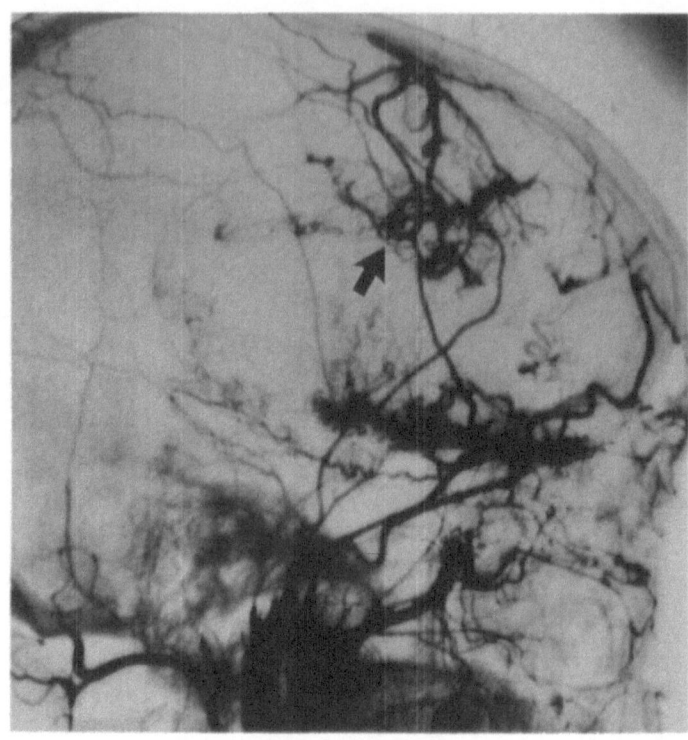

Figure 17.3. An advanced case (stage 6). Right carotid angiograms [AP (left) and lateral (right) views] show complete occlusion of the internal carotid artery, complete disappearance of basal moyamoya, and pial anastomosis of middle meningeal and superficial temporal arteries (vault moyamoya indicated by arrow).

Table 17.1. Angiographic staging of moyamoya disease.[12]

Stage	Characteristic
1	Narrowing of cartoid bifurcation
2	Beginning of moyamoya
3	Intensification of moyamoya
4	Minimization of moyamoya
5	Reduction of moyamoya
6	Disappearance of moyamoya

extension of the occlusive process to the anterior and middle cerebral arteries and development of leptomeningeal collaterals in association with intensification of the "moyamoya" formation (stage 3) (Fig. 17.1). In the later stages of the disease, there may be severe stenosis and/or complete occlusion of the internal carotid arteries, at which time the "moyamoya" vessels may be minimized (stages 4 and 5) (Figs. 17.9 and 17.10), and cerebral circulation may depend completely on leptomeningeal anastomoses when "moyamoya" vessels disappear (stage 6 with vault moyamoya) (Fig. 17.3). In some cases during the late stages of moyamoya disease, stenosis and/or occlusion of either the proximal or distal portion of the posterior cerebral artery has been reported to occur[21]. There have been few reports concerning chronological changes of the disease in adults[11].

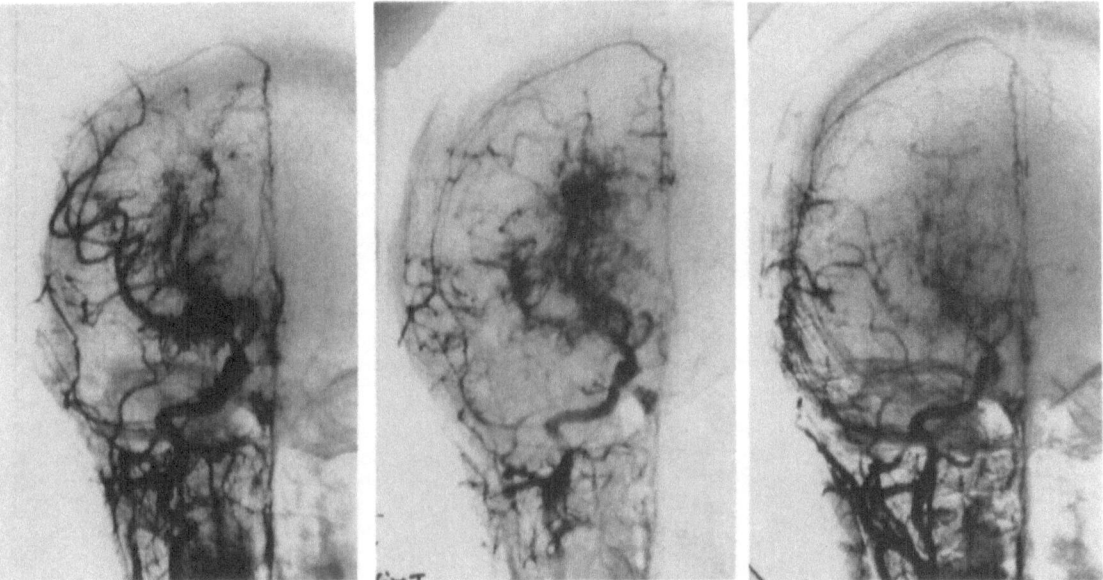

Figure 17.4. Angiograms illustrating rapid progression of moyamoya disease in a 5-year-old boy. *Left*: On admission, there is stenosis of terminal portion of the internal carotid artery and proximal portion of the middle cerebral artery the right. Note also the development of moyamoya vessels along the base of the brain (stage 2). *Center*: Six months after admission, one sees severe stenosis of the middle cerebral artery and increase in the basal moyamoya formation (stage 3). *Right*: Angiography performed 3 months after EDAS (8 months after onset) shows reduction in moyamoya vessels concomitant with revascularization of the middle cerebral artery

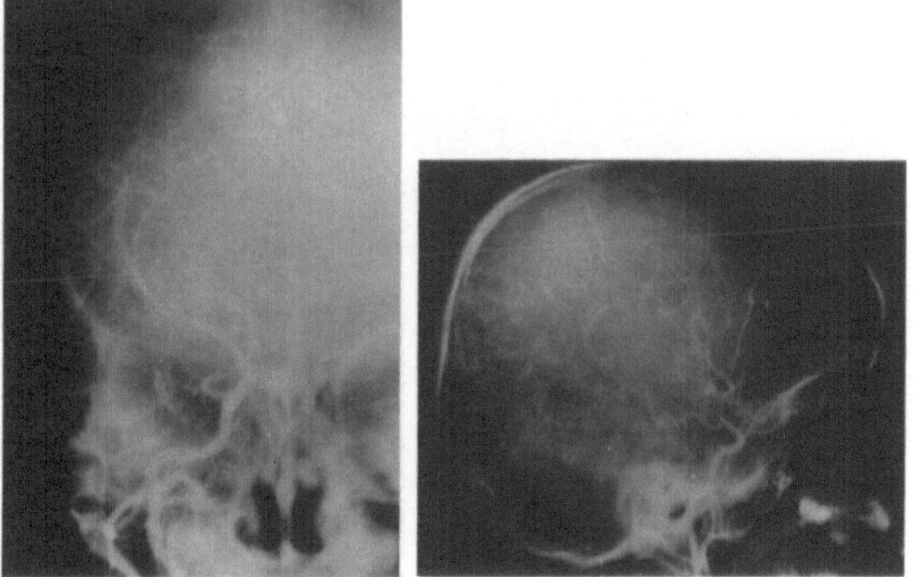

Figure 17.5. (A) Angiograms of a 3-year-old girl with moyamoya disease show early stages of moyamoya vessel development along the base of the brain (stage 2). (B) CT scans of the same patient 10 years after onset show multiple cerebral infarctions. (C) Angiograms before (top left, AP views; lower left, left lateral view, stage 6) and 3 months after (top right, AP view; lower right, left lateral view) EDAS. They show good revascularization in the areas including the posterior frontal and parietal lobes after surgery.

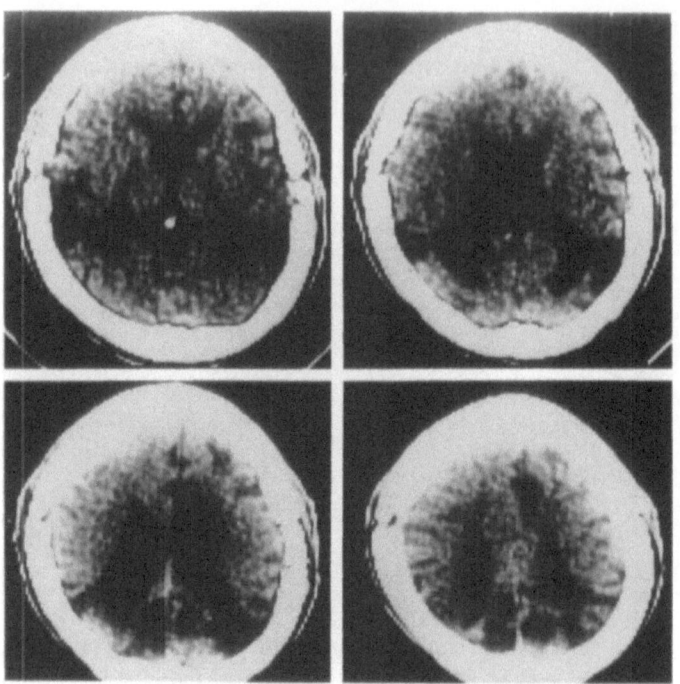

Figure 17.5B

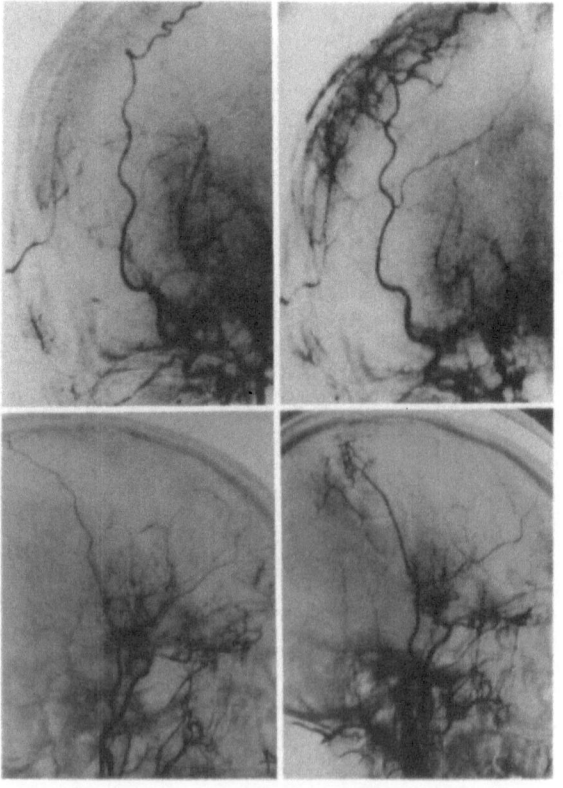

pre op.   Figure 17.5C   post op.

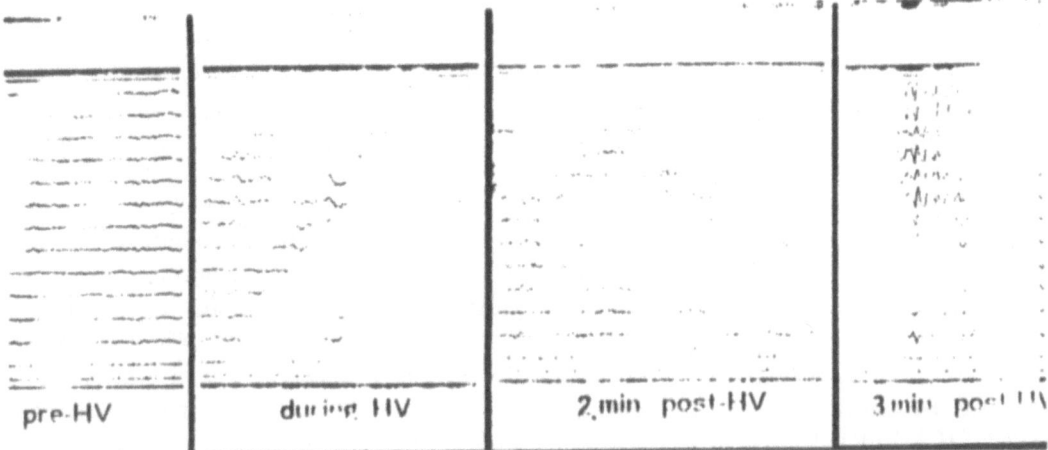

Figure 17.6. Electroencephalograms before, during, and after hyperventilation. pre-HV, Before hyperventilation; during HV, Build-up during hyperventilation; 2 min post-HV, regression of build-up 2 min after termination of hyperventilation; 3 min post-HV, rebuild-up 3 min after termination of hyperventilation.

Electroencephalographic (EEG) Features

EEG findings also are not uniform, depending on the stage of the disease. According to Kodama et al.[22], characteristic features of EEG findings in children include posterior slow, centrotemporal slow, "rebuild-up" after the cessation of hyperventilation, and sleep spindle depression. Posterior slow activity was observed mainly in EEGs recorded soon (mean, 10 months) after onset of the disease, slow activity in CT after a longer period (mean, 28 months), and diffuse low activity after far longer periods (mean, 56 months). Build-up after cessation of hyperventilation, referred to by the authors as *rebuild-up*, was reported in more than half the

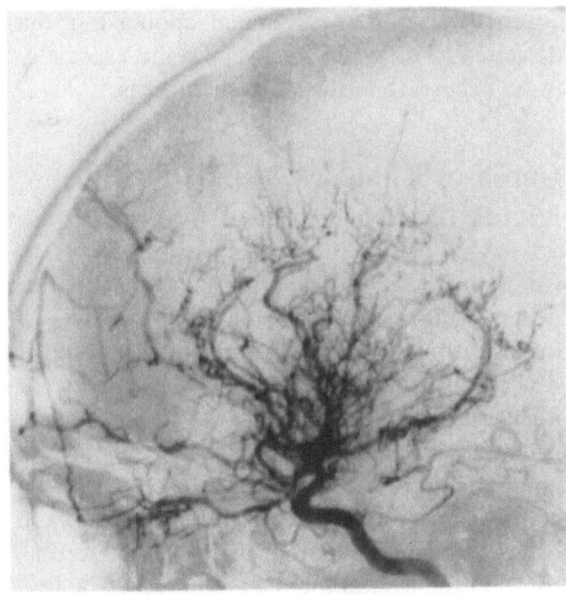
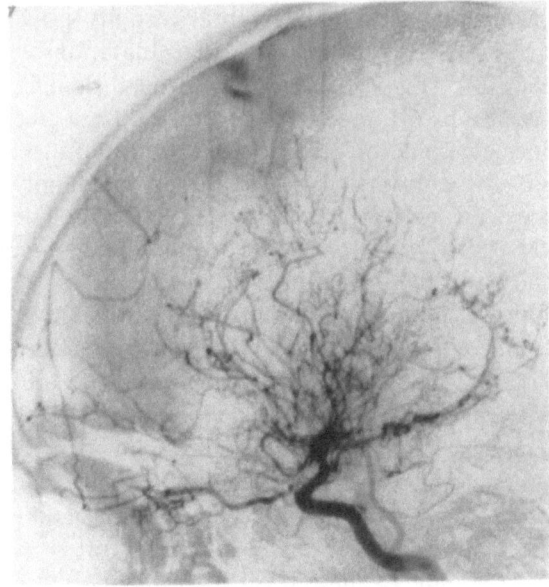

Figure 17.7. Left carotid angiograms (lateral view) before (left) and 3 min after termination of hyperventilation (right), at which time electroencephalogram indicated rebuild-up. Note marked reduction of moyamoya vessels and decrease in caliber of cerebral vessels.

cases with moyamoya disease (Fig. 17.6). In Japan, presently, it is well accepted that an EEG may be utilized as one of the screening tests for moyamoya disease where rebuild-up is considered to be diagnostic.

As illustrated in Fig 17.7, the simultaneous reduction of moyamoya and cortical vessels has been reported when angiography was performed after cessation of hyperventilation, at which time EEGs indicated build-up.[23] According to investigations involving peripheral blood gas analysis[24] and the measurement of cerebral blood flow (CBF) and cerebral metabolism rate of oxygen ($CMRO_2$) by positron emission tomography (PET)[25], build-up during hyperventilation and rebuild-up after hyperventilation ended were pathogenetically different. The build-up was thought to be due to ischemic hypoxia, and the rebuild-up to hypoxic hypoxia in addition to the preexisting ischemic hypoxia due to respiratory suppression after hyperventilation.

Neuroimaging Features

Computed tomography (CT) may reveal characteristic changes in the brain influenced by moyamoya disease. These include multiple low-density areas and cerebral atrophy associated with secondary ventricular dilatation on plain CT (Fig. 17.5B). The degree of changes revealed by CT appears to depend on the degree of stenosis and/or occlusion of the carotid fork, and the compensatory cerebral blood supply provided by the leptomeningeal collaterals. The low-density areas often are found bilaterally, and typically are multiple lesions in the brain. The gray and white matter of the frontal lobe are most frequently affected with progression of the disease, but similar lesions may extend into other parts of the brain, including the parietal, temporal, and occipital lobes. No low-density area may be observed in the basal ganglia, even when the presence of an abnormal netlike formation of vessels has been demonstrated by angiography. In addition, low-density areas also are not observed in the brainstem and cerebellum.[26–28]

Verification of carotid stenosis and/or occlu-

sion seldom is attained in CT with contrast enhancement. In the majority of cases, the main intracranial arteries are enhanced. It is unexpectedly common for moyamoya vessel not to be enhanced.[12] Takahashi et al., however, reported that curvilinear, tortuous densities due to small collateral vessels may be observed following the injection of contrast medium.[27] The foci of ischemia in the brain may be contrast enhanced when permeability of vessels in the ischemic area is increased[66] (Fig. 17.8). Needless to say, intracerebral, intraventricular, and subarachnoid hemorrhages may be detected as high-density areas by plain computed tomography.

Magnetic resonance imaging (MRI) may be considered useful for screening and follow-up examination of moyamoya disease, but not for diagnosis. Moyamoya vessels are visualized as multiple, small, round or torturous low-intensity areas extending from the suprasellar cistern to the basal ganglia in the majority of cases studied. MRI also reveals occlusive changes in the distal portion of the intracranial carotid artery and in the proximal portions of the anterior and middle cerebral arteries, collateral vessels (including arteries in the pericallosal area), and in some cases the presence of transdural leptomeningeal collaterals. MRI appears to be an improvement upon CT in the detection of ischemic cerebral lesions, especially those occurring in the watershed areas.[29–32]

Cerebral Blood Flow (CBF) and Metabolism

Changes in CBF and metabolism also appear to depend on the stages of the disease. In investigations of CBF in cases with moyamoya disease, utilizing either ^{133}Xe inhalation and/or injection, the mean CBF value in the hemisphere at rest has been reported to be low in comparison with control values. Although rCBF values in the posterior temporal and occipital regions were reported as being normal, those in the frontal lobes were found to be low. When hyperventilation was induced, however, an even reduction in regional CBF (rCBF) took place in all areas of the brain studied.[33,34]

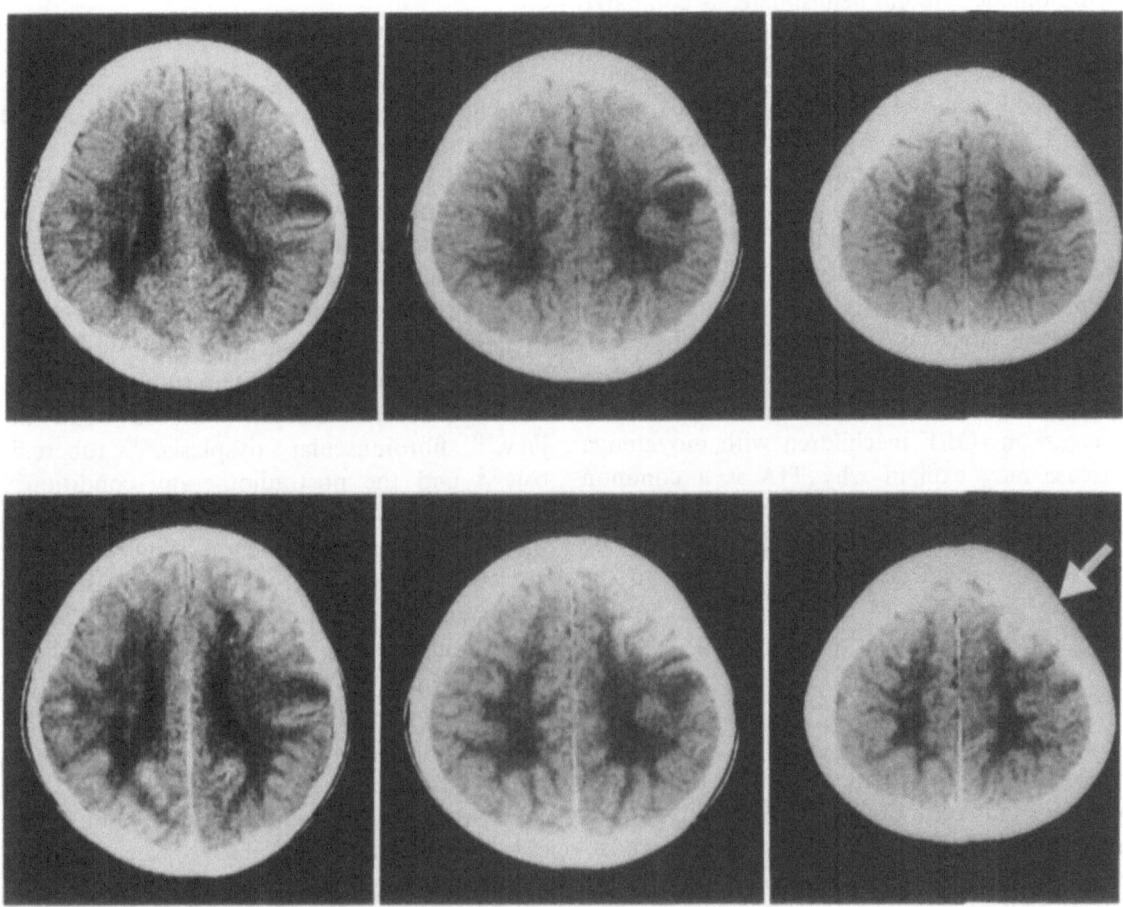

Figure 17.8. CT scans before (upper) and after (lower) contrast enhancement of 5-year-old boy admitted with TIA resulting in monoparesis of right upper extremity. Arrow indicates contrast enhancement of premotor area on the left side.

Intraoperative measurement of blood flow by means of the heat clearance method indicated that changes in the cortical surface blood flow appeared to depend on the severity of the carotid occlusion and the extent of development of ethmoidal and basal moyamoya vessel collateral blood flow.[35,36]

Changes in rCBF, regional cerebral metabolic rate of oxygen (rCMRO$_2$), regional oxygen extraction fraction (rOEF), and regional cerebral blood volume (rCBV) in cases of moyamoya disease have recently been reported by several investigators using positron emission tomography. According to Taki et al.,[37] rCBF in all gray and white matter, and basal ganglia, in subacute and chronic juvenile cases of moyamoya disease was within normal values. However, the calculated value of CBF/CBV as an index of perfusion pressure and reverse value of transit time was significantly reduced in the aforedescribed regions. In spite of the reduction of CBF/CBV, there was no significant increase in rOEF in these regions. They concluded that moyamoya disease of the ischemic type (subacute or chronic stage) appeared to be characterized by a mild decrease in perfusion pressure, dilated resistant vessels, and prolonged circulation time.[37] According to Tomura et al.,[37a] CBF and $CMRO_2$ were lower in the symptomatic cerebral hemisphere, as compared to the nonsymptomatic hemisphere. They found CBV in the lentiform nucleus to be significantly increased because of the presence of moyamoya vessels.[37a] Kuwabara et al.[38] reported a difference in cerebral hemodynamics and metabolism between children and adults: there was a more marked increase in rCBV in children than in adults, and rOEF was greater than control values in low-rCBF areas in children. There was never an increase in adults, in whom transit time was significantly prolonged relative to the control value. They speculated that an increase in rOEF in children with moyamoya disease may explain why TIA is a common symptom in this group.

The differences in the results obtained by various investigators appear to be due to the varying conditions of the individual cases of moyamoya disease they studied.

Pathology

Gross examination of cases in which infarctions occurred at different ages revealed stenosis and/or occlusion of the terminal portion of the internal carotid artery and of the proximal portions of the anterior and middle cerebral arteries.

Microscopic features of such stenotic changes have been reported to be characterized by eccentric proliferation of the connective tissue of the intima, and splitting and duplication of the internal elastic lamina.

Moyamoya vessels contributed by perforating arteries demonstrate various histologic lesions. Ruptured perforating arteries indicate dilatation, fibrin deposits in the walls, fragmented elastic laminae, and attenuated media. Non-ruptured perforating arteries are affected by microaneurysm formations, focal fibrin deposits, and marked attenuation of the wall thickness with diminution of the elastic lamina. Fundamental statistics of arteries of the vertebrobasilar system reportedly are preserved, but hypertrophy of the media, probably due to hemodynamic changes associated with progress of the disease, have been noted.[15,39-41]

Moyamoya Syndrome, Moyamoya Phenomenon, and "Unilateral" Moyamoya Disease

As bilateral stenosis and/or occlusion of the carotid bifurcation are diagnostic criteria for moyamoya disease of unknown etiology, those cases of unknown etiology in which moyamoya vessels exist unilaterally, and which are similar to moyamoya *disease*, usually are referred to as moyamoya *syndrome*, moyamoya *phenomenon*, or *unilateral* moyamoya.[42-46] Occlusion of the middle cerebral artery,[45] brain tumors,[47,48] von Recklinghausen's disease,[49] closed head injury,[50] fibromuscular dysplasia,[51] tuberculosis,[52] and the postradiotherapy condition[53] have been reported as causative factors inducing the moyamoya phenomenon. Matsushima et al.[43] recently reported two pediatric cases with occlusion of the ipsilateral internal carotid artery and posterior cerebral arteries associated with moyamoya vessels. In both cases, the etiology of the disease was not detected. The data obtained by various examinations, including positron emission tomography, in these cases were found similar to those obtained in cases of *bilateral* moyamoya disease. Consequently, they concluded that this suggested the presence of a unilateral disease lacking pathological progression to the contralateral side, although they also reported a case of moyamoya disease with progressive unilateral-to-bilateral involvement.[44]

Treatment

In a study conducted by Kurokawa et al.[54] of the prognosis of 27 children with moyamoya disease followed up for periods ranging from 4 to 15 years after onset of the disease, intellectual deterioration and neurological deficits reportedly increased with time. The outcome included no sequelae in 19% of the patients, occasional TIAs or headache alone in 33%, mild intellectual and/or motor impairment in 26%, requirement for special schooling or care by parents or institution after the age of 10 in 11%, continuous 24-hr care in 7%, and death in 3%. It was pointed out that poor prognosis was correlated with age at early onset and hypertensions. These observations strongly suggest that early revascularization of the ischemic brain associated with this disease is mandatory.

In medical therapy for moyamoya disease, vasodilators, antiplatelet agents, corticosteroids, and low-molecular-weight dextran have been used, but their efficacy is not known. Various surgical therapies have been attempted for patients with recurrent or progressive focal ischemia. Fixation of dura to the surface of the brain by Tsubokawa et al.,[55] and removal of the cervical sympathetic nerve by Suzuki et al.,[56] were pioneer works, but these procedures have not been widely accepted. Karasawa et al.[57-59] reported their experiences with surgical treatment of 17 patients in whom a series of 23 superficial temporal artery–middle cerebral artery (STA-MCA) anastomoses and 7 encephalo-myosynangiosis (EMS) (in which the temporal muscle is transpositioned onto the brain surface of the affected side) anastomoses were performed. Excellent outcomes were achieved with recovery of neurological deficits and disappearance of TIAs in nine cases, and good outcome with improvement of neurological deficits and reduction of TIAs in the remaining cases.

Krayenbuhl[9] and Amine et al.[60] then each, independently, reported a case of moyamoya disease also treated by STA-MCA anastomosis with clinical and angiographic improvement. Thereafter, omental transplantation,[61] encephalo-duro-arterior-synangiosis (EDAS), in which the superficial temporal artery is transpositioned together with galea aponeurotica to the brain surface,[62] encephalo-galeo-synangiosis,[63] and a combination of STA-MCA anastomosis and indirect revascularization techniques as described above[64] are now widely used to revascularize the ischemic brain.

STA-MCA anastomosis is seldom performed for infants because of the technical difficulty in anastomosing small arteries, and EMS or EDAS, in particular, are preferred.[65,66] The former procedure has a disadvantage in that spontaneous development of leptomeningeal anastomosis may be disturbed by an intraoperative incision of the superficial temporal artery as well as the dura mater, which cannot be avoided in performing the surgery[65].

According to Matsushima et al.,[67] 70 to 80% of patients treated with any of the indirect revascularization techniques (EMS, EDAS, or a combination of both), were found, in postoperative angiograms, to have good revascularization and disappearance of such clinical symptoms as TIA, reversible ischemic neurological deficits, and/or involuntary movements. In order to elucidate whether EDAS or EMS was the more effective procedure in terms of revascularization of the ischemic brain, Fujita et al.[68] treated seven patients in whom EDAS was performed on one side and EMS on the other. Postoperative angiography and rCBF studies revealed more revascularization from the external carotid artery on the EDAS side. On the basis of these results, they concluded that EDAS was the more effective technique for indirect EC-IC anastomosis in moyamoya disease. Although it is generally accepted at present that EDAS is the best therapy for pediatric cases of moyamoya disease,[65,66,69-71] Miyamoto et al. suggested that STA-MCA anastomosis, with or without additional indirect revascularization procedures, is necessary for prevention of stroke in cases refractory to indirect nonanastomotic revascularization as the initial treatment.[72]

We have treated 10 pediatric and 8 adult cases of moyamoya disease during the past 10 years, performing the EDAS surgical technique, with and without the Matsushima modification. Early in our experience, we treated 10 cases using Matsushima's oriiginal EDAS procedure, in which apposition of the posterior branch of the superficial temporal artery was extended onto the affected side of the brain surface. Postoperative angiography at 3 months revealed that, even though adequate revascularization could be achieved in the posterior areas frontal and parietal areas of the frontal and revascularization in the prefrontal areas was comparatively poor (Fig. 17.9). In consideration of these observations regarding our patients, and the reports of other investigators that the value of rCBF in the anterior portion of the frontal area tended to be lower than that in any other part of the brain before[33] and after revascularization procedures,[34] in the remaining seven cases to which EDAS was applied apposition of the

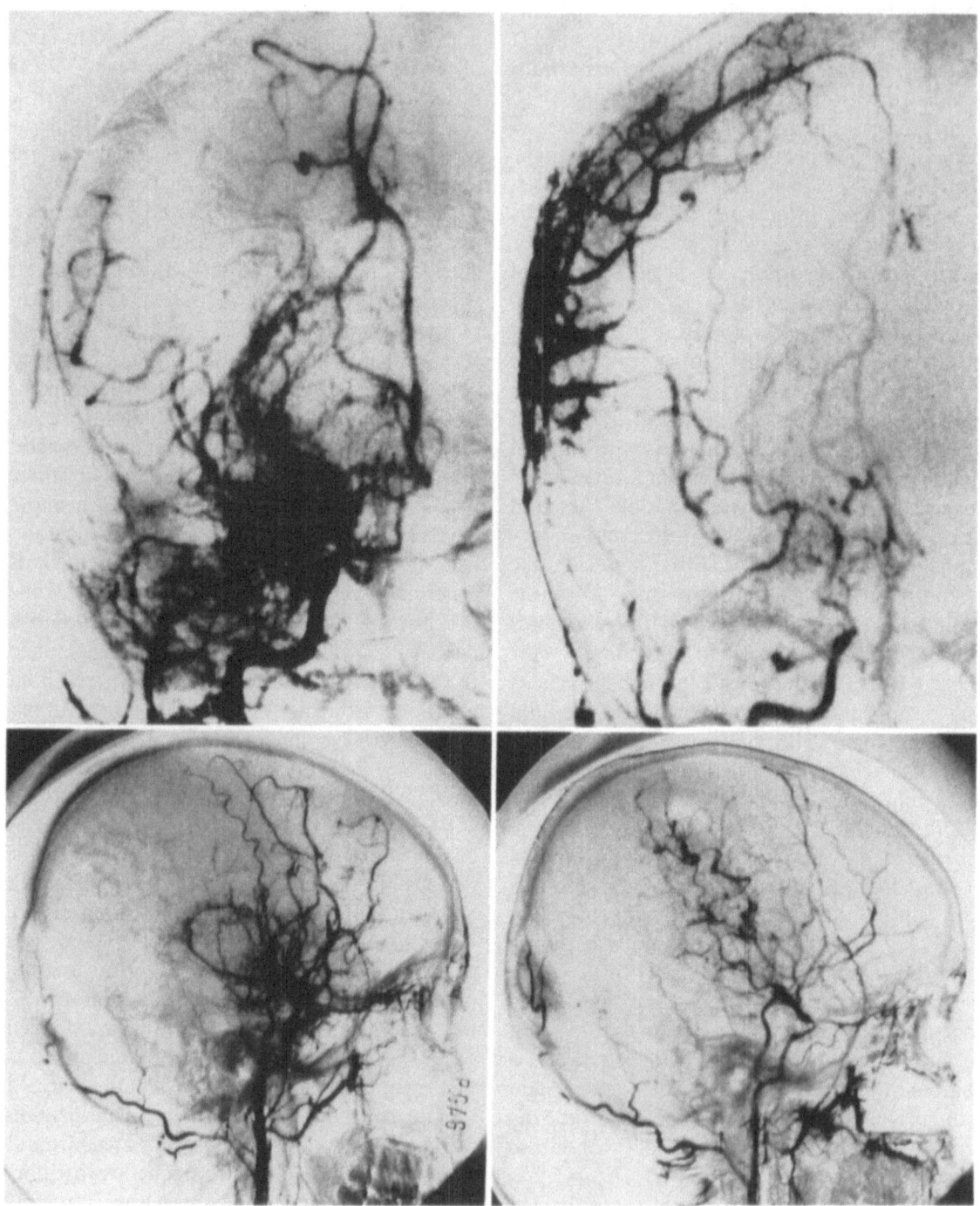

Figure 17.9. Angiograms before (top left, AP view; lower left, right lateral view, stage 4) and 3 months after (top right, AP view; lower right, right lateral view) EDAS. They show marked revascularization in the posterior frontal and anterior parietal areas and lack of same in the right prefrontal area.

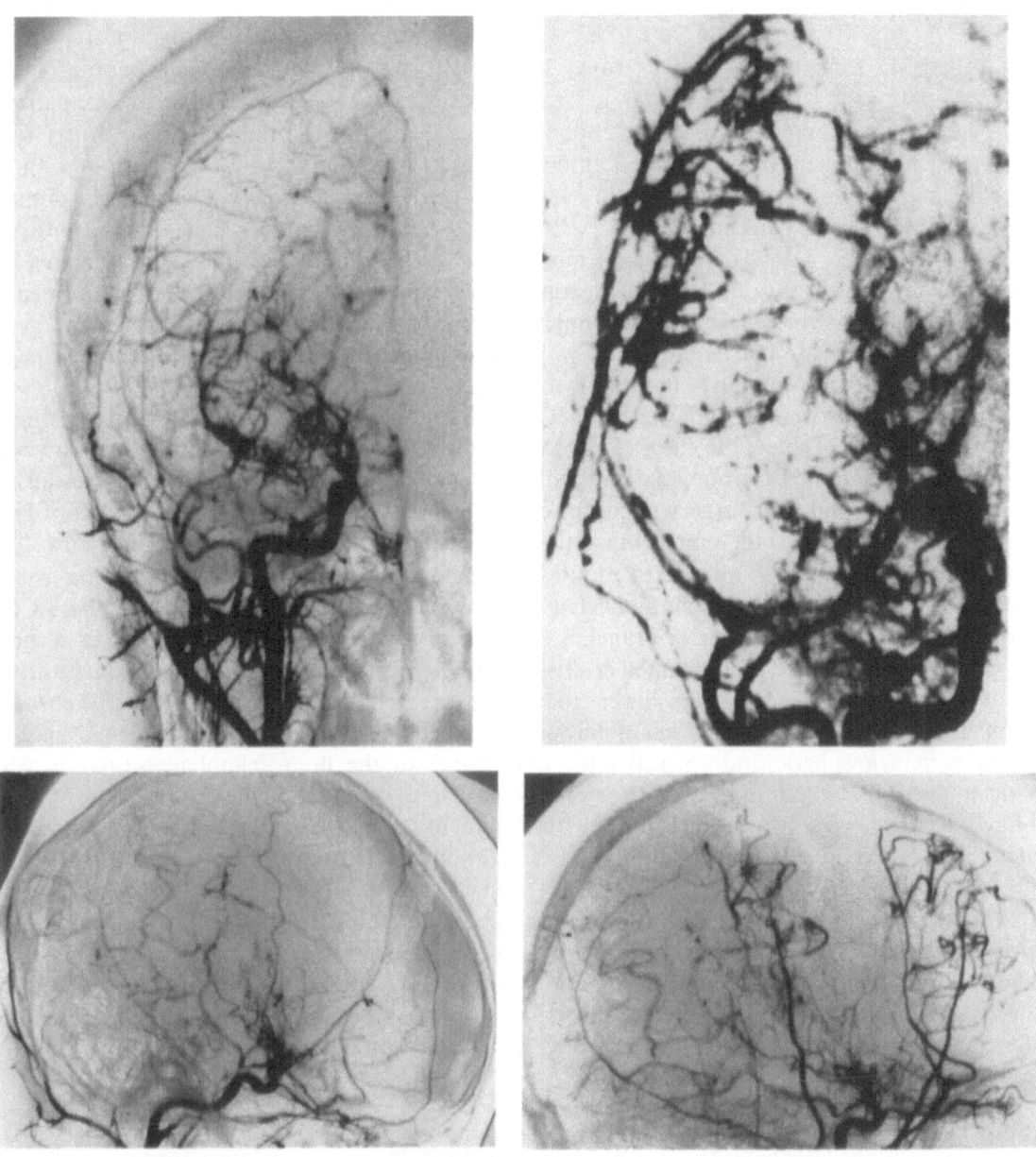

Figure 17.10. Angiograms before (top left, AP view; lower left, right lateral view, stage 5) and 3 months after (top right, AP view; lower right, right lateral view) EDAS, using the modification in which the anterior branch of the superficial temporal artery was appositioned on the surface of the prefrontal area. They show marked revascularization in prefrontal and other areas of the brain.

anterior branch of the superficial temporal artery was additionally extended to the prefrontal area. In these cases, good revascularization in the prefrontal as well as other areas of the brain was achieved (Fig. 17.10). Clinical improvement and excellent revascularization were thus obtained with utilization of the EDAS procedure in all cases of patients under the age of 40, including severely affected cases. Revascularization usually was poor in patients older than 40, in our experience.

Prognosis

Using the EMS technique, Ishii[73,74] treated 20 children with moyamoya disease. In the preoperative stage, a more marked reduction in the intelligence quotient (IQ) was found among the older patients, and the patients with low IQs in general showed, by means of the ^{133}Xe inhalation method, a tendency toward more marked depression of mean CBF. Postoperatively, a significant improvement of IQ was noted in 10, no change in 3, and deterioration in 2 cases. An increase in mean CBF, thought to be correlated with improvement of the patients' IQ, also was noted. To evaluate the effect of EDAS, Suzuki et al.[75] examined 21 young patients with the disease before and after surgery by means of angiography and the cold xenon inhalation method. Carotid stenosis continued to progress after EDAS, although angiography indicated a marked increase in the number of branches of the middle cerebral artery via implanted arteries. Preoperative cortical CBF was lower than normal. Postoperatively, there were significant increases in hemispheric and cortical CBF in patients with TIA but not in those with cerebral infarction. The increase in cortical flow at the site of EDAS was already noted within 2 weeks after surgery.

Moritake et al.[76] reported a follow-up investigation of 51 moyamoya disease patients who did/did not undergo revascularization surgery. Seven of 16 patients with clinical onset after age 16 suffered intracranial bleeding, resulting in the death of 2 of them. In contrast, no pediatric patient suffered bleeding or death. Young patients below the age of 5 at the time of clinical onset tended to suffer poor daily living activity (DLA) at the time of hospital admission, and were found to remain unchanged in terms of DLA at the time of follow-up assessment if they had not been treated by revascularization surgery. The majority of the remaining young patients who had been treated with revascularization procedures, including STA-MCA anastomosis, EMS, and/or omentum transplantation, were found to have clinical improvement in terms of DLA at the time of follow-up assessment. Worthy of note is that one case treated by surgery developed malignant hyperthermia caused by the anesthetic procedure, which exacerbated the postoperative course and resulted in deterioration of the patient's DLA[77]. Twelve of 14 pediatric patients older than 5 at the time of clinical onset were found to have improved either with or without revascularization surgery. On the basis of these observations, the authors stated that reconstructive surgery improves the clinical course of moyamoya disease patients when performed at an early stage of the disease, especially in the case of patients under 5 at the time of clinical onset.

Sato et al.[26] reported a follow-up assessment of CBF in moyamoya disease patients, who were treated either by EDAS or EMS, by means of dynamic ranging using N-isopropyl-p[^{123}I]iodoamphetamine–single photon emission CT. It was found that revascularization of the frontal lobe was poor, which was evidenced by a CBF image of a low-perfusion state with a noninfarcted ischemic pattern demonstrated in the same region. They speculated that this chronic, low-perfusion state of the frontal lobe may be related to the poor school performance, with impaired cognitive function of 70% of their patients after the revascularization procedure, although the disappearance of TIA in all cases and excellent DLA of 62% of their patients had been noted. They suggested that additional revascularization procedures may be required for such patients. These observations appear to support the modified EDAS procedure as described by Shimoji et al.[71]

References

1. Shimizu K, Takeuchi K: Dysplasia of the bilateral internal carotid arteries. Oral presentation at the 14th meeting of the Japan Neurosurgical Society, Wakayama, 1955.
2. Suzuki J, Takaku A: Cerebrovascular moyamoya disease. Disease showing abnormal net-like vessels in base of brain. Arch Neurol 20:288–299, 1969.
3. Kudo T: Juvenile occlusion of the circle of Willis. Clin Neurology 5:607–627, 1965.
4. Nishimoto A, Takeuchi S: Abnormal cerebrovascular network related to the internal carotid arteries. J Neurosurg 29:255–260, 1968.

5. Suzuki J, Takaku A, Asahi M, Kowada M: Disease showing the "Fibrille"-like vessels at the base of brain. No To Shinkei 17:767–776, 1965.

6. Takeuchi K, Shimizu K: Hypoplasia of the bilateral internal carotid arteries. No To Shinkei 9:37–43, 1957.

7. Kudo T: Spontaneous occlusion of the circle of Wills. A disease apparently confined to Japanese. Neurology 18:485–496, 1968.

8. Weidner W, Hanafee W, Markham CH: Intracranial collateral circulation via leptomeningeal and rate mirabile anastomosis. Neurology 15:39–48, 1965.

9. Krayenbuhl HA: The moyamoya syndrome and neurosurgeon. Surg Neurol 4:353–360, 1975.

10. Taveras JM: Multiple progressive intracranial occlusions: A syndrome of children and young adults. AJR 106:235–268, 1969.

11. Nishimoto A: Moyamoya disease. Neurol Med Chir 19:221–228, 1979.

12. Suzuki J, Kodama N: Moyamoya disease. A review. Stroke 14:104–109, 1983.

13. Adams HP Jr, Kassell NF, Wisoff HS, Drake CG: Intracranial saccular aneurysm and moyamoya disease. Stroke 10:174–179, 1979.

14. Nagamine Y, Takahashi S, Sonobe M: Multiple intracranial aneurysms associated with moyamoya disease. J Neurosurg 54:673–676, 1981.

15. Yamashita M, Oka K, Tanaka K: Histopathology of the brain Ovascular network in moyamoya disease. Stroke 14:50-58, 1983.

16. Fukuyama Y: Clinical and cerebral angiographic evolutions of idiopathic progress occlusive disease of the circle of Willis ("moyamoya" disease) in children. Brain Dev 7:21–37, 1985.

17. Kitahara T, Ariga N, Yamaura A, Makino H, Maki Y: Familial occurrence of moyamoya disease: Report of three Japanese families. J Neurol Neurosurg Psychiatry, 42:208–214, 1979.

18. Kitahara T, Okumura K, Semba A, Yamaura A, Makino H: Genetic and immunologic analysis on moyamoya. J Neurol Neurosurg Psychiatry 45:1048–1053, 1982.

19. Nishimoto A, Takeuchi S: Moyamoya Disease. In: Vinken PJ, Bruyn GW (eds.) Handbook of Clinical Neurology. American Elsevier Publishing Company, New York, 1972, pp 352–382.

20. Miyamoto S, Kikuchi H, Karasawa J, Nagata I, Ikota T, Takeuchi S: Study of the posterior circulation in moyamoya disease. Clinical and Neuroradiological evaluation. J Neurosurg 61:1032–1037, 1984.

21. Sato S, Shibuya H, Matsushima Y, Suzuki S: Analysis of the angiographic findings in cases of childhood moyamoya disease. Neuroradiology 30:111–119, 1988.

22. Kodama N, Aoki Y, Hiraga H, Wada T, Suzuki J: Electroencephalographic findings in children with moyamoya disease. Arch Neurol 36:16–19, 1979.

23. Takahashi A, Fujiwara S, Suzuki J: Cerebral angiography following hyperventilation in moyamoya disease. In reference to the "re-build up" phenomenon on EEG. No Shinkei Geka 13:255–264, 1985.

24. Ohyama H, Niizuma H, Fujiwara S, Suzuki J: EEG findings in moyamoya disease in children with special reference to the genesis of "re-build" up. No Shinkei Geka 13:727–733, 1985.

25. Kameyama M, Shirane R, Tsurumi Y, Takahashi A, Fujiwara S, Suzuki J, Ito M, Ido T: Evaluation of cerebral blood flow and metabolism in childhood moyamoya disease. An investigation into "re-build-up" on EEG by positron CT. Childs Nerv Syst 2:130–133, 1986.

26. Sato H, Sato N, Tamaki N, Matsumoto S: Chronic low-perfusion state in children with moyamoya disease following revascularization. Childs Nerv Syst 6:166–171, 1990.

27. Takahashi M, Miyauchi T, Kowada M: Computed tomography of moyamoya disease: Demonstration of occluded arteries and collateral vessels as important diagnostic signs. Radiology 134:671–676, 1980.

28. Takeuchi S, Kobayashi K, Tsuchida T, Imamura H, Tanaka R, Ito J: Computed tomography in moyamoya disease. J Comput Assist Tomogr 6:24–32, 1982.

29. Bruno A, Yuh WTC, Biller J, et al: Magnetic resonance imaging in young adults with cerebral infarction due to moyamoya. Arch Neurol 45:303–306, 1988.

30. Fujisawa I, Asato R, Mishimura K, Kogashi K, Itoh K, et al: Moyamoya disease. MR imaging. Radiology 164:103–105, 1987.

31. Fujita K, Shirakuni T, Kojima N, Matsumoto S: Magnetic resonance imaging. No Shinkei Geka 14:324–330, 1986.

32. Rolak LA, Rokey R: Magnetic resonance imaging in moyamoya disease. J Child Neurol 1:67–70, 1986.

33. Ogawa A, Nakamura N, Sakurai Y, Kayama T, Wada T, Suzuki J: Cerebral blood flow in moyamoya disease. No To Shinkei 39:199–203, 1987.

34. Takeuchi S, Tanaka R, Ishii R, Tsuchida T, Kobayashi K, Arai H: Cerebral hemodynamics in patients with moyamoya disease. A study of

regional cerebral blood flow by the ^{133}Xe inhalation method. Surg-Neurol 23:468–474, 1985.

35. Nakao K, Yamada K, Hayakawa T, Tagawa T, Yoshimine T, Ushio Y, Mogami H: Intraoperative measurement of cortical blood flow and its CO_2 response in childhood moyamoya disease. Neurosurgery 21:509–14, 1987.

36. Tatemichi TK, Prohovink I, Mohr JP, Correll JW, Quest DO, Jarvis I: Reduced hypercapnic vasoreactivity in moyamoya disease. Neurology 38:1575–1581, 1988.

37. Taki W, Yonekawa Y, Kobayashi A, Ishikawa M, Kikuchi H, Nishizawa S, Senda M, Yonekawa Y, Fukuyama H, Harada K, et al: Cerebral circulation and oxygen metabolism in moyamoya disease of ischemic type in children. Childs Nerv Syst 4:259–262, 1988.

37a. Tomura N, Kanno I, Shishido F, Higano S, Fujita H, Inugami A, Tabata K, Uemura K, Sayama I, Yasui N: Vascular responses in cerebrovascular "Moyamoya" disease evaluated by positron emission tomography. No To Shinkei 41:895–904, 1989.

38. Kuwabara Y, Ichiya Y, Otsuka M, Tahara T, Gunasekera R, Hasuo K, Masuda K, Matsushima T, Fukui M: Cerebral hemodynamic change in the child and the adult with moyamoya disease. Stroke 21:272–277, 1990.

39. Nishimoto A, Takeuchi S: Moyamoya Disease. In: Vinken PJ, Bruyn GW (eds.) Handbook of Clinical Neurology, American Elsevier Publishing Company, New York, 1972, pp 352–383.

40. Ohtoh T, Iwasaki Y, Namiki T, Nakamura K, Sakurai Y, Ogawa A, Wada T: Hemodynamic characteristics of the vertebrobasilar system in moyamoya disease. A histometric study. HumPathol 19:465–470, 1988.

41. Oka K, Yamashita M, Sadoshima S, Tanaka K: Cerebral hemorrhage in moyamoya disease at autopsy. Virchows Arch Pathol Anat 392:247–261, 1981.

42. Gomez CR, Hogan PA: Unilateral Moyamoya disease in an adult. A case history. Angiology 38:342–346, 1987.

43. Matsushima T, Fukui M, Fujii K, Fujiwara S, Nagata S, Kitamura K, Kuwabara Y: Two pediatric cases with occlusions of the ipsilateral internal carotid and posterior cerebral arteries associated with moyamoya vessels. "Unilateral" moyamoya disease. Surg Neurol 33:276–280, 1990.

44. Matsushima T, Take S, Fujii K, Fukui M, Hasuo K, Kuwabara Y, Kitamura K: A case of

moyamoya disease with progressive involvement from unilateral to bilateral. Surg Neurol 30:471–475, 1988.

45. Takeuchi K: Moyamoya syndrome and Moyamoya disease. No To Shinkei 30:1183–1191, 1978.

46. Wilms G, Marchal G, Van Fraeyenhoven L, Demaerel P, Casaer P, Van Elderen S, Baert AL: Unilateral moyamoya disease. MRI findings. Neuroradiology 31:442, 1989.

47. Ishikawa M, Handa H, Mori K, Matsuda I: Moyamoya vessels on the tumor in the seller region. Arch Jap Chir 48:639–644, 1979.

48. Tsuji N, Kuriyama T, Iwamoto M, Shizuki K: Moyamoya disease associated with craniopharyngioma. Surg Neurol 21:588–592, 1984.

49. Hilar SK, Solomon GE, Gold AP, Carter S: Primary cerebral arterial occlusive disease in children. Part II. Neurocutaneous syndromes. Radiology 99:87–94, 1974.

50. Yashon D, Johnson A B, Jane JA: Bilateral internal carotid artery occlusion secondary to closed head injuries. J Neurol Neurosurg Psychiatry 27:547–552, 1964.

51. Pilz P: Fibromuscular dysplasia and multiple dissecting aneurysms of intracranial arteries. A further cause of moyamoya syndrome. Stroke 7:393–398, 1976.

52. Bingham WFB, Beguin EA, Ramirez-Lassepas: Moyamoya disease in pregnancy. Wis Med J 79:21–25, 1980.

53. Rajakulasingam K, Cerullo LJ, Raimondi AJ: Childhood moyamoya syndrome. Childs Brain 5:467–475, 1979.

54. Kurokawa T, Tomita S, Ueda K, Narazaki O, Hanai T, Hasuo K, Matsushima T, Kitamura K: Prognosis of occlusive disease of the circle of Willis (moyamoya disease) in children. Pediatr Neurol 1:274–277, 1985.

55. Tsubokawa T, Kikuchi M, Asano S, Itoh H, Urabe M: Surgical treatment for intracranial thrombosis. Case report of "Durapexia". Neurol Med Chir 6:428–429, 1964.

56. Suzuki J, Takaku A, Kodama N, Sato S: An attempt to treat cerebrovascular moyamoya disease in children. Childs Brain. 1:193–206, 1975.

57. Karasawa J, Kikuchi H, Furuse S: A surgical treatment of "moyamoya" disease "encephalomyo-synangiosis". Neurol Med Chir 17:30–37, 1977.

58. Karasawa J, Kikuchi H, Furuse S, Kawamura J, Sasaki T: Treatment of moyamoya disease with STA-MCA anastomosis. J Neurosurg 49:679–688, 1978.

59. Takeuchi S, Kikuchi H, Karasawa J, Yamagata S, Nagata I: Regional cortical flow during extra-intracranial bypass surgery in young patients with moyamoya disease. Neuro Med Chir 29:10–14, 1989.

60. Amine ARC, Moody RA, Meeks W: Bilateral temporal middle cerebral artery anastomosis for moyamoya syndrome. Surg Neurol 8:3–6, 1977.

61. Karasawa J, Kikuchi H, Kawamura J, Sakaki T: Intracranial transplantation of the omentum for cerebrovascular moyamoya disease. A two year follow-up study. Surg Neurol 14:444–449, 1980.

62. Matsushima Y, Fukai N, Tanaka K, Tsuruoka S, Inaba Y, Aoyagi M, Ohno K: A new surgical treatment of moyamoya disease in children. A preliminary report. Surg Neurol 15:313–320, 1981.

63. Ichikawa A, Tanaka R, Takeuchi S, Koike T, Ishii R: Reconstructive vascular surgery in children with moyamoya disease. Neurol Med Chir 29:106–112, 1989.

64. Nakagawa Y, Gotoh H, Shimoyama M, Ohtsuka K, Mabuchi S, Sawamura Y, Abe H, Tsuru M: Reconstructive operation for moyamoya disease. Surgical indication for the hemorrhagic type, and preferable operative methods. Neurol Med Chir 23:464–470, 1983.

65. Matsushima Y, Inaha Y: Moyamoya disease in children and its surgical treatment. The introduction of a new surgical procedure and its follow up angiograms. Childs Brain 11:155–170, 1984.

66. Olds MV, Griebel RW, Hoffman HJ, Craven M, Chuang S, Schutz H: The surgical treatment of childhood moyamoya disease. J Neurosurg 66:675–680, 1987.

67. Matsushima T, Fujiwara S, Nagata S, Fujii K, Fukui M, Kitamura K, Hasuo K: Surgical treatment for paediatric patients with moyamoya disease by indirect revascularization procedures (EDAS, EMS, EMAS). Acta Neurochir 98:135–140, 1989.

68. Fujita K, Tamaki N, Matsumoto S: Surgical treatment of moyamoya disease in children: which is more effective procedure. DEAS or EMS? Childs Nerv Syst 2:134–138, 1986.

69. Eller TW, Pasternak JF: Revascularization for moyamoya disease. Five-year follow-up. Surg Neurol 28:463–467, 1987.

70. Matsushima Y, Inaba Y: The specificity of the collaterals to the brain through the study and treatment of moyamoya disease. Stroke 17:117–122, 1986.

71. Shimoji T, Sato K, Ito M: Cerebral revascularization for moyamoya disease. Usefulness of EDAS Nervous System in Children. 15:161–168, 1990.

72. Miyamoto S, Kikuchi H, Karasawa J, Nagata I, Yamazoe N, Akiyama Y: Pitfalls in the surgical treatment of moyamoya disease Operative techniques for refractory cases. J Neurosurg 68:537–543, 1973.

73. Ishii R, Takeuchi S, Kobayashi K, Tanaka R: Intelligence in children with moyamoya disease. Evaluation after surgical treatments with special reference to changes in cerebral blood flow. Stroke 15:873–877, 1984.

74. Takeuchi S, Tsuchida T, Kobayashi K, Fukuda M, Ishii R, Tanaka R, Ito J: Treatment of moyamoya disease by temporal muscle graft encephalo myo synangiosis. Childs Brain 10:1–15, 1983.

75. Suzuki R, Matsushima Y, Takada Y, Nariai T, Wakabayashi S, Tone O: Changes in cerebral hemodynamics following encephalo-duro-arterio-synangiosis (EDAS). In young patients with moyamoya disease. Surg Neurol 31:343–349, 1989.

76. Moritake K, Handa H, Yonekawa Y, Taki W, Okuno T: Follow-up study on the relationship between age at onset of illness and outcome in patients with moyamoya disease. No Shinkei Geka 14:957–963, 1986.

77. Bingham RM, Wilkinson DJ: Anaesthetic management in moyamoya disease. Anaesthesia 40:1198–1202 (68), 1985.

CHAPTER 18

Acute Hemiplegia and Migraine

W. Isler

Migraine probably represents the most frequent condition in acute transient nontraumatic hemiplegia in the young age group. Hemiplegic migraine is a complex form of migraine characterized by the sudden onset of hemiparesis. Associated symptoms may include unilateral sensory loss and aphasia. Contralateral hemicranial, bilateral diffuse, or rarely ipsilateral headache usually follows but commonly precedes the neurological deficit. Other symptoms such as nausea and/or vomiting are common. The natural history of the migrainous hemisyndrome is usually benign, but permanent neurological sequelae may occur secondary to cerebral infarction.

Definitions

> *Common migraine* migraine without neurological aura
> *Classical migraine*: migraine with visual (eventual sensory) aura
> *Complex migraine*: migraine with neurological aura (sensory, motor, aphasia)
> *Complicated migraine*: neurological deficit prolonged beyond duration of headache

There is general agreement regarding the inherited predisposition of migraine. The mode of inheritance is uncertain; it is probably multifactorial, involving several genes.[1,2] A positive family history is reported in 40 to 90%.[3-7] The prevalence of migraine in general childhood populations is documented in only a few studies. Under the age of 10 years, 2.5 to 3% have been found, with a slight preponderance in

boys. In the 13 to 15-year age group, frequency is reported to be 4 to 8% in boys and 6.5 to 15% in girls.[3,8,9] Another study, ascertaining the prevalence on less strict migraine criteria, reports higher figures.[10]

The frequency of hemiplegic migraine in children is not precisely known, varying from 5 to 30% in general.[6,7,11-14] The wide range in these figures may be explained by the use of more extensive or more restrictive definitions of hemiplegic migraine (i.e., inclusion or exclusion of unilateral sensory symptoms in the absence of motor involvement) and/or by selective referral of the investigated patients.

Hemiplegic Migraine

The age of onset is most often in adolescence, but numerous reports concern children older than 10 years.

In the great majority of cases the unilateral neurological signs and symptoms occur as a manifestation of the aura and they are confined to this phase of the migraine attack. It has been customary to refer to this generally benign and relatively common type of hemisyndrome confined to the aura as *type I*.[7,15-17] This is in contrast to the less common but more serious group referred to as *type II*. In this variety, hemiparesis continues into the headache phase or develops during the period of headache. The motor hemisyndrome and/or aphasia may persist well after the headache has subsided and may last for a prolonged time span (several days).[7,11,15,17]

It is characteristic for the hemiplegic migraine attack to begin with sensory symptoms. In about half of the patients initial visual symptoms in the ipsilateral field of vision (scintillating or simple scotomata, hemianopia) precede unilateral sensory symptoms (numbness, tingling). Remarkably, these paresthesias evolve over a period of several minutes in a gradual spread over the face, arm and leg, most often starting in the hand and then extending to the leg. In about half of the reported children with *hemiplegic migraine* the neurological symptoms are only sensory, sometimes combined with aphasia but without motor deficits. Unilateral motor symptoms follow, but never precede, the sensory hemisyndrome, with slow progression of weakness in the arm and leg. Typically, the hemiparesis is most accentuated in the hand or arm and often confined to the upper extremity. Facial palsy is rarely reported. Dysarthria and/or aphasia (receptive or expressive) accompanies the neurological deficit in more than half of the patients. Impaired consciousness, varying in degree frequently accompanies the hemiplegic migraine attack. The neurological deficit confined to the aura (type I) rarely lasts more than half an hour, sometimes a few hours. The neurological symptoms are replaced by diffuse, contralateral, or rarely ipsilateral, headache, which is often but not always reported as throbbing in quality. The migraine attack commonly resolves with sleep but may occasionally continue for a few days. Hemiparetic attacks without headache may occur in the same individual. Many children also suffer attacks of common or classic migraine. As a rule hemiplegic migraine shows a relapsing course, mostly with random alteration of the side of the hemisyndrome. Often, hemiplegic migraine attacks cease in adulthood, being replaced by other forms of migraine.[18]

In a minority of patients the neurological deficit continues into the headache phase or develops during or following the headache period. In this group (type II), the duration of the neurological deficit is prolonged compared to that in type I. The neurological symptoms may persist for several days and may continue well after the headache has subsided, and it often proceeds to full hemiplegia. Nevertheless, complete recovery is the rule.

Familial Hemiplegic Migraine

This is a peculiar form of hemiplegic migraine in which most of the various family members present a stereotyped pattern of unilateral symptoms, often affecting the same side.[11,15,16,18–20]

Basilar Artery Migraine

This type of migraine is now recognized as an entity,[21,22,23] and the constellation of symptoms corresponds to a dysfunction of those structures supplied by the vertebrobasilar arterial system, including the visual system. Estimations of the incidence in childhood diverge greatly, (2.5 to 24% of the series comprising all forms of migraine).[6,7,23,24] The discrepancy results from differences in the definition. A more restricted definition requires more than just vertigo, because attacks of common or classical migraine in childhood are frequently accompanied by vertigo, an ambiguous complaint closely related to dizziness, giddiness, or unsteadiness.

The age of onset may range from early childhood through adolescence. In the young age group there is no sex preponderance, whereas from puberty onward there is a strong female predominance. The clinical features vary greatly from patient to patient, with symptoms of neurological dysfunction consisting of aura preceding the headache phase.

Visual symptoms usually appear first. They typically involve both fields of vision and consist of dimming, amblyopia, or hemianopia, often as positive manifestations (flashes of light). Early in the attack specific symptoms appear: truncal or appendicular ataxia, often accompanied by vertigo. Bilateral sensory symptoms (numbness, tingling) in the face and hands, or feet, are common. Weakness, related to the bulbocorticospinal system, frequently develops (hemiparesis, diplegia, quadriparesis), often combined with cranial nerve impairment (vestibular, auditory, oculomotor, abducens, facial, glossopharyngeal). Altered consciousness (lethargy, stupor, profound sleep) accompanies the attack in nearly half the patients.

The specific neurological symptoms resolve within a fraction of an hour in most patients, but may occasionally persist for many hours or a few days. Headache, as a rule, follows the neurological symptoms, often after an interval of minutes or half an hour. The headache phase is usually combined with prostrating nausea and vomiting. Prognosis is excellent, mild residual impairment very rare.

Migraine-Related Stroke

Many reports attest to cerebral infarction in the course of migraine attacks in young adults[25–30] and to stroke accounting for 15 to 25% in patients below 30 to 50 years, with a marked preponderance of women.[30–32] Fatal brain infarction resulting from migraine was reported in a 16-year-old girl[33] and in 28-year-old man.[34] In the pediatric age group, only 13 cases with migraine-related stroke may be found in the literature.[7,25,27,30,31,35,36] Eleven of these children, 7 boys and 5 girls, aged 6 to 16 years, suffered previously from attacks of migraine (common, classic, or complicated) and the family history for migraine was positive in all. The diagnosis of brain infarction was based on clinical symptomatology in five children, and on computed tomography (CT) or angiography in six. Follow-up is reported in nine of these children with full recovery in six and partial deficits remaining in three. Recurrent stroke occurred in one boy. Studies on the functional outcome and stroke recurrence in patients with migraine-related cerebral infarction are scarce. Prognosis in young adults is remarkably favorable and relapses are rare.[31]

In my personal series of 84 patients (45 girls and 39 boys, aged 3 months to 16 years), with angiographically proven cerebral arterial occlusion, the cause of obstruction is unknown in 36 patients. Some of these children presented with headache during the stroke episode, sometimes accompanied by mild nausea. In none of these patients was migrainous stroke accepted, because the previous and follow-up histories did not yield evidence for a migraine symptomatology. Stroke in childhood caused by migraine seems extremely rare.

Alternating Hemiplegia of Childhood

This very rare syndrome represents an entity of a peculiar paroxysmal disorder starting very early in life and progressing with gradual mental and motor deterioration. The development of the child is normal until the onset of the disease, generally before 18 months but as early as 3 months. Repeated attacks of hemiplegia affecting alternate or both sides of the body last from a fraction of an hour to a few days, occasionally a few weeks. A striking feature is the association with acute dystonia and/or tonic fits on the affected side. Acute discomfort and often autonomic disturbances (pallor, vasomotor changes, air regular respiration), and frequently oculomotor abnormalities (strabismus, nystagmus), accompany the attack. The frequency and severity of the attacks are variable, but become less frequent and severe as the child gets older.

Remarkably, there are few or no characteristic symptoms of migraine reported in patients with the typical syndrome, either during or between the attacks. Siblings are not affected with acute hemiplegia and there is no evident relationship with familial hemiplegic migraine, in which the onset is at a much later age.

The cause of this bizarre syndrome is obscure. The hypothesis of a vascular or an epileptic disorder has never been substantiated from numerous investigations, including electroencephalography (EEG), CT, and angiography. All attempts at treatment with anticonvulsant and antimigraine drugs have failed. Surprisingly, flunarazine, a calcium entry-blocking agent, gave promising results in the majority of the tested patients.[37–41]

Pathomechanism

The pathomechanism of migraine-induced focal neurological deficit is not known. Based on the classic theory of a primary vascular disorder of migraine, the hypothesis of ischemic functional loss due to vasospasm in major cerebral arteries was widely accepted.[42] Numerous angiographic studies yielded controversial findings. Spasm of large cerebral arteries was documented by serial arteriograms before, during, and after the aura had been demonstrated in a single patient suffering from hemiplegic migraine.[43] These angiograms showed normal cerebral vasculature before the migraine attack, and after the disappearance of visual aura symptoms, the latter at the time of typical headache. During the aura, a progressive decrease in caliber with filling of the intracranial carotid system and reflux into the posterior cerebral artery was present. At this point, the patient complained of bilateral scotomata. Therefore, the spasm was inconsistent with the area of the neurological deficit. However, after the headache phase was over, and after a symptom free interval of 15 min, the patient became hemiparetic with rapid recovery within 1 hr. During the last event no angiogram was made.

Normal angiographic findings in patients with migraine-related stroke[11,25,27,30–32,44,45] exceed by far the number of cases with pathological angiograms (branch occlusion, vasospasm).[25–27,30,31,33,35,46] However, it must be recognized that delayed arteriography might miss transient spasm or stenosis, and that a negative study does not exclude occlusion in smaller cerebral branch vessels not visualized by angiography. Migraine-related cerebral infarction occurs in the posterior hemispheres in a large proportion of patients.[31,32] In many of the angiographic studies the vertebrobasilar system has not been examined.

Evidence against the traditional theory of spasms in major cerebral arteries in classic and hemiplegic is provided by repeat measurements of regional cerebral blood flow (rCBF) with high spatial resolution techniques.[47–49] Studies revealed reduced rCBF in the occipital lobe during classic migraine attacks, gradually moving forward across the cortex and not confined to the territory of supply of one or more major cerebral arteries. This *spreading oligemia* was observed in patients presenting hemiplegic migraine, a finding that correlates by its rate of spread almost exactly with the aura of classical hemiplegic migraine. The parallel to Leao's spreading depression is obvious.[48,50,51] This animal experimental phenomenon is characterized by a spreading depression of cortical activity with transient but severe disruption of neural activity.[52]

Another proposed mechanism causing prolonged focal cerebral symptoms in complicated migraine is the hampering of blood flow due to increased platelet aggregability.[53,54] This platelet abnormality is found in most migraine patients, especially in the complicated migraine type. Decreased cerebral circulation due to spreading oligemia could enhance platelet accumulation in low-flow areas.[55,56]

It seems likely that migraine is a primary neuronal dysfunction with related vascular changes. The basic defect is unknown, but metabolic disorders certainly are involved.[7,55]

Associated Neurological Disorders and Symptoms

Epilepsy

A common pathophysiology between migraine and epilepsy has long been asserted by many reports claiming a higher incidence of epilepsy in migraine patients.[12,57,58] However, many other studies oppose such a relationship.[59–63] The incidence of seizures in patients presenting migraine is 3% in a combined series of several reports.[7]

Electroencephalographic changes are more frequent in patients with migraine than in nonmigraine children. There is general agreement upon the absence of specific EEG abnormality in migraine. Reports on the incidence differ considerably from what can be explained in part by selection of patients, and in part by the recent change in the concept of abnormality in the juvenile EEG.

The most frequent EEG abnormality observed *between* paroxysms consists of slow waves in the posterior regions, occurring in 40 to 70% of migraine children. Epileptic discharges have been reported with a 10 to 20% frequency in juvenile migraine.[7] The EEG *during* the paroxysms of complicated migraine, where a transient neurological deficit occurs, shows abnormality in almost 100%. The usual finding is lateralized or focal high-amplitude slowing, occasionally localized depression of brain activity. The focus is usually consistent with the clinical signs, although the EEG change is more often widespread than the clinical signs would suggest. EEG return to the interictal pattern in patients with complicated migraine attacks outlasts as a rule the resolution of clinical signs by hours, days, and occasionally weeks. Prolonged slow-wave foci relate either to edema or may reflect infarction.[2]

In basilar artery migraine, the ictal EEG shows posterior slow waves, whereas the resting EEG is usually normal. These EEG characteristics separate a peculiar syndrome from the entity of basilar artery migraine. It is characterized by almost continuous occipital spike-wave discharges, suppressed by eye opening and by infrequent generalized or focal seizures, announced by a visual aura, often with nausea and vomiting and mostly followed by postictal headache. The prognosis is benign.[64–67]

Diagnosis and Differential Diagnosis

There are neither specific symptoms and signs, nor specific tests to prove that the phenomena are migrainous. A generally accepted clinical definition of migraine is not available. The principal feature of migraine is paroxysmal occurrence of headache with symptom-free intervals. Additional criteria separate migraine from other headache disorders. These include nausea and/or vomiting, neurological aura symptoms, hemicrania, throbbing quality of headache, and positive family history for migraine.[4,59,68] Yet, this definition of migraine des not exclude migraine-like attacks triggered by underlying disorders (symptomatic migraine). A clinically safer and simpler diagnostic alternative accepts recurrent paroxysmal headache as migraine if there is return to full health, both mental and physical, between the attacks, and that other causes of headache have been excluded.[69]

It must be emphasized that a cerebral dysfunction or an insult to the brain of any cause can trigger an attack of migraine on a basis of constitutional predisposition. Most migraine attacks apparently occur spontaneously. By far, the most frequent factors related to migraine paroxysms are psychological troubles (stress, anxiety, emotional upset). Various precipitants

of migraine are well documented. Banal *head trauma* can induce a migraine attack in children. There is typically a latent interval of a fraction of an hour or more before onset of the aura (hemiparesis, loss of vision, aphasia, confusion) and the neurological deficit often persists for several hours and is accompanied by migrainous headache.[70–74] Occasionally, focal seizures follow the neurological deficit, especially in younger children with good prognosis.[71] Other well-known migraine precipitants are visual stimulation,[59,75] exposure to sun,[76] fasting, hypoglycemia,[7] and food factors.[7,69]

Migraine, and particularly complicated migraine, can be a symptomatic expression of intracranial disease. A serious diagnostic challenge is presented in patients with an attack of complex migraine as a first manifestation of migraine. Extensive investigations, including CT, are required in the following conditions:

    Migraine attacks with neurological symptoms persisting after recovery from headache during or following the headache phase
    Paroxysmal headache accompanied by focal seizures
    Incomplete return to normal health after an attack
    Recent school failure or change in behavior

The chance of an underlying organic cerebrovascular disease in such a case is higher than the probability of idiopathic migraine. In my experience, ischemic infarction caused by cerebral arterial disease or systemic thromboembolism is more frequent than hemorrhagic stroke caused by vascular malformation (84 children with cerebral arterial occlusion, 46 children with intracranial hemorrhage from cerebral vascular malformations, and an additional 20 children without hemorrhage from the vascular anomaly).

In the context of stroke, there is a discussion on migraine as a risk factor in patients with prolapse of the mitral valve. The enhanced platelet aggregability, associated with migraine, could be an important contributory factor to formation of emboli.[7] However, a prospective study on migraine stroke in young adults matched with a control group revealed no significant correlation.[32]

Cerebrospinal Fluid

Cerebrospinal fluid (CSF) showing mild pleocytosis is an occasional finding in hemiplegic or complex migraine.[77-82] Modest transient elevation of CSF protein can result from severe and prolonged juvenile migraine headache, especially by complex symptomatology.[7] Unexplained *fever* of brief duration and confined to the time period of the migraine episode was observed,[7] but there are no systematic studies.

Diagnosis of migraine is by exclusion and by a reasonable period of observation. The following observation by the author may illustrate the latter point. A 12-year-old girl experienced her first classical migraine attack, initiated by visual aura. Recurrent similar paroxysms occurred every 2 to 3 months. Mother and maternal grandmother suffered from classical migraine. Seven months after the initial migraine attack the girl developed cerebellar signs and chronic increased intracranial pressure was identified. Since the removal of a cerebellar astrocytoma no further migraine episodes occurred during a follow-up of 9 years.

Treatment

Treatment begins with establishing the diagnosis. It is my firm impression that improvement frequently begins with reassurance of patient and parents of the presence of a principally benign disorder, although temporarily annoying and incapacitating. Medication depends on the severity and frequency of attacks. If they are prolonged and associated with neurological deficit, preventive treatment should be considered; if they are severe and recur several times a month, prophylactic treatment is recommended.

Drug Treatment of the Acute Attack

Early treatment provides best results. Relief may be obtained by *analgesics* (aspirin, paracetamol).

Ergotamine is claimed to be the most effective agent in adolescents and adults. Newer studies no longer recommend its use in childhood.[5,69] Positive results have been obtained with *diazepam* in combination with analgesics, and with *chlorpromazine*; however, controlled studies are not available.[69]

Prophylactic Treatment. The most widely used drug at the present time is *propranolol*, a β-adrenergic blocking agent, the value of which in children is not established.[83-86] The same statement applies to *clonidine*, a drug that alters central vasomotor regulation.[87] *Methysergide*, a serotonin antagonist, may be used in older children who are refractory to other remedies (intermittent application for no more than 3 months).[7] This drug is not recommended for use in young children because of side effects.

Calcium Channel Blockers. *Flunarazine* is at the present time both on trial and widely used. Reported positive results do not yet allow a definitive judgment.[88] *Verapamil*, *nimodipine*, and *nifedipine* have been tested in adults with positive effect.[89,90]

Antiepileptic Drugs. *Phenobarbitone* and *phenytoin* have been proven useful in the prophylaxis of childhood migraine.[4,7] However, their efficacy is not yet tested in double-blind trials.

Pharmacotherapy in childhood migraine too often is not satisfactory. There is no medication effective in all children and there are patients refractory to all remedies.[69]

Psychological factors play an important role in triggering migraine headache in children. This fact must be considered in planning the program of treatment. In my experience, many migrainous children benefit more from a regular life style (bedtime, arising, meals) and from avoidance of overload in daily activities in school and leisure than from medication. Optimal treatment may not result from medication, but each case must be considered individually.

References

1. Devoto M, Lozito A, Staffa G, et al.: Segregation analysis of migraine in 128 families. Cephalalgia 6:105–105, 1986.

2. Dalessio DJ (ed.): Wolff's Headache and other Head Pain, 5th Ed. Oxford University Press, Oxford, 1987.

3. Bille BO: Migraine in school children. Acta Paediatr Scand 51 (Suppl 136):14–151, 1962.

4. Prensky AL: Migraine and migrainous variants in pediatric patients. Pediatr Clin North Am 23:461–471, 1976.

5. Congdon PJ, Forsythe WI: Migraine in childhood: a study of 300 children. Dev Med Child Neurol 21:209–216, 1979.

6. Ritz A, Jacobi G, Emrich R: Komplizierte Migrääne beim Kind. Monatsschr Kinderheilk 129:504–512, 1981.

7. Barlow CF: Headaches and migraine in childhood. Clin Dev Med 91:XX–XX, 1984.

8. Dalsgaard-Nielsen T, Engberg-Pedersen H, Holm HE: Clinical and statistical investigations of the epidemiology of migraine. Danish Med Bull 17:138–148, 1970.

9. Sillanpáá M: Changes in the prevalence of migraine and other headaches during the first seven school years. Headache 23:15–19, 1983.

10. Deubner DC: An epidemiologic study of migraine and headache in 10–20 year olds. Headache 17:173–180, 1977.

11. Bradshaw P, Parsons M: Hemiplegic migraine, a clinical study. Q J Med 34:65–85, 1965.

12. Prensky AL, Sommer D: Diagnosis and treatment of migraine in children. Neurology 29:506–510, 1979.

13. Jay GW, Tomasi, LG: Pediatric headaches: a one year retrospective analysis. Headache 21:5–9, 1981.

14. Whitty CWM: Familial hemiplegic migraine. In: Vinken, PJ, Bruyn GW, Klawans HL, et al. (eds.), Headache. Handbook of Clinical Neurology, Vol. 48, Ch. 11. Elsevier, Amsterdam, 1986, pp. 141–153.

15. Whitty CWM: Familial hemiplegic migraine. J Neurol Neurosurg Psychiatry 16:172–177, 1953.

16. Blau JN, Whitty CWM: Familial hemiplegic migraine. Lancet 2:1115–1116, 1955.

17. Ross RT: Hemiplegic migraine. Can Med Assoc J 78:10–16, 1958.

18. Jensen TS, Olivarius T de F, Kroft B, et al. Familial hemiplegic migraine—a reappraisal and long term follow-up study. Cephalalgia 1:33–39, 1981.

19. Glista GG, Mellinger JF, Rooke ED: Familial hemiplegic migraine. Mayo Clin Proc 50:307–311, 1975.

20. Rosenbaum HE: Familial hemiplegic migraine. Neurology 10:164–167, 1960.

21. Bickerstaff ER: Basilar artery migraine. Lancet 1:15–17, 1961; 2:1057–1059, 1961.

22. Golden GS, French JH: Basilar artery migraine in young children. Pediatrics 56:722–726, 1975.

23. Hockaday JM: Basilar migraine in childhood. Dev Med Child Neurol 21:455–463, 1979.

24. Lapkin ML, Golden GS. Basilar artery migraine. Am J Dis Child 132:278–281, 1978.

25. Connor RCR: Complicated migraine. A study of permanent neurological and visual defects caused by migraine. Lancet 2:1072–1075, 1962.

26. Hungerford GD, du Boulay GH, Zilkha KJ: Computerized axil tomography in patients with severe migraine: a preliminary report. J Neurol Neurosurg Psychiatry 39:990–994, 1976.

27. Dorfman LJ, Marshall WH, Enzmann DR: Cerebral infarction and migraine: clinical and radiologic correlations. Neurology 29:317–322, 1979.

28. Spaccavento LJ, Solomon GD: Migraine as an etiology of stroke in young adults. Headache 24:19–22, 1984.

29. Featherstone HJ: Clinical features of stroke in migraine: a review. Headache 26:128–133, 1986.

30. Rothrock JF, Walicke P, Swenson MR, et al.: Migrainous stroke. Arch Neurol 45:63–67, 1988.

31. Broderick JP, Swanson JW: Migraine-related strokes. Clinical profile and prognosis in 20 patients. Arch Neurol 44:868–871, 1987.

32. Bogousslavsky J, Regli F, Van Melle G, et al.: Migraine stroke. Neurology 38:223–237, 1988.

33. Buckle RM, Du Boulay G, Smith B: Death due to cerebral vasospasm. J Neurol Neurosurg Psychiatry 27:440–444, 1964.

34. Guest IA, Woolf AL: Fatal infarction of brain in migraine. Br Med J 1:225–226, 1964.

35. Castaldo JE, Anderson M, Reeves AG: Middle cerebral artery occlusion with migraine. Stroke 13:308–311, 1982.

36. Dunn DW: Vertebrobasilar occlusive disease and childhood migraine. Pediatr Neurol 1:252–254, 1985.

37. Casaer P: Flunarazine in alternating hemiplegia in childhood. An international study in 12 children. Neuropediatrics 18:191–195, 1987.

38. Krägeloh I, Aicardi J: Alternating hemiplegia in infants: report of 5 cases. Dev Med Child Neurol 22:784–791, 1980.

39. Hosking GP, Cavanagh NPC, Wilson J: Alternating hemiplegia: complicated migraine of infancy. Arch Dis Child 53:656–659, 1978.

40. Verret LS, Steele JC: Alternating hemiplegia in childhood: a report of eight patients with complicated migraine beginning in infancy. Pediatrics 47:675–680, 1971.

41. Aicardi J: Alternating hemiplegia of childhood. Int Pediatr 2:115–119, 1987.
42. Wolff HG: Headache and Other Head Pain. Oxford University Press, New York, 1963.
43. Dukes HT, Vieth RG: Cerebral arteriography during migraine prodrome and headache. Neurology 14:636–639, 1964.
44. Pearce JMS, Foster JB: An investigation of complicated migraine. Neurology 15:333–340, 1965.
45. Fisher CM: Cerebral ischemia—less familiar type. Clin Neurosurg 18:267–335, 1971.
46. Murphy JP: Cerebral infarction in migraine. Neurology 5:359–361, 1955.
47. Olesen J, Larsen B, Lauritzen M: Focal hyperemia followed by spreading oligemia and impaired activation of rCBF in classic migraine. Ann Neurol 9:344–352, 1981.
48. Lauritzen M, Olesen J: Regional cerebral blood flow during migraine attacks by xenon-133 inhalation and emission tomography. Brain 107:447–461, 1984.
49. Olesen J: The ischemic hypotheses of migraine. Arch Neurol 44:321–322, 1987.
50. Pearce JMS: Is migraine explained by Leao's spreading depression? Lancet 2:763–766, 1985.
51. Blau JN: Migraine pathogenesis: the neural hypothesis reexamined. J Neurol Neurosurg Psychiatry 74:437–442, 1984.
52. Leao AAP: Spreading depression of activity in the cerebral cortex. J Neurophysiol 7:359–390, 1944.
53. Kalendovsky Z, Austin JH: "Complicated migraine," its association with increased platelet aggregability and abnormal plasma coagulation factors. Headache 15:18–35, 1975.
54. Jones RJ, Forsythe AM, Amess JAL: Platelet aggregation in migraine patients during the headache-free interval. Adv Neurol 33:275–278, 1982.
55. Welch KMA: Migraine. A biobehavioral disorder. Arch Neurol 44:323–327, 1987.
56. Hachinski V: The nature of migraine. Arch Neurol 44:327, 1987.
57. Lennox WG, Lennox MA: Borderlands of Epilepsy. Little, Brown, Boston, 1960.
58. Basser LS: The relation of migraine and epilepsy. Brain 92:285–300, 1969.
59. Bille B: Migraine in school children. Acta Paedol 51 (suppl 136):1–151, 1962.
60. Lees F, Watkins SM: Loss of consciousness in migraine. Lancet 2:647–750, 1963.
61. Slatter KH: Some clinical and EEG findings in patients with migraine. Brain 91:85–98, 1968.
62. Klee A: A Clinical Study of Migraine with Particular Reference to the Most Severe Cases. Munksgaard, Copenhagen, 1969.
63. Ziegler DK, Wong G: Migraine in childhood: clinical and EEG study of families. Epilepsia 8:171–187, 1967.
64. Camfield PR, Metrakos K, Andermann F: Basilar migraine, seizures and severe epileptiform EEG abnormalities. Neurology 28:584–588, 1978.
65. Panayiotopoulos CP: Basilar migraine, seizures, and severe epileptic EEG abnormalities. Neurology 30:1122–1125, 1980.
66. Gastaut H: A new type of epilepsy: benign partial epilepsy of childhood with occipital spike-waves. Clin Electroenceph 13:13–22, 1982.
67. Deonna T, Ziegler AL, Despland PA: Paroxysmal visual disturbances of epileptic origin and occipital epilepsy in children. Neuropediatrics 15:131–135, 1984.
68. Vahlquist B: Migraine in children. Int Arch Allerg 7:348–355, 1955.
69. Hockaday JM: Migraine in Childhood. Butterworths, London, 1988.
70. Haas DC, Pineda GS, Lourie H: Juvenile head trauma syndromes and their relationship to migraine. Arch Neurol 32:727–730, 1975.
71. Oka H, Kako M, Matusushima M, et al.: Traumatic spreading depression syndrome. Review of particular type of head injury in 37 patients. Brain 100:287–298, 1977.
72. Snoek JW, Minderhoud JM, Wilmink JF: Delayed deterioration following mild head injury in children. Brain 107:15–36, 1984.
73. Eldridge PR, Punt JAG: Transient cortical blindness in children. Lancet 1:815–816, 1988.
74. Matthews WB: Footballer's migraine. Br Med J 2:326–327, 1972.
75. Maratos J, Wilkinson M: Migraine in children: a medical and psychiatric study. Cephalalgia 2:179–187, 1982.
76. Vijayan N, Gould S, Watson C: Exposure to sun and precipitation of migraine. Headache 20:42–43, 1980.
77. Rossi LN, Vassella F, Bajc O, et al.: Benign migraine-like syndrome with CSF pleocytosis in children. Dev Med Child Neurol 27:192–198, 1985.
78. Bartleson JD, Swanson JW, Whisnant JP: A migrainous syndrome with cerebrospinal fluid pleocytosis. Neurology 31:1257–1262, 1981.
79. Kremnitzer M, Golden GS: Hemiplegic migraine: cerebrospinal fluid abnormalities. J Pediatr 85:139, 1974.
80. Novum MJ: Migraine and CSF pleocytosis. Neurology 32:1073–1074, 1982.

81. Schraeder PL, Burns RA: Hemiplegic migraine associated with an aseptic meningeal reaction. Arch Neurol 37:377–379, 1980.
82. Ferrari MD, Buruma OJ, van Laar-Ramaker H, et al.: A migrainous syndrome with pleocytosis. Neurology 33:813, 1983.
83. Forsythe WI, Gillies A, Sills MA: Propranolol (Inderal) in the treatment of childhood migraine. Dev Med Child Neurol 26:737–741, 1984.
84. Ziegler DK, Hurwitz A, Hassanein RS, et al.: A comparison of propranolol and amitriptyline. Arch Neurol 44:486–489, 1987.
85. Rosen JA: Observations on the efficacy of propranolol for the prophylaxis of migraine. Ann Neurol 13:92–93, 1983.
86. Bille B, Ludvigsson J, Sanner G: Prophylaxis of migraine in children. Headache 17:61–63, 1977.
87. Sills M, Congdon P, Forsythe WI: Clonidine and childhood migraine—a pilot and double-blind study. Dev Med Child Neurol 24:837–841, 1982.
88. Sorge F, De Simone R, Marano E, et al.: Flunarazine in prophylaxis of childhood migraine. Cephalalgia 8:1–6, 1988.
89. Solomon GA, Steel G, Spaccavento LJ: Verpamil prophylaxis of migraine. A double-blind, placebo-controlled study. JAMA 250:2500–2502, 1983.
90. Rascol A, Montastruc JL, Rascol O: Flunarazine versus pizotifen: a double-blind study in the prophylaxis of migraine. Headache 26:83–85, 1986.

Index